Life Cycle Nutrition
Conception through Adolescence

Life Cycle Nutrition
Conception through Adolescence

Linda Kelly DeBruyne   Sharon Rady Rolfes
Eleanor Noss Whitney, editor

West Publishing Company

ST. PAUL   NEW YORK   LOS ANGELES   SAN FRANCISCO

Composition: Carlisle Communications
Copyediting: Susan Ecklund
Cover and Interior Design: Roslyn Stendahl, Dapper Design
Cover Image: *Family Group* by Henry Moore. 1948-49. Bronze.
    Photo by Lee Boltin. Reproduced with permission from the
    Hakone Open-Air Museum, Kanagawa-ken, Japan.
Illustrations: Ted Bollmann and Rolin Graphics

COPYRIGHT ©1989   By WEST PUBLISHING COMPANY
                  50 W. Kellogg Boulevard
                  P.O. Box 64526
                  St. Paul, MN 55164-1003

Printed in the United States of America
96 95 94 93 92 91 90 89   8 7 6 5 4 3 2 1 0
Library of Congress Cataloging-in-Publication Data

DeBruyne, Linda K.
    Life cycle nutrition : conception through adolescence / Linda
  Kelly DeBruyne, Sharon Rady Rolfes : edited by Eleanor Noss Whitney.
        p.   cm.
    Bibliography: p.
    Includes index.
    ISBN 0-314-46971-0
    1. Children—Nutrition.   2. Pregnancy—Nutritional aspects.
  I. Rolfes, Sharon Rady.   II. Whitney, Eleanor Noss.   III. Title.
  RJ206.D43 1989
  613.2'088054—dc19

                                                          88-30457
                                                          CIP

PHOTO CREDITS
Chapter 2   **60** Petit Format/Nestle/Photo Researchers, Inc.; **61** Petit Format/ Nestle/Photo Researchers, Inc.; **62** Petit Format/Nestle/Photo Researchers, Inc.;
Focal Point 2   **99** Dr. James Hanson/University of Iowa Hospitals and Clinics;
Chapter 3   **124** Elizabeth Crews; **125–126** From "The Breast-feeding Guide for Working Mothers" courtesy of Mead Johnson Nutritionals; **134** Elizabeth Crews;
Chapter 5   **209** Anthony M. Vannelli.

CREDITS FOR CHAPTER OPENING SCULPTURES
Chapter 1   *Couple* (Dans la nuit) by Gaston Lachaise. 1935. Bronze. 31 × 88½ × 41 inches. Courtesy of the National Trust for Historic Preservation, Nelson A. Rockefeller Collection.
Chapter 2   Nayarit (Pre-Columbian) pottery vessel of pregnant woman. Photograph from the Lee Boltin Picture Library.
Chapter 3   Detail of *Fountain of the Seasons* by Christian Petersen. 1940. Limestone. Courtesy of Iowa State University.
Chapter 4   *Father and Son* by Paul T. Granlund, sculptor-in-residence at Gustavus Adolphus College in St. Peter, Minnesota. 1968. 30 inches.
Chapter 5   *Children* by Paul T. Granlund. 1963. 22 inches.
Chapter 6   *Girl on a Swing* by Richard Fleischner. 1966–67. Polyester resin, Fiberglas, and polypropylene rope. 69½ × 15 × 30¼ inches. Courtesy of the National Trust for Historic Preservation, Nelson A. Rockefeller Collection.

This book focuses on the nourishment of individuals and families, but all of its concerns fall within the larger context of the whole human family—of over five billion individuals and the earth that nourishes us all. We therefore dedicate this book to the Earth herself in the hope that all who read it will remember to take care of her as she cares for us.

To the loves of my life—Tom, Zachary, and Tyler—you inspire, sustain, and delight me every single day. To mom, whose love and laughter I cherish, and whose confidence in me gives me strength and happiness. To Ellie, whose wisdom, energy, and unselfish dedication to making the world a better place is simply remarkable. And to Sharon, my friend, my partner, the mother of my children's best friends, and the best coauthor anyone could ever have.

Linda

To Sitto Della and Jiddo Tony and to Sitto Futha and Jiddo Tom, the parents of my parents, who have given me through their lives the pride of honoring a heritage, an appreciation for living healthfully, and the joy of loving others.

Sharon

Contents

▶ Preface

The information in this book is derived from over a thousand scientific research articles. Each one contributes to the understanding of how nutrition influences people throughout their lives. In relaying this wealth of knowledge, we have tried to maintain a writing style and organization that is both educational and enjoyable to read.

A life cycle nutrition book is about science applied to people. This book makes the effort to recognize that both science and people are changing. It contains the most recent available scientific information. It also addresses the new roles people in the family and society are playing. The traditional family of mother, father, and children, with father going off to work while mother tends to the home and children is the exception, rather than the rule. Men and women are sharing the tasks of parenting and earning family income; children are attending day-care at an earlier age. The children of a family may be biological, adoptive, or step-children; the parents may be single or married. In some cases, the caretaker is not a parent; this book uses the terms parent and caretaker interchangeably.

The chapters of this book present the life cycle in chronological sequence. Chapter 1 begins the life cycle story with a look at the needs of a prospective mother and the factors that surround reproduction and conception. Chapter 2 describes the changes that come with pregnancy. Chapter 3 presents information on breastfeeding and formula feeding and on how to decide between the two. Chapter 4 tells of infant growth and development. Chapters 5 and 6 continue the story through childhood and adolescence. So it is that life's cycle completes itself, for at adolescence, people are physically capable of beginning the cycle anew for the next generation.

The Focal Points provide a detailed look at specific topics relevant to phases in the life cycle. By standing apart from the chapters, they receive the attention they deserve. Focal Point 1 describes inborn errors of metabolism and how diet therapy can make a difference even prior to conception. Focal Point 2 tells of the devastating effects that alcohol intake during pregnancy can cause. Focal Point 3 provides the details of tooth development and current research on the cariogenicity of foods. Focal Point 4 discusses some of the common nutrition-related disorders that most children experience at one time or another—infections and fever, diarrhea, and constipation. Focal Point 5 explores obesity—its development, effects, and treatment—with a special focus on children. Focal Point 6 examines the role drugs, alcohol, and tobacco play in the lives of teenagers and in relation to nutrition.

The Practical Points apply nutrition knowledge to peoples' lives. They provide "how to" information on such topics as breastfeeding, finding financial assistance, and eating fast food.

Appendixes provide easy reference. Notice especially Appendix A, which presents many tables, figures, and forms to assist in preparing and understanding a nutrition assessment. Appendix B provides the RDA and RDI and the Canadian RNI tables; Appendix C describes the Four Food Group Plan; Appendix D presents a table of infant formula composition; Appendix E offers tables of vitamin and mineral supplements; and Appendix F lists nutrition resources.

This book was conceived shortly after our first children were born. Now, several years later, they—and their siblings—have grown and developed into healthy, happy children and the book has finally completed its gestation! We wrote this book from knowledge gained through both research and experience with the intent to offer you the understanding of both conceptual and practical aspects of nutrition through the life cycle. We hope it serves you well.

Linda Kelly DeBruyne
Sharon Rady Rolfes
November 1988

▶ Acknowledgments

We must begin our thank you list with Gary Woodruff for his encouragement to write this book in the first place and Ellie Whitney for her many contributions to its content and style. Our editors, Peter Marshall, Becky Tollerson, and Laura Mezner Nelson deserve a round of applause for the care they gave this book in coordinating its review and production. We are grateful to Linda Patton for her efficient library research work and to Ted Bollmann for his skilled artistry.

We give thanks daily for our children, Lyle, Zak, Tyler, and Marni, who have given us many experiences that brought the information in this book to life. We appreciate the love and enthusiastic support of "the Toms", and of our associates Fran and Ellie in helping us to complete this project.

Finally, we thank our reviewers for enhancing the quality and accuracy of this text:

Kathryn Anderson
Florida State University

Dee Baxter
Georgia State University

Sarah Burroughs
California Polytechnic State
University—San Luis Obispo

Christine Condit
Appalachian State University

Gail Disney
University of Tennessee

Karen Hauersperger
Presbyterian Hospital, School of
Nursing—Charlotte, NC

Michael Jenkins
Kent State University

Bernice Kopel
Oklahoma State University

Edith Lerner
Case Western Reserve University.

Nina Mercer
University of Guelph

Sam Smith
University of New Hampshire

Anne Smith
University of Utah

Virginia Utermohlen
Cornell University

Prepregnancy: Nutrition and Conception

1

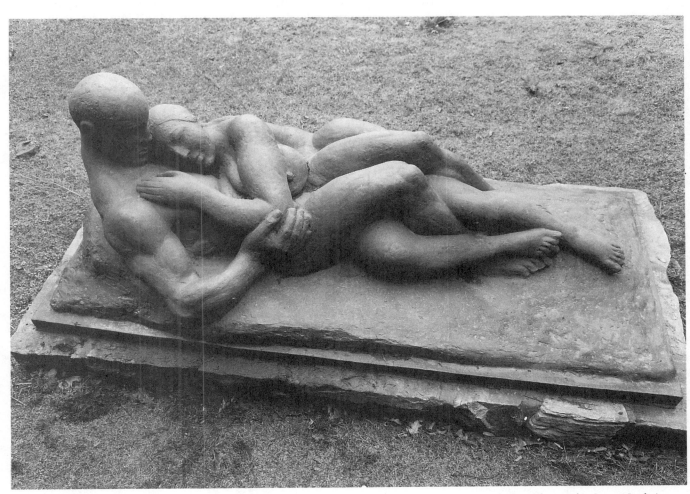

Couple (Dans la nuit) by Gaston Lachaise.

1

Each person enters this world in a human body that carries the person through the years—from birth to death. Each human body receives a unique genetic map that determines the primary route physical and mental characteristics will take throughout life. A person must accept many of these characteristics without option for change, but can change others for better or worse within genetically defined limits. One of several ways a person can affect the growth, maintenance, and general health of the body is through proper nutrition. Food intake, and the ways the body handles the nutrients in that food, share in determining the nutritional health of a body. Ideally, nutrients supplied by the diet will at least adequately cover the requirements and losses incurred by the physiological demands of growth, reproduction, lactation, disease, and aging.

Each day, people make dietary choices. Each choice to some extent improves or impairs the body's later health and performance. The health of a woman's body prior to conception influences her fertility, the health of an infant she may later conceive and bear, and her health later in life. The union of an ovum and spermatozoon in the creation of a zygote begins the development of a human being, and a multitude of new experiences for the parents. The time prior to this moment provides a unique opportunity for a woman to prepare herself physically, mentally, and emotionally for the many changes to come. To prepare the mother's body as the most suitable environment in which a fetus will develop requires establishing healthful habits.

A discussion on prepregnancy nutrition must, by its nature, focus primarily on women prior to and between pregnancies. Their needs are different from those of men, from those of pregnant and lactating women, and from those of women after menopause. Men's nutrition may affect their fertility and possibly the genetic contributions that they make to their children; it is discussed where appropriate. The physiological changes and hormonal shifts women experience create special nutrient needs. The better a woman takes care of herself nutritionally before and between pregnancies, the more successful her pregnancies are likely to be.

This chapter begins with women's nutrition in general as a background for special topics related to prepregnancy. Where necessary, it looks ahead to explain a few details about pregnancy itself, in order to illustrate why nutrition *prior* to pregnancy is so important. The miniglossary defines some of the terms health care providers and researchers commonly use to describe women and infants, and the events and times surrounding a pregnancy and birth. Figure 1–1 places some of these terms on a time line.

conception: the union of the male spermatozoon and the female ovum; fertilization.

fertility: the capacity of a woman to produce a normal ovum periodically and of a man to produce normal spermatozoa; the ability to reproduce.

ovum (OH-vum): the female reproductive cell, capable of developing into a new organism upon fertilization, commonly referred to as an egg; *ova* is the plural.
ovum = egg

spermatozoon (sper-mat-oh-ZOH-on): a male reproductive cell, capable of fertilizing an ovum; *spermatozoa* is the plural.
spermatos = seed
zoon = life

zygote: the term for the product of the union of ovum and spermatozoon for the first two weeks after fertilization.

Women's Nutrition Prior to Pregnancy

Dietary recommendations for the general public are applicable in limited ways to everyone, but individual subgroups of the population also need specific recommendations of their own. In the case of the recommendations being made today for the general public, many are not tailored to women's needs. Of course, some recommendations, such as to eat a variety of foods, to exercise, and to maintain a healthy body weight, are appropriate for both genders. Others, however, are not.

Miniglossary of Pregnancy and Birth Terms

These terms describe a woman's pregnancy status before, during, and after:

pregravid: before pregnancy.
pre = before
gravid = pregnant

gravid (GRAV-id): pregnant. A **gravida** (GRAV-ih-da) is a pregnant woman; **gravidity** (gra-VID-ih-tee) is pregnancy. A woman during her first pregnancy is a **primigravida** (pry-me-GRAV-ih-da). A woman who has been pregnant two or more times is a **multigravida** (MUL-tee-GRAV-ih-da).

postpartum: after childbirth.
post = after
partus = birth

These terms describe the number of a woman's pregnancies from the smallest to the largest:

nullipara (nul-LIP-ah-ra): a woman who has borne no children; the adjective is **nulliparous** (nul-LIP-ar-us).
null = none
parere = to bear

primipara (pry-MIP-ah-ra): a woman who has had or who is giving birth to her first child; the adjective is **primiparous** (pry-MIP-ah-rus).

multipara (mul-TIP-ah-ra): a woman who has borne more than one infant, regardless of infant survival; the adjective is **multiparous** (mul-TIP-ar-us).

These terms describe the time surrounding birth:

prenatal: before birth.
pre = before
natal = birth

perinatal: the time preceding, during, or after birth.
peri = around

neonatal: concerning the first four weeks after birth; a newborn infant is a **neonate**.
neos = new

postnatal: occurring after birth.
post = after

These terms describe an infant's gestational age at birth:

preterm: an infant born prior to the 38th week of gestation; also referred to as a **premature** infant.

term: an infant born between the 38th and 42nd weeks of gestation.

post term: an infant born after the 42nd week of gestation. (The term **gestation** refers to the period from conception to birth; for human beings, normal length of gestation is from 38 to 42 weeks.)

Figure 1–1   Terms for Stages Surrounding Pregnancy and Birth

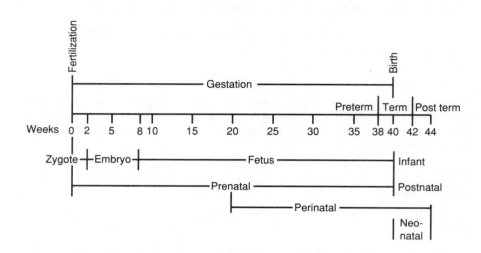

A major aim of many dietary recommendations today is to prevent disease. Much attention focuses on preventing cardiovascular disease in particular, the number one killer of men. To this end, current guidelines recommend avoiding too much fat and sodium and advocate a diet that limits high-fat foods such as red meats and dairy products.

The recommendations to limit fat and sodium might benefit everyone threatened with cardiovascular disease, but women have other specific needs in their reproductive years, and their hormones help to protect them to some extent from this particular disease. If they need to limit fat and sodium, they need to do so in a different way from men. Men may benefit from limiting red meats and dairy products, but women may suffer iron and calcium deficiencies following such advice. In short, some of the nutrition- and diet-related problems men and women face are as different as their bodies. A task force for the American Dietetic Association (ADA) has therefore developed a set of Nutrition Recommendations for Women to promote health and prevent disease specifically for women (see Practical Point: Nutrition Recommendations for Women).[1] Any woman wanting to do all that she can to make a future pregnancy possible and healthy should review these recommendations with an eye to improving her diet wherever necessary. Appendix C describes the Four Food Group Plan for diet planning.

At first glance, these recommendations appear similar to the *Dietary Guidelines for Americans* developed by the U.S. Department of Agriculture (USDA), which are shown here for contrast. A close look reveals differences. The Nutrition Recommendations for Women specify *how to* attain appropriate body weight, encourage women to include calcium- and iron-rich foods in the daily diet, and suggest that they restrict vitamin and mineral supplements to specific circumstances. They also address general health concerns beyond nutrition, with recommendations on exercise and smoking. These are worthy of attention, for they speak to the particular needs of women and, if followed, they will especially protect prepregnant women.

Nutrition Recommendations for Women: a set of dietary guidelines designed by the ADA specifically to meet the needs of women.

Dietary Guidelines for Americans:

1. Eat a variety of foods daily.
2. Maintain desirable weight.
3. Avoid too much fat, saturated fat, and cholesterol.
4. Eat foods with adequate starch and fiber.
5. Avoid too much sugar.
6. Avoid too much sodium.
7. If you drink alcoholic beverages, do so in moderation.

difference b/t USDA and ADA

Nutrition Recommendations for Women

1. Eat a variety of foods daily from all major food groups:

   ▶ 3 to 4 servings of low-fat dairy foods.

   ▶ 2 servings of low-fat meat/meat alternates.

   ▶ 4 servings of vegetables/fruits.

   ▶ 4 servings of whole-grain breads/cereals.

2. Maintain a healthy body weight.

   ▶ For adults to lose weight, if necessary, safely and effectively, do not go below 10 kcalories per pound of present weight, do not skip meals, and increase physical activity (exercise).

   ▶ Gain weight, if necessary, by increasing kcaloric intake and exercising in moderation.

3. Exercise regularly (three days per week).[a]

4. Limit total fat to no more than one-third of daily kcalories:

   ▶ Select a variety of fat sources: saturated, polyunsaturated, and monounsaturated.[b]

   ▶ Limit nonfood-group foods, such as margarine, butter, cooking oils, salad dressings, cookies, cakes, and cream.

   ▶ Choose low-fat selections of meat and milk food groups.

5. Eat at least one-half of daily kcalories from carbohydrates:

   ▶ Select complex carbohydrates, such as beans, peas, pasta, vegetables, seeds, and grains.

6. Eat a variety of fiber-rich foods:

   ▶ Make daily selections from fresh fruits with skin, vegetables, legumes (navy, pinto, and kidney beans), and whole grains (brown rice, oatmeal, and oat and wheat bran).

   ▶ Increase intake of fiber gradually.

   ▶ Avoid excess fiber intake, especially from one source.

7. Include 3 to 4 daily servings of calcium-rich foods:

   ▶ Consume low-fat milk, yogurt, and cheese.

   ▶ Increase milk in cooking.

   ▶ Eat broccoli, sardines with bones, canned salmon with bones, and collard greens.

---

[a] Chapter 6 expands on the benefits of regular exercise.
[b] The American Heart Association recommends a total fat intake of 30 percent of total kcalories, with 10 percent coming from each type of fat (saturated, monounsaturated, and polyunsaturated).

8. Include plenty of iron-rich foods:

   ▸ Make daily selections from lean meat, liver, prunes, pinto and kidney beans, spinach, leafy green vegetables, enriched and whole-grain breads/cereals.

9. Limit intake of salt and salt-containing foods:[c]

   ▸ Limit addition of salt in food preparation.

   ▸ Limit use of saltshaker.

10. Rely on foods for necessary nutrients, using vitamin and mineral supplements only under specific circumstances.

11. If you drink alcoholic beverages, limit alcohol intake to one to two drinks daily.[d]

12. Avoid smoking.

13. Adjust diet, exercise, and other health promotional behaviors to correspond with your own identified risk factors:

    ▸ Diet is only one risk factor.

    ▸ Heredity, lifestyle, and environment are other factors.

    ▸ Consult a physician with questions about risk factors.

14. If you have questions about the adequacy of your diet, consult a registered dietitian.

Source: Adapted from The American Dietetic Association's Nutrition Recommendations for Women, Copyright The American Dietetic Association. Reprinted by permission from *Journal of the American Dietetic Association* Vol. 86: 1663, 1986.

---

[c]Omit foods that are high in salt such as pickles, luncheon meats, sardines, potato chips, and soy sauce. Sodium restriction recommendation omitted in light of the finding that salt specifically, and not sodium-containing products, raises blood pressure; T. W. Kurtz, H. A. Al-Bander, and C. Morris, "Salt-sensitive" essential hypertension in men: Is the sodium ion alone important? *New England Journal of Medicine* 317 (1987): 1043–1048.

[d]Focal Point 6 discusses alcohol metabolism and the health risks associated with drinking alcoholic beverages. Focal Point 2 highlights the dangers associated with alcohol use during pregnancy.

The sections on undernutrition and overnutrition on pages 33 and 35 describe the impact of prepregnancy weight on pregnancy.

10-kcalorie rule: a rule presented in the ADA Nutrition Recommendations for Women that establishes the number of kcalories a woman should consume to achieve gradual weight loss and dietary adequacy—10 kcalories per pound of present body weight.

Appropriate Body Weight

The ADA recommendation to maintain healthy body weight is old advice that includes a valuable new concept—that of body weight being described as "healthy" rather than as "ideal" or "desirable." This concept suggests that there is a weight (more likely a range) at which the body is most healthy. Prior to pregnancy, a woman determining her appropriate body weight needs to consider her optimal health, not cultural norms which may be unrealistic. The ADA advises the woman losing weight to follow a specific rule of thumb—a "10-kcalorie rule" (see Practical Point: 10-kCalorie Rule). A woman consuming 10 kcalories per pound (of her present body weight) can gradually lose

10-kCalorie Rule

If, in order to lose weight, a woman wants to know what her energy intake should be, she has two options. One is to use the traditional method of estimating total energy expenditure and subtracting a number of kcalories per day from that to arrive at a desired rate of weight loss. The other is to use a simpler, often safer, alternative suggested by the ADA—the 10-kcalorie rule.[a]

Consider the first alternative, using a sedentary woman who weighs 135 pounds (61 kg). To estimate her energy expenditure, you will need to combine estimates for her basal metabolism and voluntary muscular activity. To estimate basal metabolic energy output for a woman, use the factor 0.9 kcalories per kilogram body weight per hour:

$$61 \text{ kg} \times 0.9 \text{ kcal/kg/hr} \times 24 \text{ hr/day} = 1318 \text{ kcal/day.}$$

To approximate energy output for physical activity for a sedentary person, add 50 percent of the estimate for basal metabolism:

$$1318 \text{ kcal/day} \times 50\% = 659 \text{ kcal/day.}$$

Her total estimated energy output, then, is:

$$1318 \text{ kcal/day} + 659 \text{ kcal/day} = 1977 \text{ kcal/day.}$$

Next, pick a rate of weight loss. For each pound of weight loss per week, subtract 500 kcalories per day. The woman in this example wants to lose 2 pounds per week, so she calculates:

$$1977 \text{ kcal/day} - 1000 \text{ kcal/day} = 977 \text{ kcal/day.}$$

This method provides no guidelines to ensure a safe rate of weight loss or minimum number of kcalories, but guidelines are often offered along with it: "Do not lose more than 1 to 2 pounds per week"; or "Eat no less than 1200 kcalories per day." The woman therefore chooses to eat 1200 kcalories per day.

Now compare the 10-kcalorie rule for weight loss for another sedentary, 135-pound woman:

$$10 \text{ kcal/day} \times 135 \text{ lb} = 1350 \text{ kcal/day.}$$

On this intake, the woman will lose between 1 and 2 pounds per week. Her energy intake and rate of weight loss will not be much different from those of the first woman, but she arrived at them differently. The first woman picked a rate of weight loss and adjusted energy intake accordingly; the second picked an energy intake and the rate of weight loss adjusted accordingly. The 10-kcalorie rule limits weight loss to the maximum

difference in the two methods [handwritten]

Conversion Factors
1 kg = 2.2 lb.
1 lb body fat = 3500 kcal.

---

[a] The American Dietetic Association's Nutrition Recommendations for Women, *Journal of the American Dietetic Association* 86 (1986): 1663–1664.

safe rate. It requires <u>smaller women to lose weight less rapidly,</u> for safety's sake, and it permits <u>more rapid weight loss at higher body weights.</u> For example, for a 110-pound woman, the 10-kcalorie rule provides 1100 kcalories per day, an amount that would permit her to lose at the rate of 1 pound per week. For a 220-pound woman, the 10- kcalorie rule provides 2200 kcal/day, which would enable her to lose 2 pounds per week. Each weight-loss rate is safe for the individual concerned, and each energy intake is high enough to be realistically achievable and to provide dietary adequacy.

Appendix A discusses diet history and other assessment techniques.

weight and at the same time, with the appropriate food selections, can meet her nutrient needs.

The ADA's purpose in offering a minimum number of kcalories for weight loss is to ensure that a woman can make a selection of foods that will deliver all nutrients in adequate amounts. As the upcoming section on preconceptual influences discusses, a woman's prepregnant nutrition status is important to the outcome of any future pregnancies. Dietary habits are easy to observe, and a woman attempting to lose weight has an opportunity to evaluate hers prior to pregnancy. A dietary history taken by a dietitian or a dietary intake recorded by the woman and assessed by a dietitian can determine where improvements are possible.

By learning to eat nutrient-dense foods prior to pregnancy, a woman can establish, in advance, eating habits that will support a healthy pregnancy later without excessive weight gain. Most women cannot eat many high-kcalorie, low-nutrient foods such as candy and chips without exceeding their energy needs and gaining unneeded fat. For underweight women and for women whose energy needs are extraordinarily high, adding high-kcalorie foods to a well-balanced diet may be appropriate.

Problem Nutrients

The diets women typically eat provide some nutrients in ample quantities. Vitamin C and protein are examples. Other nutrients seem harder to get—notably, calcium, iron, vitamin B_6, folacin, magnesium, and zinc. The ADA recommendations specifically address two of these—calcium and iron.

Calcium   Ninety-nine percent of the body's calcium resides in the skeletal system. Bone may appear to be static but, like other body tissues, it is always changing—being broken down and reformed. Bone continuously exchanges calcium with its surrounding fluids. During times of inadequate calcium intake, the bones serve as a source of calcium for the tissues' needs. With repeated withdrawals, the calcium stores become depleted, threatening the integrity of the bones.

Figure 1–2 shows the three phases of bone development throughout life. From birth to approximately age 20, the bones are actively growing by modifying their length, width, and shape. This rapid growing phase overlaps with the next period of peak bone mass development that occurs between the ages of 12 and 40. During this next period, skeletal mass increases. Bones grow both thicker and denser by remodeling, a maintenance and repair process involving the loss of existing bone and the deposition of new bone. The final

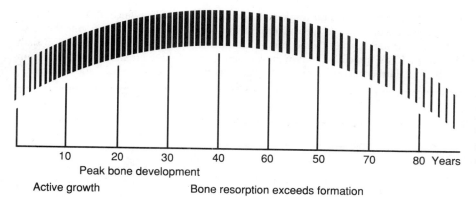

10   20   30   40   60   50   70   80 Years
Peak bone development

Active growth   Bone resorption exceeds formation

Figure 1–2   Phases of Bone Development throughout Life
The bones actively grow from birth to approximately age 20. The active growth phase overlaps with the next phase of peak bone mass development that occurs between the ages of 12 and 40. The final phase, when bone resorption exceeds formation, begins between ages 30 and 40 and continues throughout life.

phase, which begins between 30 and 40 years of age and continues throughout life, finds bone loss exceeding new bone formation.

Bone loss is a natural process that women cannot completely prevent, but they can minimize its impact by achieving maximal bone mass before and during the childbearing years. One of the many factors determining a woman's bone mass is dietary calcium; therefore, she needs an adequate calcium intake throughout her early life. Because milk and other dairy products are the primary sources of calcium, and because drinking milk is a habit best learned early, Chapter 5, Childhood, discusses solutions to such problems as milk dislikes, milk allergies, and lactose intolerance.

The average calcium intake of females of childbearing age is consistently less than the recommended intake, as Figure 1–3 illustrates. It is clear, then, that the calcium intake of many individuals is even lower than the average and that they may be maintaining their blood calcium concentrations at the expense of bone losses. Our society's emphasis on thin bodies has prompted many females to adopt low-kcalorie diets, which are often low in milk products. Others mistakenly believe that adults no longer need calcium after they have stopped growing—that bones remain strong without further deposits.

Not only do many women's daily calcium intakes fail to meet their recommendations, but for women facing future pregnancies, calcium needs will intensify. Women require additional calcium throughout pregnancy, even though most of it does not transfer to the fetus until the last trimester. Even with the adaptive mechanisms that favor calcium retention, infants born to mothers on low-calcium diets have suboptimal bone density.[3] Evidently, to avoid such occurrences, women need to put away greater calcium stores *before* pregnancy in order to meet the increased demands of pregnancy.

To help maximize calcium stores before the start of pregnancy, females should eat calcium-rich foods regularly or take supplements if circumstances require. The ADA recommendation suggests that a woman eat 3 to 4 servings of calcium-rich foods daily. To consume enough calcium from dairy products without exceeding energy intake limits requires careful selection of low-fat items. Table 1–1 lists various foods according to their calcium content per average serving size and per 100 kcalories. Canned sardines with bones are an excellent source of calcium, but with a high-kcalorie price tag. Some vegetables such as bok choy cabbage, turnip greens, and spinach appear to offer an advantage by providing more calcium per kcalorie than do dairy products or

Chapter 2 discusses calcium needs, transfer, and adaptive mechanisms during pregnancy.

Figure 1–3   Daily Calcium Intakes of Females Compared to Their RDA
Not only are women's average calcium intakes below recommendations, but they also
fall lower throughout life. Some authorities favor a still higher recommendation than
that of the RDA, indicating that many women may be falling far short of their calcium
needs. The dotted line indicates the higher calcium need of pregnancy and lactation.

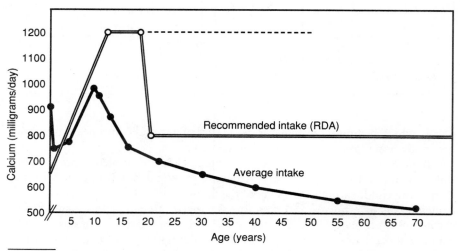

Source: Adapted from National Center for Health Statistics, *Dietary Intake Source Data:
United States, 1976–1980,* DHHS Publication No. (PHS) 83-1681, March 1983.

Table 1–1   Calcium in Foods

Foods Ranked by Calcium per Serving	Calcium per Serving (mg)	Energy per Serving (kcal)	Calcium per 100 kCal (mg)
Sardines, canned w/bones (3 oz)	371	175	212
Kefir (1 c)	350	160	219
Shrimp, boiled (3.5 oz)	320	109	595
Romano cheese (1 oz)	302	110	275
Nonfat milk or yogurt (1 c)	302	86	351
1% lowfat milk (1 c)	300	102	294
Whole milk (1 c)	291	150	194
Buttermilk (1 c)	285	99	288
Chocolate milk, whole (1 c)	280	210	133
Swiss cheese (1 oz)	272	107	254
Spinach, cooked (1 c)	244	41	595
Cheddar cheese (1 oz)	204	114	179
Muenster cheese (1 oz)	203	104	195
Oysters, raw (1 c)	202	160	126
Turnip greens, cooked (1 c)	198	29	683
Broccoli, cooked (1 c)	178	46	387
Salmon, canned w/bones (3 oz)	167	120	139
Beet greens, cooked (1 c)	165	40	413
Bok choy cabbage, cooked (1 c)	158	20	790
Cottage cheese, lowfat 2% (1 c)	155	205	76

sardines. However, the fiber and oxalates in them impair calcium absorption. The results of studies suggest that the reduced calcium absorption negates the increased calcium from the vegetables.[4] These foods are nutritious for many reasons, but not for their calcium contributions. The upcoming section on supplements describes calcium supplement usage, absorption, and risks.

Iron Iron functions as a component of hemoglobin, myoglobin, and several enzymes. Iron stores complete the body's total iron content. With inadequate iron intake, the stores serve as a source of iron to meet the body's needs. Only after the depletion of iron stores do hemoglobin concentrations begin to fall. Therefore, iron depletion progresses quite far before this standard blood test can diagnose it.

During the procreative years, women are in a precarious state with respect to iron sufficiency. Their normal iron losses exceed those of men because of repeated menstrual blood losses. In addition, the average iron intake of women is consistently less than the recommended intake as Figure 1–4 illustrates. The combination of inadequate iron intake and the natural iron loss that occurs in the procreative years makes attaining iron sufficiency a challenge. It is not uncommon for women to enter pregnancy with depleted iron stores.

With a pregnancy, the increase in blood volume and the fetal requirements drain the iron stores further. It is important to realize that fetal withdrawals of iron are made regardless of the mother's iron status. Thus, the hemoglobin concentration in a newborn may be normal even when the mother's stores are low. However, if her diet has been inadequate and her stores are depleted when fetal withdrawals are made, then both mother and fetus will have low

Appendix A describes iron assessment techniques and provides laboratory test values.

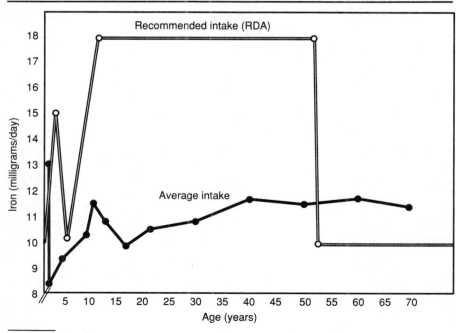

Figure 1–4 Daily Iron Intakes of Females Compared to their RDA
Women's average iron intakes fall below recommendations.

Source: Adapted from National Center for Health Statistics, *Dietary Intake Source Data: United States, 1976–1980,* DHHS Publication No. (PHS) 83-1681, March 1983.

hemoglobin values. The implications of maternal iron deficiency are evident in an increased risk of poor pregnancy outcome—fetal death, preterm birth, low birthweight, and medical abnormalities.[5]

A woman planning to become pregnant can benefit from a nutrition assessment to determine her iron status. If deficient, she will want to remedy the problem before she becomes pregnant. Otherwise, the stress of iron-deficiency anemia can seriously impair her physical health and emotional adjustment.

The best way to *prevent* iron deficiency is to eat iron-rich foods regularly. The best way to *treat* iron deficiency may be to combine iron-rich foods and supplements. (A discussion of iron supplements follows this section.) Table 1–2 ranks various foods by their iron content per serving size and per 100 kcalories. The iron content of a food provides only a rough estimate of a person's actual iron intake, though, for iron absorption is a complex process that is influenced by the intestinal mucosa, the type of iron in the food (whether it is heme or nonheme), and other dietary factors. The body absorbs heme iron more efficiently than nonheme iron. Meat, fish, poultry, and vitamin C-rich foods eaten at the same meal with foods that contain nonheme iron enhance nonheme iron absorption.

Appendix A explains how to calculate iron absorbed from meals.

Other nutrients The ADA recommendations include special mention of calcium and iron, but other nutrients may also be lacking in the diets of many women. The average vitamin B_6, folacin, magnesium, and zinc intakes of

Table 1–2 Iron in Foods

Foods Ranked by Iron per Serving	Iron per Serving (mg)	Energy per Serving (kcal)	Iron per 100 kCal (mg)
Oysters, raw (1 c)	16.80	160	18.60
Sirloin steak, lean (8 oz)	7.68	480	1.60
Spinach, cooked (1 c)	6.42	41	15.66
Lima beans, cooked (1 c)	5.90	260	2.27
Beef liver, fried (3 oz)	5.30	185	2.86
Peach halves, dried (10)	5.28	311	1.70
Navy beans, cooked dry (1 c)	5.10	225	2.27
Soy beans, cooked dry (1 c)	4.90	235	2.09
Hamburger patty, bun (4 oz)	4.84	445	1.09
Kidney beans, canned (1 c)	4.60	230	2.00
Parsley, chopped fresh (1 c)	3.72	20	18.60
Sauerkraut, canned (1 c)	3.47	44	7.89
Peas, dry split, cooked (1 c)	3.40	230	1.48
Blackeyed peas, cooked (1 c)	3.30	190	1.74
Green peas, cooked (1 c)	3.15	67	4.70
Beef pot roast, lean (3 oz)	3.14	232	1.36
Prune juice, bottled (1 c)	3.02	181	1.67
Baked potato, whole (1)	2.75	220	1.25
Beet greens, cooked (1 c)	2.74	40	6.85
Sardines, canned (3 oz)	2.60	175	1.49

women between the ages of 19 and 55 range between 50 and 75 percent of the Recommended Dietary Allowances (RDA).[6]

Foods rich in vitamin B_6 are bok choy cabbage, turnip greens, and spinach. The very vegetables that were rejected earlier as calcium sources are ideal for providing vitamin B_6. These vegetables, and many others, are also rich in folacin. Similarly, many of the foods that provide a woman with iron are equally rich in zinc. These observations illustrate that a wise selection of foods can offer substantial quantities of more than one nutrient to rectify several problems with one solution. However, no one food or food group can correct for all inadequacies. Eating a variety of foods from each of the food groups emerges as the best plan.

The inadequacy of the magnesium intake of women may reflect a spuriously high recommendation rather than a true deficiency problem. The recommendation bases its requirement on a limited number of balance studies and on usual daily intakes. Actual magnesium deficiency symptoms, however, are seen only in pathological conditions such as alcohol abuse, protein-energy malnutrition, and malabsorption diseases. In any case, a woman who varies her diet to obtain the other nutrients will receive adequate magnesium. Many vegetables, beans, peas, and seeds are rich in magnesium.

Supplements

The ADA recommendations urge women to rely on foods for necessary nutrients, using vitamin and mineral supplements only under specific circumstances. The following list acknowledges that specific conditions may justify the taking of supplements by prepregnant women, including:[7]

▶ Women with low energy intakes, such as habitual dieters.

▶ Women who eat bizarre or monotonous diets, such as some food faddists.

▶ Women with illnesses that take away the appetite.

▶ Women with illnesses that impair absorption of nutrients—including diseases of the liver, gallbladder, pancreas, and digestive system.

▶ Women taking medications that interfere with the body's use of specific nutrients (see Table A–3 in Appendix A).

▶ Women who have diseases, infections, or injuries, or who have undergone surgery resulting in increased metabolic needs.

▶ Strict vegetarians.

Women can get all the nutrients they need (except iron during pregnancy) by eating a varied diet of whole foods. Unfortunately, many do not eat this way, for one reason or another. To determine whether an individual is at risk for a nutrient deficiency requires a complete nutrition assessment. When such an assessment so indicates, a health care provider can recommend an appropriate supplement. Single nutrient supplements correct for specific nutrient deficiencies. Women who do not eat well enough to receive the nutrients they need may benefit from multivitamin-mineral supplements. A reliable rule of thumb when selecting a supplement is to find one that provides all of the RDA nutrients in amounts smaller than, equal to, or very close to the RDA for that person.

Appendix A describes nutrition assessment techniques.

Ca supplementation

As mentioned earlier, inadequate calcium intake does contribute to age-related bone loss. However, calcium supplementation has yet to be proven effective in preventing osteoporosis and is not unanimously accepted by the medical community.[8] Nevertheless, supplementation may be the only way some women can meet their calcium needs. To the previous list of justifications for supplement use, add:

▶ Women whose calcium intakes are too low to forestall extensive bone loss.

Most healthy people absorb calcium equally well from calcium carbonate, calcium acetate, calcium lactate, calcium gluconate, and calcium citrate, as from whole milk.[9] A consumer could refine the choice among these by comparing other variables such as cost and number of tablets to be ingested. Calcium carbonate contains the highest percentage of calcium (40 percent) and therefore can meet daily needs with the smallest number of tablets. Consumers should avoid calcium-rich preparations of bone meal or dolomite (limestone) because they may contain unsafe levels of contaminants such as lead, arsenic, cadmium, or mercury. Consumers using calcium supplements combined with vitamin D must keep track of the quantity of vitamin D they are taking in order to avoid toxic doses.

Iron is like calcium and all other nutrients in that foods meet the body's requirements better than supplements do. Still, many women are unable to meet their iron requirements with foods alone and might benefit from supplements providing the recommended 18 milligrams.[10] The body absorbs the ferrous form of an iron supplement efficiently and taking the supplement before meals enhances absorption.[11] A final addition to the previous list of circumstances that may justify the taking of a supplement:

▶ Women who bleed excessively during menstruation.

The taking of individual mineral supplements requires caution. Minerals compete for binding sites and thus interfere with each others' bioavailability. For example, the calcium phosphate dibasic supplement inhibits magnesium absorption. If it is fortified with magnesium, then it interferes with both calcium and iron absorption.[12] Calcium carbonate and calcium hydroxyapatite supplements also interfere with iron absorption when taken with meals.[13] Likewise, iron supplements may impair folacin, zinc, copper, and selenium status, although research findings conflict.[14]

In addition to adversely affecting the bioavailability of other nutrients, supplement use can cause other problems with varying degrees of severity. Calcium phosphate dibasic causes calcium deposition in the kidneys of rats.[15] For this reason, people susceptible to kidney stones would be wise to avoid using this supplement. Iron supplements cause heartburn and constipation in some people. These side effects diminish if the iron is taken in small doses after meals.

For the best possible health prior to pregnancy, women need to pay attention to their food and nutrient intakes as described above. Hand in hand with these goes another lifestyle factor that enhances health—exercise.

Exercise

The ADA task force on women's recommendations recognizes the health advantages of regular exercise. Exercise burns kcalories and, if a balanced program is chosen, improves muscular strength, endurance, and flexibility. In addition, aerobic exercises such as jogging, swimming, cycling, and dancing provide the added benefits of improving cardiovascular and respiratory endurance and resistance to disease. Regular exercise provides psychological benefits as well. These include a positive self-image, a sense of well-being, and a positive attitude in general—all important to a person whose body is about to be temporarily transformed by a pregnancy.

In addition, exercise improves a woman's nutrition status. Bones do not passively accumulate calcium from foods; they store calcium and become dense, strong, and able to carry more weight in response to physical activity. Physical activity also develops the lean body tissue that serves as a storage site for iron and other nutrients. In pregnancy, a healthy circulatory system developed in response to exercise will be critical in transporting nutrients through the maternal body and to the fetus.

A healthy woman, conditioned to physical activity prior to pregnancy, can enjoy exercising throughout her pregnancy. Most obstetricians recommend that a woman can continue to exercise during pregnancy at her prepregnant level of intensity and frequency until she becomes uncomfortable. When she becomes pregnant, a woman is advised not to overexert herself or to attempt unfamiliar exercises. For example, a runner will run a shorter distance, less often or at a slower pace, as the pregnancy progresses. She must be running regularly prior to her pregnancy; conception is not a good time to begin. (It is, however, a good idea for a pregnant woman who has not been regularly active to start a *moderate* exercise program such as walking or swimming.)

In summary, a woman who wants to be physically active when she becomes pregnant needs to become physically active *beforehand*. She must establish a baseline of exercise intensity, duration, and frequency that will represent the maximum for the duration of any future pregnancy. Women who are physically active prior to and throughout pregnancy find it much easier to resume an exercise regimen after recovery from the birth. The physically active woman will be grateful that she has already made the effort to establish regular exercise habits prior to conception. They will sustain her during the pregnancy and after the infant arrives.

Women's Cycles and Nutrition

As stated in the introductory remarks, women's nutrient needs differ in each phase of life. The following section focuses on the first phase—the nonpregnant, reproductive time in a woman's life—a time of menstrual cycles. Then, because many women use contraceptive devices and methods during these years, this section continues with a look at the nutrition implications of contraception.

The Menstrual Cycle

The average woman experiences 500 menstrual cycles in her lifetime, losing more than 17 liters of blood and 6500 milligrams of iron.[16] No doubt, the physical losses incurred by menstrual cycles impose tremendous needs of all

menarche (men-ARK): the onset of menstruation; the first menstrual period, usually occurring between the ages of 11 and 14.
men = month
arche = beginning

ovaries (OH-vah-rees): the two glands that produce ova and female hormones.

uterus (YOU-ter-us): the muscular organ within which the embryo and fetus develop from the time of implantation to birth.

menopause: the time in a woman's life when menstrual activity ceases, usually between the ages of 35 and 55.
pause = cessation

follicle: a small, saclike structure in the ovary, consisting of an ovum surrounded by epithelial cells that secrete estrogen.

FSH or **follicle-stimulating hormone:** a hormone from the pituitary gland that stimulates the growth of follicles.

LH or **luteinizing** (LOO-tin-eye-zing) **hormone:** a hormone from the pituitary gland that stimulates development of the ruptured follicle into the corpus luteum and signals ovulation.

ovulation: the ripening and rupturing of the mature follicle and subsequent release of the ovum.

nutrients, not only of iron. Furthermore, the constantly changing hormonal and metabolic activity of the cycle has a great impact on women's energy needs, as this section reveals. An understanding of the interrelationships between the hormones and organs involved in a typical menstrual cycle will lay a foundation for understanding the nutrition needs of women during this phase of life.

During puberty, a woman's monthly cycles begin—an event known as menarche. Hormones synchronize and coordinate the events of the monthly menstrual cycle. These hormones elicit responses from each other, from the sex organs, and from the body's other organs and tissues. Figure 1–5 illustrates how their fluctuating concentrations account for the events of the month.

The most dramatic physical changes occur in the ovaries and the uterus. Female infants are born with about one million ova in each ovary. Of these ova, relatively few will reach maturity and participate in a menstrual cycle. Fewer still will undergo fertilization and develop into new lives. Most ova will degenerate over the years, leaving none at the time of menopause.

In the ovary, an ovum, surrounded by a layer of follicular cells, enlarges and develops into a mature follicle. The hormone FSH (follicle-stimulating hormone), which dominates the beginning of the cycle, encourages the growth of the follicle. When the follicle reaches maturity, a sharp rise in the hormone LH (luteinizing hormone) triggers its rupture, thus releasing the ovum. This event, ovulation, occurs approximately 14 days prior to the next menstrual flow. The process of follicle development takes approximately two weeks and

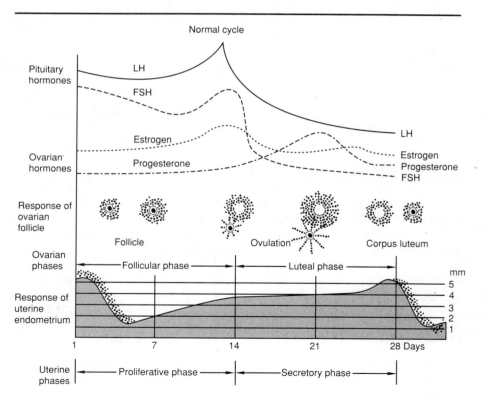

Figure 1–5 The Menstrual Cycle
Changes in hormone concentrations elicit ovarian follicle development and changes in the uterine lining during the menstrual cycle.

Miniglossary of Menstrual Cycle Phases

Several names apply to the phases of the menstrual cycle. One set of names reflects the events occurring within the ovaries; another, those occurring in the uterus. The ovary's follicular or preovulatory phase coincides with menstrual flow and with the uterus's proliferative phase. Similarly, the ovary's luteal or postovulatory phase coincides with the uterus's secretory phase (see Figure 1–5).

follicular phase: ovarian events of follicle development prior to ovulation; coincides with uterine menstrual flow and proliferative phase.

menstrual flow: the periodic discharge of blood, disintegrated endometrial cells, and gland secretions from the uterus.

proliferative phase: uterine events of endometrium development prior to ovulation; coincides with ovarian follicular phase.

luteal phase: ovarian events of corpus luteum development from ovulation to menstrual flow; coincides with uterine secretory phase.

secretory phase: uterine events of endometrium disintegration from ovulation to menstrual flow; coincides with ovarian luteal phase.

---

is called the follicular phase of the menstrual cycle (see Miniglossary of Menstrual Cycle Phases).

In response to the high levels of LH, the ruptured follicle transforms into a structure known as the corpus luteum. Without ovum fertilization, the corpus luteum gradually develops to maturity and then rapidly degenerates. (If pregnancy does occur, the corpus luteum remains active.) The process of corpus luteum development and degeneration takes roughly 10 to 14 days and is called the luteal phase of the menstrual cycle.

Both the follicle and the corpus luteum secrete estrogen. The time of maximum activity of these two structures is evident in the two rises in estrogen concentration during the cycle (see Figure 1–5). During the last half of the follicular phase, the rapidly rising levels of estrogen signal the pituitary to reduce FSH production (negative feedback) and to increase LH production (positive feedback). During the luteal phase, the rise in estrogen does not stimulate the surge of LH as it did in the follicular phase. This is because the corpus luteum is secreting progesterone, as well as estrogen. The progesterone-estrogen combination inhibits FSH and LH release, thus preventing follicle development. With corpus luteum degeneration, progesterone and estrogen levels diminish, FSH and LH levels begin to rise, and the cycle repeats itself.

In the uterus, profound changes occur in response to progesterone and estrogen. The rising levels of estrogen during the first half of the menstrual cycle stimulate the growth of the uterine lining, the endometrium. The endometrium thickens and develops an extensive vascular system in preparation for the implantation of the ovum, should fertilization occur. The proliferative phase of endometrium development lasts about 10 days, ceasing with ovulation. Without fertilization, the endometrium begins to disintegrate—the secretory phase. Finally, the endometrium lining begins to slough. Menstrual "blood" is the endometrium lining, which leaves the body

corpus luteum (CORE-pus LOO-tee-um): a mass of glandular tissue that develops from a ruptured follicle and secretes hormones.
corpus = body
luteum = yellow

estrogen (ESS-tro-jen): one of the female sex hormones produced in the ovaries, responsible for sexual development and for regulation of the menstrual cycle.

progesterone (pro-JESS-teh-rone): a female hormone produced in the ovaries responsible for changes in the uterine endometrium in the luteal phase of the menstrual cycle.

endometrium (en-doe-MEE-tree-um): the membrane lining the inner surface of the uterus.

implantation: the stage of development in which the zygote embeds itself in the wall of the uterus and begins to develop, during the first two weeks after conception.

within four or five days. At the end of menstruation, the endometrium has returned to its minimal state.

The average menstrual cycle lasts 28 days, give or take a few days. The days are usually counted from the first day of bleeding because it is easy to detect.

Many physiological activities support the menstrual cycle's many events and have nutrition implications. Basal body temperature and basal metabolic rate fluctuate with the changing events of the menstrual cycle. Basal body temperature drops during the follicular phase and rises during the luteal phase.[17] The temperature begins its rise with the surge in LH. It continues to climb after the LH peak, coinciding with the increase of serum progesterone concentrations, which raise body temperature. Secretion of progesterone during the menstrual cycle also coincides with changes in basal metabolic rate.[18]

These changes in basal body temperature and basal metabolic rate may affect food intake and body weight changes. Women tend to eat more food per day for the half month after ovulation (prior to menstruation) than during the half month before ovulation (after menstruation). One study noted that mean energy intake prior to menstruation was 500 kcalories per day greater than after menstruation.[19] A follow-up study revealed that the source of the additional kcalories was carbohydrate-rich foods.[20] Another study found that basal metabolic rates have the same variation pattern through the menstrual cycle as the energy intake reported in the first study, but the kcaloric difference was only 350 kcalories.[21] This 150 kcalorie difference may be at least partially explained by recognizing that the first study examined the food intake patterns of women in normal life situations, whereas the second study examined energy expenditures in a metabolic unit. Other variables, such as activity patterns, affect the kcaloric differences reported by any study.

These studies suggest that it may be unrealistic for a woman to maintain a constant daily energy intake throughout the month. Eating more food prior to menstruation may be a woman's most appropriate response to an elevated basal metabolic rate. If there is a harm related to responding to increased premenstrual energy needs by eating extra food, the harm comes from ignoring the postmenstrual decline. Energy needs change, and therefore a woman's energy intakes can also change without her having to feel guilty about eating more on some days than on others. Instead, a woman can respond to her body's signals by carefully selecting a well-balanced diet that provides additional energy prior to menstruation and returns to a lower energy intake following menstruation.

Premenstrual Syndrome

During the past decade, interest in women's health issues heightened, and premenstrual syndrome became a popular news item—even though its existence preceded its name by centuries. As is often the case when health problems make a news splash, companies and clinics were quick to offer "solutions" before scientific research could provide answers to the possible causes and treatments of PMS.

Premenstrual syndrome (PMS) is a cluster of physical, emotional, and psychological symptoms that some women experience prior to their menstrual

premenstrual syndrome (PMS): a cluster of physical, emotional, and psychological symptoms that occur prior to menstruation and diminish during or after menstruation.

cycles. Specific PMS symptoms and combinations of symptoms vary from woman to woman. The distinguishing feature of PMS is the timing of the symptoms with a woman's menstrual cycle. Most women begin to experience symptoms seven to ten days prior to menstruation, during the luteal phase of their cycles. Symptoms disappear, or at least diminish significantly, with menstruation.

Exactly how many women have PMS is unknown primarily because its diagnosis depends solely on a woman's description of her symptoms. By keeping a symptom diary, a woman can see how her physical and emotional well-being fluctuate in relation to her menstrual cycle. Physicians may conduct diagnostic tests to eliminate the possibility that a woman's symptoms derive from another disorder, but not to confirm the diagnosis of PMS. For some women, an underlying physical or emotional disorder (such as migraine headaches or depression) surfaces premenstrually and blurs the distinction between PMS and other problems. Some women recognize a few symptoms prior to their menstrual periods as a signal, not a problem. Others become incapacitated. The intensity of the symptoms and the woman's perception of them differs for each woman.

The cause or causes of PMS remain undefined, although researchers generally agree that the hormonal changes of the menstrual cycle must be responsible.[22] Following the trail of these hormones requires masterful detective work. The hormones involved in the menstrual cycle influence the activities of a number of other hormones and neurotransmitters, with a multitude of effects on physical, emotional, and psychological health. Even successfully identifying the path of changes does not solve the mystery, for not all women experience PMS.

Without a full understanding of the ways PMS arises, treatment efforts flounder. In some instances, physicians prescribe remedies for specific symptoms, such as tranquilizers for anxiety. Others attempt to treat the syndrome as a whole. One obstacle researchers encounter in their efforts to find a treatment is that many women with PMS respond favorably to placebo treatments.

Unproven treatments for PMS include hormones (most often, progesterone), drugs that alter hormone actions, and various nutrient supplements. In addition, over-the-counter medicines provide temporary relief of some symptoms: diuretics for fluid retention, caffeine for fatigue, and aspirin, acetaminophen, and ibuprofen for headaches.

The nutrients receiving most of the PMS attention are vitamin B_6, vitamin A, vitamin E, magnesium, zinc, and omega fatty acids. In each case, weak links connect these nutrients with PMS, yet none provides enough evidence to support its use. Women wanting to take vitamin and mineral supplements to relieve PMS need to be forewarned that the benefits are uncertain and the risks of toxicity are possible.

Some women find that improvements on their general health benefit their PMS. They lose weight, eat a nutritious diet, exercise regularly, avoid using tobacco, and avoid drinking alcohol and caffeine beverages in excess. In addition, relaxation techniques help women to cope with the stresses of PMS. No question that these changes are advantageous to a woman's health; perhaps PMS, whatever its cause, becomes more tolerable when the body is healthier.

Suggested Rx healthier living

Common PMS Symptoms:

▸ Headache.

▸ Breast swelling and tenderness.

▸ Water retention.

▸ Weight gain.

▸ Irritability.

▸ Anxiety.

▸ Fatigue.

▸ Depression.

▸ Appetite changes and food cravings.

▸ Backache.

▸ Acne.

▸ Constipation.

placebo: an inert drug or treatment used for its psychological effect.

Contraception

Each menstrual cycle presents a woman and her partner with the responsibility for making a choice of whether to start a pregnancy. Many personal factors influence the decision—their ages and status of their relationship, the age spread between children, the number of children wanted, career commitments, family support, financial status, and philosophical views. These concerns take a high priority when couples discuss their futures; another concern is even more important to the health of a future pregnancy—the woman's physical, as well as emotional, condition. The spacing of pregnancies and contraceptive methods used should complement her health needs. Couples are in the best position to select from the several contraceptive methods available with the consultation of their health care providers. An examination of the nutrition implications of some contraceptive methods may help a couple in their decision. The two selected here are those that have a known nutrition impact—oral contraceptives and intrauterine devices.

Oral contraceptives   Millions of women use oral contraceptives, popularly known as the "pill", to prevent pregnancy. In its 30-year history, the pill has become the most studied drug in the United States.[23] The identification of a number of risk factors has prompted changes in the dosages and formulations of the pill to produce an effective contraceptive with a wide margin of safety. The pills of the 1980s contain one-fifth the estrogen and one-tenth the progesterone originally in the pills of the 1960s, making them as risk free as possible, yet still effective.[24]

In addition to low hormone concentrations, the concentrations may vary throughout the month to roughly simulate the hormone changes that normally occur during a menstrual cycle. Such pills are known as multiphasic pills and may avert some minor side effects, such as breakthrough bleeding, or even more serious ones, such as blood lipid changes in some women.[25] Some manufacturers claim that multiphasic pills are a more natural product or one that is physiologically superior to fixed-dose pills, however, this is fallacious .[26] After all, the purpose of oral contraceptives is to alter the natural events of the menstrual cycle.

There are two types of oral contraceptives—the combination pill and the minipill. Of the women using oral contraceptives in the United States, 99 percent take the combination type pill which contains synthetic versions of the hormones estrogen and progesterone.[27] Recall from the discussion on the menstrual cycle that the ovaries naturally produce estrogen after ovulation, to suppress ovulation until after the next menstruation. The estrogen in the combination pills prevents pregnancy the same way—by suppressing ovulation.

The other type of oral contraceptive, the minipill, contains only synthetic progesterone, known as progestin. The progestin in the minipill makes the mucus surrounding the uterine opening (the cervix) less penetrable to spermatozoa and may deactivate them. It also interrupts the normal preparation of the uterine endometrium so as to prevent zygote implantation.

Oral contraceptives not only prevent pregnancy, but also benefit a woman's reproductive system physiologically. (Table 1–3 lists the positive and negative side effects of oral contraceptives.) Apparently, the suppression of

Table 1–3   Side Effects of Oral Contraceptives

Reduced risk of:	Increased risk of:
Benign breast disease[a]	Coronary artery disease
Endometrial cancer	Gallbladder disease
Ovarian cancer	Glucose intolerance
Ovarian cysts	High blood pressure
Painful menstrual periods	
Premenstrual syndrome	
Pregnancy	

[a]The effect of oral contraceptives on breast cancer is inconclusive; it appears that oral contraceptive use is not a risk for breast cancer.

Source: Adapted from B. D. Shephard, Oral contraceptives—An overview, *Journal of the Florida Medical Association* 73 (1986): 763–767; E. L. Marut, Oral contraceptives—Who, which, when, and why?, *Postgraduate Medicine* 82 (1987): 66–70; G. R. Huggins and P. K. Zucker, Oral contraceptives and neoplasia: 1987 update, *Fertility and Sterility* 47 (1987): 733–761; D. R. Miller and coauthors, Breast cancer risk in relation to early oral contraceptive use, *Obstetrics and Gynecology* 68 (1986): 863–868; R. Russell-Briefel and coauthors, Cardiovascular risk status and oral contraceptive use: United States, 1976–1980, *Preventive Medicine* 15 (1986): 352–362; P. B. Moser and coauthors, Carbohydrate tolerance and serum lipid responses to type of dietary carbohydrate and oral contraceptive use in young women, *Journal of the American College of Nutrition* 5 (1986): 45–53; R. Russell-Briefel and coauthors, Impaired glucose tolerance in women using oral contraceptives: United States, 1976–1980, *Journal of Chronic Diseases* 40 (1987): 3–11; J. K. Williams, Oral contraceptives—The long-term perspective, *Journal of the Florida Medical Association* 73 (1986): 769–771; B. L. Strom, Oral contraceptives and other risk factors for gallbladder disease, *Clinical Pharmacology and Therapeutics* 39 (1986): 335–341.

ovulation reduces the likelihood of ovarian cancer, ovarian cysts, painful menstrual periods, and premenstrual syndrome.[28] The reduced risk of ovarian cancer is seen in women who use the pill for as little as three months, and continues for 15 years after their use ends.[29] The progesterone in the pill offers protection against endometrial cancer and benign breast disease.[30] The protective effect against endometrial cancer is seen in women who use the pill for at least 12 months, and persists for 15 years after pill cessation.[31]

The effect of oral contraceptives on breast cancer is inconclusive, primarily because breast cancer may correlate with an event, such as menarche, that occurred three to four decades earlier, and the pill has been available for less than three decades. For now, it appears that even long-term oral contraceptive use in a young, prepregnant woman is not a risk for breast cancer.[32]

The pill presents negative side effects as well, most in response to its progesterone content. Progesterone is thought to be the culprit in altering blood lipids and raising the risk of coronary artery disease for pill users. Most oral contraceptives elevate total cholesterol and triglyceride concentrations and lower HDL concentrations, tipping the balance toward cardiovascular disease.[33] The risk is greatest for women after age 35 who smoke and for all women over age 45.[34] These women should find alternative contraceptive methods. For young, healthy women who do not smoke, the association between oral contraceptives and coronary artery disease disappears.[35] The progesterone in the pill is also responsible for high blood pressure in some users, especially women who are older, multiparous, and obese. This high blood pressure reverts to normal when users stop taking the pill.[36]

The progesterone in oral contraceptives alters carbohydrate metabolism.[37] Glucose tolerance diminishes and blood glucose and insulin levels are high, especially in women predisposed to diabetes.[38] For most women, the changes in carbohydrate metabolism are minimal and return to normal with cessation of pill use.[39] Because these metabolic effects are transient and reversible, the risk of diabetes is small compared to other nonreversible factors, such as genetics.[40]

One risk, that of gallbladder disease, has a dose-response relationship with the estrogen content of oral contraceptives. This risk appears to be greater for young women than for women over age 40.[41] The risk of gallstone formation in oral contraceptive users stems from the progesterone-caused changes in cholesterol metabolism mentioned earlier.[42]

Oral contraceptives reduce menstrual blood flow and thereby conserve for the body all nutrients normally lost in menstrual blood—most notably iron. They also alter the metabolism of many vitamins and minerals. Their specific effects vary with each nutrient and with the hormone concentrations of the pills. For some nutrients, oral contraceptives affect the absorption or excretion rate. For others, the rate of metabolic conversion changes the nutrient status. Whatever the mechanism, the effects on vitamins and minerals are reflected in higher or lower blood concentrations. Table 1–4 lists the effects of oral contraceptives on various nutrients.

[handwritten margin note: sum of effect of pill on nutrients]

In some cases, the effects of oral contraceptives on vitamin and mineral status may appear more positive than they are. For example, oral contraceptives raise plasma retinol concentrations but lower liver retinol concentrations. This suggests a possible redistribution of retinol in the body, and not necessarily the improved status that high plasma values might seem to imply. In other cases, concentrations of vitamins or minerals in the body are low, reflecting an increased demand in metabolic pathways, impaired absorption, increased excretion, or altered tissue distribution. However, the clinical significance of these reductions in nutrient concentrations is minor in the overall picture of factors affecting women's nutrition status.

The use of supplements to correct the nutrient fluctuations incurred by oral contraceptive use is inappropriate. If nutrient deficiencies and excesses are evident in women taking oral contraceptives, the remedy is to improve the diet. Oral contraceptive users should refrain from taking large doses of individual vitamin supplements unless advised to do so for medically valid reasons by a health care provider. Most women will find that a nutritionally sound diet is all that is needed. Any woman suspected of having borderline deficiencies for any reason may benefit from a multivitamin-mineral supplement that does not exceed the RDA, in addition to a well-balanced diet. Supplements are indicated only if deficiency symptoms are apparent and not correctable by diet alone.[43]

Experimental evidence supports the contention that the routine use of supplements is unnecessary for women using oral contraceptives. In one study, researchers compared the adverse effects of oral contraceptives on vitamin metabolism in three groups of women.[44] One group took two multivitamin supplements a day for one week each month, another group took one multivitamin supplement every day, and the other took a placebo each day. The data demonstrated that routine use of multivitamin supplementation in women on oral contraceptives is unjustified.

Temporary water retention, seen in many women around the time of their menstrual periods, may add a few pounds on the scale. Oral contraceptives

Table 1–4 Nutrient Effects of Oral Contraceptives

Nutrient	Effect on Blood Concentrations and Metabolism
Energy-Yielding Nutrients	
carbohydrate	elevated fasting glucose elevated insulin
protein	elevated coagulating proteins lowered albumin
lipid	elevated triglycerides elevated LDL cholesterol lowered HDL cholesterol
Vitamins	
vitamin A	elevated retinol (lowered liver stores) elevated retinol-binding proteins lowered carotene
vitamin E	no effect
vitamin K	elevated clotting factors (and lowered response to anticoagulants)
vitamin C	lowered in leukocytes, thrombocytes, and platelets
riboflavin	lowered (in some studies) impaired enzyme activity (in some studies)
vitamin B_{12}	lowered in serum; normal in red blood cells
vitamin B_6	lowered
folacin	lowered (in some studies)
Minerals	
copper	elevated
iron	elevated
zinc	lowered
Water	retained temporarily

Source: The information in this table is compiled from a number of studies, including D. Dimperio, Effect of oral contraceptives on nutrient status, an address presented at the Conference on Nutrition for Pregnancy, Lactation, and Infancy on 13 February 1987, in Gainesville, Florida and L. B. Tyrer, Nutrition and the pill, *Journal of Reproductive Medicine* 29 (1984): 547–550.

seem to produce the same fluid retention effect. This has led some women to believe that fat gain is a side effect of oral contraceptive use. Fear of fat gain may deter women from using oral contraceptives. One study found no difference in the weight gain of females using oral contraceptives when compared with those using other contraceptive methods.[45] A woman who does gain fat during the initial months of oral contraceptive use should first check her diet and exercise habits and then consult her physician about switching to another type of pill or method.

If a lactating mother wants to use the pill, she is wise to wait until after she has weaned her infant and to use another method of contraception in the meantime. Standard oral contraceptive pills contain estrogen, which reduces milk volume and protein content of breast milk.[46] The lower milk volume does not appear to impair infant growth or behavior when the mother is well nourished and lactation is well established.[47] Progestin-only contraceptive pills do not affect milk volume and are preferable for women wishing to use oral contraceptives, especially if maternal nutrition is inadequate. The hormones of oral contraceptives also reach the infant via the breast milk, but the concentrations are low and the effects, if any, are probably transient.

Intrauterine device (IUD)   The intrauterine device (IUD, or coil) is a small piece of molded plastic or plastic and metal that is inserted into the uterus. One type of IUD contains progestin. The IUD's effectiveness is not completely understood. Apparently, it induces a change in the uterine lining that interferes with the implantation of a zygote.

IUDs cause increased blood loss. Heavy menstrual bleeding can be inconvenient and distressing, but rarely signifies a serious disorder. It does entail a nutrition risk, however: the development of iron-deficiency anemia due to loss of blood. Therefore, the iron status of a woman using an IUD requires regular assessment.

The hormonal changes of the menstrual cycle and of contraception affect a woman's health. The changes that accompany pregnancy affect not only her health, but that of her progeny.

Appendix A discusses assessment of iron status.

Conception and Implantation

In nourishing themselves well early in life, a young man and woman are not only engaging in self-care, but are also helping to provide healthy environments for the development of the special cells that will transmit the characteristics of earlier generations to the next generation. To understand the importance of nutrition to normal conception and fetal development, it is necessary to understand the basics of three processes: inheritance, fertilization, and implantation.

Inheritance

gamete (gam-EAT): a mature male or female reproductive cell; the spermatozoon or ovum.
gamein = to marry

chromosomes: the bodies within each cell that contain the genetic material (deoxyribonucleic acid, or DNA).

genes: the basic units of hereditary information, made of DNA, that are passed from parent to offspring in the chromosomes of the gametes. Each gene codes for a protein.

A female gamete, an ovum, packs within it a set of 23 chromosomes containing all of the genetic information necessary to make a human being. Each chromosome bears along its length thousands of genes, and each gene consists of coded instructions for making a single working protein—an enzyme, a structural protein, a muscle protein, or some other body protein. Each protein will determine, or help to determine, traits for the new person, such as eye color, hair color and texture, maximum height, and brain size. The exact combination of these and many other characteristics makes each individual unique. These are the characteristics that a person must accept without option for change.

When a man's body makes a spermatozoon, it too contains 23 chromosomes bearing sets of instructions for the same characteristics. When the ovum and spermatozoon merge at fertilization to form a single cell, the chromosomes from each parent line up side by side within that cell. Now there are not 23 chromosomes but 23 *pairs*—46 chromosomes in all (see Figure 1–6). There-

Figure 1–6   Gametes and Chromosomes

Human body cells contain 23 pairs of chromosomes, and gametes contain one member of each pair, or 23 single chromosomes. In these cells, only 2 pairs are shown. These pairs separate when the gametes are formed, and each gamete receives only one member of each pair (2 chromosomes in this diagram).

When the gametes join in fertilization to form a zygote, new pairs of chromosomes are formed. Each contains one member from the male and one from the female. Thus the zygote has a full set of 46 chromosomes like the parent cells (4 are shown in this diagram).

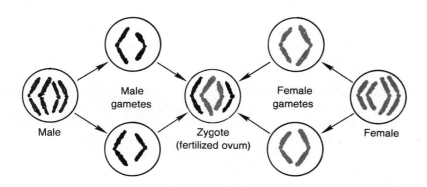

after, as the zygote splits into two new cells, and those cells split again, all 46 chromosomes are faithfully copied at each division so that every new cell inherits the entire set of 46 chromosomes. To be strictly accurate, each of the somatic cells (that is, every cell in the body except the germ cells) contains the full complement of 46 chromosomes. But when the individual has become sexually mature, then divisions of the germ cell line in the gonads produce cells with just 23 chromosomes once again. These are, of course, the gametes, the special cells through which the individual will contribute one member of each of its pairs of chromosomes to the *next* generation. Thus, a parent passes along some chromosomes from its father, and some from its mother, to its child.

For each chromosome inherited from the father, an offspring inherits a corresponding chromosome from its mother. It always, therefore, inherits two sets of genes, or instructions for making each piece of molecular machinery. In many cases, simple duplication occurs—both genes code for the same product. In some cases, differences exist between the two products—both are produced, and the resulting trait is a blend. In a few cases, one of the two genes may be altered by mutation and will produce no product or a defective product that will not function—but the other will produce a product that will function. (The inheritance of two sets of instructions gives the new individual two chances to "get it right," in a sense.)

Occasionally, two defective genes come together in an individual, and the result is the malfunction or absence of some gene product altogether. One such case may present no problem if the characteristic governed by that gene product is not essential to life or health. Another such case may cause a major biochemical defect in an organism, known as an inborn error of metabolism

somatic cells: the nonreproductive cells or tissues of the body.
soma = body

germ cells: an informal term for the cells in the ovary and testis that produce gametes.
germinate = to begin life

gonads (GO-nads): the primary sex organs containing the germ cells; testes in the male and ovaries in the female.
gone = seed

inborn error of metabolism: an inherited flaw in a structural or functional characteristic of a person evident as a disorder or disease present from birth.

(see Focal Point 1). Many such cases are lethal, leading to spontaneous abortions and stillbirths.

The result of mixing two sets of genes is that some of the new individual's traits may be identical to the father's, some to the mother's, and some intermediate between the two. Some brand-new traits will emerge, also: for example, traits determined by genes on chromosomes donated by the grandparents—genes that were hidden but not expressed within one or the other parent. New traits may also arise from unique combinations of gene products occurring for the first time in this new individual.

The simplest genetic arrangement to understand is the type governed by a single gene pair—the arrangement for eye color, for example. A gene on one of the chromosomes from the mother and a gene on the same location on the corresponding chromosome from the father govern this characteristic. The two genes may or may not be identical; the combination determines what the actual eye color will be.

Say, for example, that the father's gene specifies that the person should make blue-eye pigment, but the one from the mother carries information for brown pigment. Brown pigment colors eyes brown, whether blue-eye pigment is present or not; that is, the gene for brown eyes is dominant, and the gene for blue eyes is recessive. That means the person who inherits one copy of each will have brown eyes.

In another instance, a mother's ovum does not carry the message for brown eyes but contains the recessive message for blue eyes, just as the father's spermatozoon does. (Remember, the mother also inherited two genes for eye color; she can pass along either one.) Since no dominant brown-eye genes are present to rule, the normally recessive genes are expressed, and the person turns out to be blue-eyed.

Two brown-eyed people can thus have a blue-eyed child, if both the father and the mother pass along a blue-eye gene to the child. Both parents are brown-eyed because both possess a dominant, brown-eye gene; but both can also carry a blue-eye gene and pass that one along to their offspring. This is one way in which "new" traits emerge in new generations.

The way an infant's gender is determined is a variation on this theme. Many years ago, people thought that a mysterious characteristic about some women made them producers of girls or boys. A king could even divorce or behead his queen if she failed to produce a male heir for him. The truth is that the king's gametes, not the queen's, determine the sex of the infant. One of the 23 pairs of chromosomes, known as the X-Y, or sex, chromosomes, carries the sex-determining genes. People can either inherit two Xs, in which case they are female, or an X and a Y, in which case they are male. No one ever gets two Y chromosomes because mothers, being female, have two Xs and can only donate Xs to their offspring. Males donate X chromosomes to half of their offspring, on the average, and Y chromosomes to half—thus, boys and girls are born in equal numbers. In the race to fertilize the ovum, the spermatozoon that swims best or that gets through the ovum's outer covering first is the winner—and is the one that determines the infant's gender (see Figure 1–7).

It is unlikely that the diet's composition strongly influences the determination of an infant's sex at conception. Researchers, however, have proposed that the woman's diet may somewhat affect the odds in favor of conceiving a boy or a girl.[48] The fluid in the vagina, through which spermatozoa swim to the waiting ovum, normally favors neither those carrying the X, nor those

dominant gene: a gene that produces a product whose effect is expressed in the appearance or functioning of the organism.

recessive gene: a gene that produces no product, or a product whose effect is not expressed when the product from a dominant gene is present.

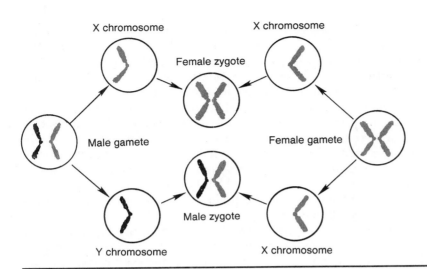

Figure 1–7   Sex Inheritance
One of the 23 pairs of chromosomes, known as the X–Y, or sex, chromosomes, carries the sex-determining genes. Males contain an X and a Y; females contain two Xs. Males donate X chromosomes to half of their offspring, on the average, and Y chromosomes to half—thus, boys and girls are born in equal numbers.

carrying the Y, chromosome. However, the two kinds of spermatozoa have somewhat different reactions to their environments, and if the fluid in which they are swimming changes, its composition may favor one over the other in the race to fertilize the ovum. The woman's diet, in turn, can influence the composition of the vaginal fluid. Researchers attempting to find out what dietary characteristics might influence sex determination claim to have managed, in one study, to correctly predict the sex of about 80 percent of babies just by analyzing the mothers' diets.[49] In another study, mothers' diets were adjusted in an effort to influence the sex of their babies. Diets high in the minerals sodium and potassium were 80 percent successful in producing boy babies, while those high in the minerals calcium and magnesium produced girls equally successfully.[50] Foods, not supplements, were used in the studies, so it is possible that some other factor present in the foods along with those minerals was responsible for the effect, or even that something that was *missing* brought about the difference. Therefore, these studies do not suggest that taking mineral supplements is an appropriate strategy for a person who wishes to conceive a baby of a particular sex. In fact, some minerals can be toxic to developing gametes.

The studies mentioned here were preliminary, but they were seized upon by a public eager to choose the sexes of their babies. Some irresponsible publications suggested tampering with women's nutrition with no regard for their nutrient needs and no proof that megadoses of any kind would not be harmful to their developing gametes. This was, of course, sensationalism—the premature drawing of conclusions from scientific findings before their implications are fully known.

Nutrition and Inheritance

With this basic understanding, it should be possible to see how nutrition relates to conception and heredity. Genes are normally copied with amazing accuracy. This is important, for they contain instructions that are crucial to the correct making of an organism. A set of parental genes is copied each time a gamete

mutation: a change in a cell's genetic material (DNA).

mutagens: agents or events that cause genetic mutations.
mutare = to change
genesis = to produce

drug: a substance that can modify one or more of the body's functions.

birth defects: congenital abnormalities (present in an individual from birth), often caused by somatic mutations.

teratogens (teh-RAT-oh-gens): agents that cause somatic mutations that lead to abnormal fetal development and birth defects.
terat = monster

is made. The genes are copied from the parent's germ cell into the set of 23 chromosomes that make up the hereditary material contained in the gamete. Then, after the male and female gametes have been united to form a zygote, all 46 chromosomes are copied over and over again as the zygote divides and redivides to form the billions of cells of the adult organism.

As a cell duplicates its genetic material in preparation for dividing to form two cells, every now and then it makes a mistake—a mutation. Such mistakes arise in the average gene about once in every 100 million copies. Most are immediately corrected by way of an intracellular system of comparing copies with the original, destroying defective ones, and recopying, but a few mistakes slip by. Once a mutation has occurred and has been transmitted to a new cell, it will then be as faithfully copied as the original was, and it will be transmitted to all future offspring of that cell.

Agents that cause mistakes (mutations) in the genetic material are known as mutagens. Mutagens include both chemical and physical agents. Among the chemical agents are the tars in tobacco, toxins produced by bacteria, many pesticides, heavy metals and other poisons, and many drugs, including both illegal and legal (prescription and over-the-counter) varieties. Among the physical agents are several forms of radiation, including the sun's ultraviolet rays and radioactivity. (Irradiated food, however, does not contain mutagens; it has been exposed to radiation, but it does not contain any substances that, themselves, give off radiation.) The mutations that mutagens can cause include not only those leading to inborn errors, but others leading to birth defects, cancer, possibly atherosclerosis and diabetes, and probably other diseases as well. The special class of mutagens that cause birth defects are known as teratogens.

The earlier in development a harmful influence exerts itself, the more devastating the consequences are likely to be. Mutations in the germ cells are especially harmful, for the gametes are made from these cells. Such mutations will be passed on to every cell of the offspring's body and from generation to generation through the germ cell line. They are usually recessive; typically, the gene altered by mutation produces an inactive product or no product. An individual who inherits such a defective gene will exhibit no abnormality only if the defective gene is paired with a normal gene contributed by the other parent. Such an individual is said to be a carrier of the mutation. On the rare occasion when two carriers conceive a child, and each contributes the defective member of its pair of genes for that trait to the child, the child is unable to produce a normal product (such as an enzyme), and so has an inborn error of metabolism (see Focal Point 1). Mutations in the germ cell line may persist invisibly for many generations before their effects become apparent, but should enough of them accumulate within the human genetic material, they could condemn the human race to ever-increasing disabilities. It is for this reason, more than any other, that both women and men should, throughout their reproductive lives, avoid contact with any chemical or physical agent that causes mutations. (It is for this reason, too, that accidents involving mutagenic radiation, such as the one that took place at Chernobyl in April 1986, are so frightening.)

Teratogens cause mutations, not in the germ cell line, but in somatic cells during an individual's development. These are also harmful, but they will affect only that individual and will not be passed on to future generations. They can be devastating, however. If mutations occur during the first two weeks of a zygote's development, they are likely to be lethal. The reason is that each cell in a developing zygote is destined to become a large part of the body of an adult. Major abnormalities induced in whole organ systems preclude survival. Lesser abnormalities lead to birth defects. A section at the end of this chapter describes some teratogenic effects of alcohol, drugs, and environmental contaminants. Table 2–4 in Chapter 2 identifies some common birth defects.

Clearly, practically all mutations are harmful—that is, they impair the genetic codes for normal, needed products. A gene altered by a mutation will produce defective products—for example, enzymes that work slowly, or cell-membrane proteins that fail to effectively bar unwanted chemicals from cells. Alternatively, the gene will produce no product at all, and some cellular process will not take place.

Exceptions to the rule that all mutations are unambiguously harmful are known. A famous example is that of sickle-cell anemia, in which a mutation in one of the genes for the protein hemoglobin causes the amino acid valine to replace the amino acid glutamine in one location along the protein chain. The resulting protein is an abnormal shape, which results in red blood cells of an abnormal shape. Although this causes a disabling anemia, it also confers resistance to the parasite that causes malaria—a relative advantage in the tropics. Still, 999 out of 1000 mutations are disadvantageous, and therefore all *mutagens* can be classed as unambiguously harmful.

Although inborn errors and many birth defects are known to be caused by mutations, it is never possible to look back in time and say when those mutations arose. They are, however, most likely to arise during times of cell division. Clearly, then, all of a man's adulthood is a vulnerable time, for the spermatozoa are being made. The time surrounding conception is a vulnerable time, for the chromosomes are dividing often in the formation of a zygote. Early embryonic development is a vulnerable time, for rapid cell division continues throughout that period. The entire course of a female fetus' development is a vulnerable time, for her ova are being made. Young men and women should therefore at all times avoid exposure to mutagenic radiation and contamination of food and water that might threaten the integrity of their genetic material and young offspring. To the earlier statements about obtaining a diet that is adequate, balanced, varied, and so forth should be added another descriptor: all of the foods and beverages selected should be free of contamination—in a word, safe.

Nutrition and Fertilization

Once the gametes are produced, they need to be able to meet, join, begin the production of a new individual, and settle into the uterus to develop. The meeting and joining are, of course, fertilization. The settling in is implantation (see next section). Nutrition influences both, not only in providing all the necessary building materials and energy, but also in providing the environmental chemistry and freedom from adverse influences that will support the normal course of events.

A review of the events surrounding conception may help in understanding the importance of adequate nutrition prior to this time. Sexual intercourse from 48 hours before to 15 hours after ovulation is most likely to result in

oviduct: one of two tubes extending from the uterus which serves to convey the ovum from the ovary to the uterus; also called the fallopian tube.

conception. The average life spans of the spermatozoon (48 hours) and the unfertilized ovum (10 to 15 hours) determine this time frame. During ovulation, the ovary discharges an ovum into the oviduct. The ovum works its way down the oviduct into the uterus over the next several days. (Figure 1–8 illustrates the relationship between the ovaries, oviducts, and uterus.) The short life span of the ovum requires fertilization to occur in the oviduct as illustrated in Figure 1–9.

Generalized malnutrition and fertilization   Whether fertilization can take place depends both on the health of the gametes and on their environment. Maternal malnutrition prior to conception reduces fertility. The food shortages and birthrates reported in the medical journals of Europe before, during, and after the Second World War provide valuable records for analyzing the influence of preconceptual nutrition on the fertility of women. During that war, a transportation strike restricted food supplies into Holland from September 1944 to May 1945. The resultant severe nutritional deprivation reduced fertility at a time in many people's lives when they might otherwise have conceived, as is evident from several findings.[51] The number of births declined dramatically nine months after the onset of the war-related famine. The number of births was only one-third of the expected rate.[52] With the availability of food, birthrates began to climb, indicating that starvation-caused infertility is reversible. Meanwhile, fertility did not decline in areas with adequate food supplies, even under similar conditions of war and weather.

One precondition of fertility is a woman's ability to ovulate. The women experiencing the food shortages and malnutrition in Holland had abnormal menstrual cycles. Approximately one-half of the female population stopped menstruating; only one-third of the women had normal menstrual cycles.[53]

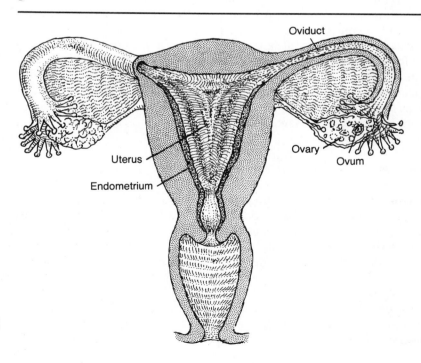

Figure 1–8   The Ovaries, Oviducts, and Uterus

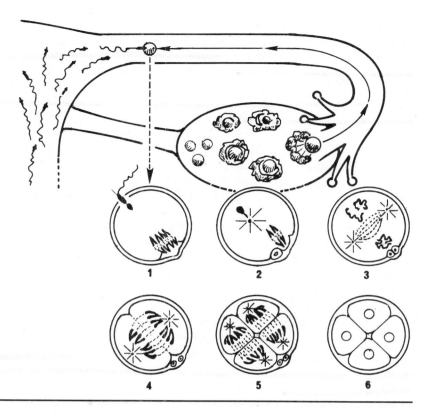

Figure 1–9 Fertilization
The union of an ovum and spermatozoon occurs in the oviduct and creates a zygote. The original cell begins its division into many cells, changing its number, but not its size.

Malnutrition is not the only factor that interferes with ovulation. Lactation also prevents ovulation; its relation to fertility is discussed in Chapter 3. Another precondition of fertility is a man's ability to produce enough viable spermatozoa. Food deprivation in men has several effects on spermatozoa, reducing their numbers, motility, and life spans.[54] Furthermore, both men and women appear to lose sexual interest during times of starvation.

These war records and other research suggest that there is a "nutritional infertility threshold."[55] Below this threshold, hormonal secretions diminish and women develop amenorrhea, becoming infertile. Between the optimal nourishment that produces a healthy infant and the starvation that causes infertility, an intermediate zone exists that offers suboptimal prospects for pregnancy.

Underweight and fertilization Many females who diet excessively or who engage in intense physical exercise are underweight and amenorrheic. Weight gain usually initiates menarche or restores regular menstrual cycles. Amenorrhea is a complex phenomenon characterized by low concentrations of estrogen. Controversy surrounds the exact causative factors.

Researchers question whether a minimal level of body fat is necessary for the onset and maintenance of regular menstrual cycles.[56] Amenorrhea occurs in women who lose 10 to 15 percent of their normal weight for height—approximately one-third of their body fat. Minimum weights for various heights necessary for the onset or restoration of menstruation have been

motility: ability to move spontaneously.

amenorrhea (a-MEN-oh-REE-ah): the absence, temporary or permanent, of menstrual periods; normal before puberty, after the menopause, during pregnancy, and during lactation; otherwise abnormal.
a = not
men = month
rhoia = flow

underweight: body weight at least 10 percent less than standard weight for height.

Chapter 6 discusses athletic amenorrhea and the amenorrhea of anorexia nervosa.

identified, but it is not known whether amenorrhea depends on body weight or percent body fat. The argument for percent body fat's being the critical factor has a sound physiological basis. Fat stores affect the menstrual cycle by serving as a site for estrogen synthesis (the major source in postmenopausal women), influencing estrogen metabolism, and altering estrogen-binding properties of cells.[57] Dietary fat correlates with estrogen concentrations which may, in turn, reflect its influence on fat stores.[58]

Whether amenorrhea occurs in response to altered metabolic signals, reduced food intake, altered body temperature, or depleted fat stores is unclear. One study found no difference in body composition or weight between women with amenorrhea and women with eumenorrhea.[59] Differences in energy intake were significant, however. The energy intake of the amenorrheic women was approximately 25 percent less than that of the eumenorrheic women, even though their energy expenditures were similar.

Amenorrhea can, of course, be due to other causes, such as psychological stress. Whatever the underlying mechanism, the amenorrhea of an underweight woman may be viewed as an adaptive response to curtail reproduction. Many animals respond to food shortages and stress with hormonal changes that diminish fertility. Thus, animals do not use reproductive energies to create offspring when the environment is not conducive to their survival.

Specific nutrients and fertilization   In some instances, malnourishment is more specific—that is, a particular nutrient deficiency or excess correlates with an infertility problem. An example of an excess is seen in the association of elevated serum carotene concentrations (carotenemia) with amenorrhea.[60] Women with amenorrhea whose carotenemia reflects a diet of predominantly raw vegetables can lower their serum carotene concentrations and restore their fertility with dietary changes.[61] Results from other research studies, however, indicate that caution is required in drawing conclusions regarding carotene and amenorrhea.[62] Carotene is only one of a multitude of components found in vegetables, and women taking carotene supplements of a nonplant origin do not experience menstrual irregularities. Perhaps it is the excessive consumption of another compound commonly associated with carotene that is to blame.

Subclinical vitamin C deficiency may be responsible for nonspecific sperm agglutination, one cause of infertility in men. Studies of men who are unable to impregnate their wives due to sperm agglutination find consistently low serum vitamin C concentrations.[63] In one study, men with this problem took a combination supplement of vitamin C, calcium, magnesium, and manganese.[64] The results were dramatic, with all twenty men successfully impregnating their wives within the study period. In an effort to isolate the specific nutrient responsible, another study provided just vitamin C supplementation of 1 gram per day.[65] Within four days, vitamin C raised both serum and semen vitamin C concentrations and lowered the percentage of agglutinated sperm to below the level that distinguishes fertility from infertility.

Nutrition and Implantation

The zygote undergoes several cell divisions while passing through the oviduct. After reaching the uterus, it floats freely for several days, receiving nourishment from the intrauterine fluid. Cell division continues.

eumenorrhea: normal menstruation.

The section on anorexia nervosa in Chapter 6 provides more details on stress-related amenorrhea.

When a single fertilized ovum completely divides into two independent organisms, the result is monozygotic (identical) twins. When two fertilized ova develop into two independent organisms, the result is dizygotic (fraternal) twins.

Simultaneously, the endometrium is preparing to receive the zygote. Conditions in the uterus at the time of conception determine whether the zygote will successfully implant and begin normal development. Failure to implant causes the loss of the zygote, possibly even before the woman knows she is pregnant.

The uterine environment can be either hospitable or hostile. With an appropriate balance of hormones and nutrients, a zygote implants and continues its development. When drugs or other toxins are present, the endometrium may reject the zygote or the zygote may be unable to attach to the lining. Even with successful implantation, the zygote may suffer damage that will become evident during later development. Ideally, nutrition is optimal and exposure to contaminants minimal during the time surrounding implantation.

During the two weeks in which implantation takes place, the zygote divides into many cells, and these cells sort themselves into three layers—the ectoderm, mesoderm, and endoderm. Little growth in size occurs at this time, but because of the rapid cell division taking place, this is, as mentioned, a vulnerable time. Authorities agree that, to provide the most nearly ideal environment possible for implantation, a woman should have been well nourished for a long time prior, should not be taking drugs of any kind, even aspirin, and should be protected from all harmful environmental exposures.

ectoderm: the outermost layer of a developing embryo, which evolves into the nervous system and skin.
ecto = outside
derm = skin

mesoderm: the middle layer of a developing embryo, between the ectoderm and endoderm, which evolves into the muscular, skeletal, circulatory, and internal organ systems.
meso = middle

endoderm: the innermost layer of a developing embryo, which evolves into the glands and linings of the digestive, respiratory, and excretory systems.
endo = inside

Prepregnant Nutrition's Effects on Pregnancy

Like conception and implantation, early embryonic development also depends both on the inherited genetic material and on the environment. Discussion of the environment in which the embryo develops might properly be postponed to the chapter on pregnancy (and it is discussed in more detail there), but a woman's lifestyle habits and exposures prior to pregnancy continue to influence her body's chemistry when she is pregnant. Thus, the choices a prepregnant woman makes can influence the course of a pregnancy she is not even planning at the time.

The environment can affect development in two ways—by altering the genes themselves (causing somatic mutation) or by altering their expression. Genes provide potential—that is, the capacity to reach a certain developmental level. That potential can fail to be fully realized, for poor nutrition, chemical damage, radiation, lack of oxygen, or other conditions can all interfere with correct gene copying or prevent the full or normal expression of the genes. Congenital abnormalities, then, can result from adverse physical or chemical conditions during development of the gametes or the fetus. Among the major adverse conditions are undernutrition, overnutrition, alcohol use, and other drug use. These subjects will all be mentioned again in the chapter on pregnancy, but their prepregnancy effects, as best they can be sorted out, are discussed here.

Undernutrition

Undernutrition prior to pregnancy can have major detrimental impacts on early embryonic development, leading to low birthweight, morbidity, mortal-

morbidity: affected by or characteristic of disease.

mortality: pertaining to death.

ity, and retarded physical and mental development. The evidence for this comes from two sources—records taken during famines, and data on women who are underweight for other reasons (such as ill-advised dieting).

Famine at conception   The recorded food shortages in Europe during the Second World War not only reduced conception rates as already mentioned, but also impaired the courses and outcomes of pregnancies when women did manage to conceive. These effects were particularly dramatic in Holland, where daily food rations for pregnant women reached a low point of 1145 kcalories and 34 grams of protein.[66] Rations for other adults were even more limited. The records showed that stillbirths and neonatal deaths were significantly higher for infants *conceived* during the famine than for those conceived prior to or following it. Apparently, many women received enough nourishment to be fertile, but not enough to have healthy infants—that is, they were in the intermediate zone referred to earlier. Conception of infants during times of limited food supplies consistently correlates with congenital malformations of the central nervous system.[67]

One of the tasks a woman's body performs at the start of a pregnancy is to develop a placenta, an organ of great importance. (The characteristics of the placenta are described in full in Chapter 2.) If a woman's nutrition status is poor early in pregnancy, then the placenta may never attain its full growth potential. It will be unable to deliver optimum nourishment to the fetus, and the infant will be born small.

If this small infant were a female, she in turn would have an elevated risk of having a poor pregnancy outcome. She would be more likely to have a miscarriage or a stillbirth, or to give birth to an infant with congenital malformations, with respiratory distress, or in need of neonatal intensive care.[68]

The intrauterine growth retardation of a female is not the only factor affecting her future reproductive performance. Her nutrition during her infancy and childhood is also of crucial importance. For example, rickets or protein-energy malnutrition in childhood may cause the development of a contracted pelvis, leading to problems in pregnancy and childbirth.

Thus, the poor development of infants may reflect adverse conditions of their mothers' own early development. A woman's nutrition before or during her pregnancy can have an impact not only on her child but on her *grandchild*.[69] In short, the effects of nutritional insults reach into future generations.

Underweight at conception   The famines that tragically affect human health normally arise during wars or natural events such as droughts. The effects of poor nutrition can also be seen, however, in women during times of peace and plenty when they intentionally starve themselves.

The health of, and outlook for, an infant at birth can be predicted by several indicators, as Chapter 2 describes in detail. One of the most reliable of these indicators is the infant's birthweight, and that is the one used here. Several characteristics of the mother's pregnancy predict infant birthweight. Maternal weight gain and length of gestation are two of the most reliable of these (see Chapter 2), but a third equally inportant one is maternal weight for height prior to pregnancy, a subject appropriate to this chapter.

An underweight woman is at high risk for giving birth not only to a low-birthweight infant but also to a preterm infant, and perinatal mortality

stillbirth: birth of a dead fetus.

miscarriage: known medically as a spontaneous abortion, the separation of the developing fetus and the placenta from the inner wall of the uterus, resulting in the unintentional termination of the pregnancy, occurring before the beginning of the twentieth week of gestation.

contracted pelvis: a pelvis whose diameter is reduced to a degree that impedes childbirth.

rates are highest for these women.[70] An underweight woman maximizes her chances of having a healthy infant by gaining weight to the standard prior to conception, or by gaining extra pounds during pregnancy.

The underweight woman who attempts to increase her weight before conceiving needs to know that weight gain is best achieved by physical conditioning combined with a high-kcalorie diet. A high-kcalorie diet alone results in fat gain, which can be more harmful than being underweight. Exercise ensures that the weight gained will be at least partly lean tissue. Strength training (such as situps, pushups, and repetitions with heavy weights) is the most efficient way to support weight gain efforts.

Energy intake must be high enough to support both exercise and weight gain, perhaps 700 to 1000 kcalories per day above the customary intakes. If a woman only eats enough to support exercise, muscles develop at the expense of body fat. To raise energy intake, a woman selects high-kcalorie foods such as milk shakes, peanut butter, and muffins. She adds sour cream to her potatoes, creamy dressings to her salads, and cream cheese to her toast. She eats quickly and frequently, beginning each meal and snack with the highest-kcalorie foods and beverages. Diet plans and nutrient recommendations for pregnancy are also appropriate for an underweight woman to follow prior to pregnancy.

Chapter 2 provides dietary recommendations for pregnancy.

Overnutrition

Approximately one of every four women between the ages of 20 and 44 is obese.[71] Studies examining the effects of obesity must state the criteria used to define obesity. Most often, researchers use 20 percent above standard body weight as a minimum definition of obesity. Researchers studying morbidly obese people may use a higher cut-off point, such as 50 percent. The complications are similar, but their rate and severity intensify with increasing weight.

obese: body weight of at least 20 percent above standard weight for height.

Like the underweight woman, the obese woman faces her own set of problems related to pregnancy and childbirth. Women who are obese at conception risk the obstetrical complications associated with hypertension, gestational diabetes, and postpartum infections.[72] (Chapter 2 discusses these obstetrical complications.) They also face the necessity of having to have labor induced by oxytocin, and infants delivered by cesarean section more often than nonobese women.

oxytocin-induced labor: use of the pituitary hormone oxytocin to stimulate the uterus to contract, thus beginning the childbirth process.

Maternal obesity affects not only mothers but their infants as well. These infants are likely to be born post term and to weigh more than 4000 grams (8.9 pounds).[73] Obese women are less likely to have premature infants, but if they do, their infants are likely to be large-for-gestational age. This may result in a misclassification of the infants as term infants, with resulting failure to recognize problems associated with prematurity.

cesarean section: removal of the fetus by an incision into the uterus, usually by way of the abdominal wall.

An overweight woman attempting to lose weight before conception will want to adopt a lifelong plan that combines changes in diet, exercise, and behavior. Weight loss is possible without exercise, but a low-kcalorie diet alone results in the loss of both lean and fat tissue. The most efficient way to lose fat while building lean tissue is to undertake and maintain a program of endurance training, such as running, swimming, or cycling.

Chapters 2 and 4 discuss the risks associated with preterm births and infants.

The 10-kcalorie rule recommended earlier in this chapter guides a woman in determining an appropriate energy level for safe weight loss. To lower energy intake, a woman selects nutrient-dense foods such as nonfat milk, vegetables, grains, and lean meats. She must design an eating plan for life—one that provides enjoyment as well as an adequate nutrient intake without excess food energy.

Traditional weight loss plans typically allow for a loss of one to two pounds per week. For people who have much weight to lose, this slow rate is unacceptable. In an effort to speed weight loss, researchers have designed very-low-kcalorie diets.[74] These diets maximize the rate of fat loss while preserving lean body tissue, normal blood chemistry, and overall good health. A very-low-kcalorie diet consists of a formula containing at least the RDA of protein; enought carbohydrate to attain approximately 400 to 500 kcalories a day; essential nutrients; fluid; and fiber. An obese person follows the very-low-kcalorie diet plan for up to three months under close medical supervision, either going off the formula at intervals to eat specified meals or, during the diet, eating one specified meal a day while using the formula for the other meals. Typical weight loss rates range from about three to five pounds a week for people having more than 50 pounds to lose and from to one to three pounds a week for people with fewer pounds to lose. Such a weight loss regimen would be most inappropriate for a pregnant woman. Therefore, women are cautioned to prevent pregnancy while on a weight loss diet.

For a few morbidly obese people, gastric bypass surgery is a treatment option. Pregnancies following gastric surgery for the treatment of obesity involve risks of their own. Nutrient deficiencies are common following gastric bypass surgery, and recent studies have linked dietary inadequacies with neural tube defects. Reports of infants with neural tube defects borne by women with gastric bypasses suggest that careful medical and dietary management of these women during pregnancy is imperative.[75] In fact, vitamin supplementation prior to and throughout pregnancy reduces the occurrence of neural tube defects.[76] With proper dietary and medical attention, pregnancy after gastric bypass can be successful.[77] The incidence of hypertension and large newborns is lower in women who have had gastric bypass surgery with adequate aftercare than in women who have remained obese.

Some women who have battled against weight gain fear the weight gain of pregnancy. Weight loss during pregnancy is unhealthy, and weight loss following pregnancy is challenging, even to a woman who does not have a weight problem. The prospect of gaining 25 pounds, having a protruding belly, and then having to get back in shape may inspire dread and even outright avoidance of pregnancy. These women might find comfort in a reminder that they will be getting *pregnant*, not *fat*. The weight gained and the distortion of the figure are necessary to meet placental, fetal, maternal, and lactation needs.

For the first time, an overweight woman will be able to see an increase on the scales as normal, even healthy. In fact, obstetricians express concern when a pregnant woman is not gaining weight. Inadequate weight gain in pregnancy compromises the growth and genetic potential of the fetus.[78] If an overweight pregnant woman eats the appropriate foods, much of her gained weight will be lost at delivery and the remainder within a few months, as her body systems return to normal.

Alcohol and Other Drugs

Alcohol abuse during pregnancy, especially early pregnancy, causes devastating birth defects. The impact of alcohol on pregnancy depends on the time,

---

morbidly obese: twice or more the average standard weight for height or 100 pounds over the standard weight.

gastric bypass surgery: a surgical procedure intended to limit food intake; a small segment of the upper stomach is closed off from the lower portion and attached to the small intestine, thus bypassing a major portion of the stomach.

neural tube defects: any of a number of defects with the orderly formation of the neural tube during early gestation, resulting in various central nervous system disorders, such as spina bifida.

Chapter 2 describes the components of weight gain during pregnancy, and patterns of weight gain appropriate for women of different prepregnancy weights.

Focal Point 2 discusses fetal alcohol syndrome.

intensity, and duration of abuse. Of particular interest to the subject of this chapter is alcohol abuse prior to conception. Even if a woman stops drinking prior to conception, her prior alcohol abuse will affect the development of her fetus. One study showed this clearly—infants born to women who had a history of alcohol abuse but abstained during pregnancy weighed less than infants born to women who did not consume alcohol.[79] Perhaps the earlier alcohol abuse led to maternal liver dysfunction and nutrient deficits that impaired fetal growth and development. This is not to say there is no point in abstaining during pregnancy. The other half of the story is that infants born to women who had a history of alcohol abuse and abstained from drinking during pregnancy weighed more than infants born to women who had a history of alcohol abuse and continued drinking.

The first month of pregnancy is a critical period of fetal development. Because pregnancy confirmation usually requires five to six weeks, a woman may not even realize she is pregnant during that critical first month. Therefore, it is advisable for women who are trying to conceive or who suspect they might be pregnant to curtail their alcohol intakes to ensure a healthy start.

Other drugs, both medical and illicit, can be harmful in similar ways. Megadoses of vitamin supplements also have druglike effects. Most medications have warnings on their labels that state, "As with any drug, if you are pregnant or nursing an infant, seek the advice of a health professional before using this product." Because this warning does not appear on all harmful substances, women must warn themselves of the potential dangers of their actions. Women considering pregnancy should include themselves along with pregnant and lactating women and heed the warning.

An example of a drug whose effects are particularly well known is Accutane. Generically known as isotretinoin, Accutane is effective in treating severe cystic acne that has been unresponsive to other treatments. Accutane bears a warning label that advises women to use an effective form of contraception beginning at least one month before the inception and continuing until one month after the termination of Accutane's use. Red stickers warn that it can cause birth defects, and pharmacists add labels that caution, "Do not become pregnant while using Accutane."

Many infants born to women taking Accutane suffer major birth defects.[80] Young women are especially vulnerable to the dangers of Accutane because they are often unwilling to admit to their dermatologists that they are sexually active. A pregnancy test two weeks prior to the onset of treatment is imperative. Some dermatologists require monthly pregnancy tests while Accutane is taken.

A list of specific drugs to discontinue prior to pregnancy is not available. However, this one example illustrates the potent effect that a drug taken near the time of conception, even one approved by the Food and Drug Administration and prescribed by a physician, can have on the outcome of a pregnancy. The effectiveness and clearance rates of different drugs vary. Even a short-term, low dose of a dangerous drug can expose a fetus to irreparable harm. Other factors influencing the nature and severity of the harm to the fetus include the time and duration of administration. Obviously, the situation requires more caution when a women is sexually active and conception is a possibility than when she is sexually abstinent or practicing contraception.

Among the drugs to discontinue if a woman wants to become pregnant are, of course, the oral contraceptives. Once a woman stops taking oral

Chapter 2 discusses drug ingestion and vitamin megadoses during pregnancy.

contraceptives, she can expect a delay of one to three months before regular ovulation and menstruation resume. If she waits for her menstrual cycle to resume before becoming pregnant, she will be able to calculate her due date. After the initial delay, conception rates become the same for these women as for others not using contraceptives. However, oral contraceptives cause no fetal damage, even if taken after conception.[81]

Much research focuses on the effects of maternal drug ingestion on conception and fetal development, but until recently, few studies had examined the effects of paternal exposure to drugs. Pregnancy begins with the union of an ovum and a spermatozoon, and it stands to reason that adverse influences on the male might affect conception. Male rats given methadone prior to mating with untreated females, sired pups with low birthweights and altered behavior patterns.[82] Neonatal mortality was also high. In human males, lead, anesthetic gases, cigarettes, and caffeine are associated with adverse effects on reproduction.[83] Drugs may alter spermatozoon formation, maturation, or motility, and this can affect fertility.[84] In addition, paternal drug ingestion might alter male hormone activity, damage the spermatozoa, or affect the intrauterine environment or the newly fertilized ovum if the drug or its metabolites pass in the ejaculate.[85]

A female's body is a remarkable vehicle. For approximately the first decade of life, her body's primary focus is on its own growth and maintenance only. Then, with menarche, her body begins to offer ova for reproduction. With the fertilization of an ovum, her body becomes a vehicle to nurture another human being and release it into this world. This is life's cycle—from infancy to childhood to adolescence to pregnancy, returning to infancy. Each of these phases of life is vital to the cycle's continuation. A woman leaves the cycle only after menopause, when she begins her journey into old age. Until then, a woman who nourishes and protects her body does so not only for her own sake, but also for future generations.

methadone: a synthetic analgesic drug widely used in the treatment of heroin abuse.

Chapter 1 Notes

1. The American Dietetic Association's Nutrition Recommendations for Women, *Journal of the American Dietetic Association* 86 (1986): 1663–1664.
2. R. P. Heaney and coauthors, Calcium nutrition and bone health in the elderly, *American Journal of Clinical Nutrition* 36 (1982): 986–1013.
3. K. A. V. R. Krishnamachari and L. Iyengar, Effect of maternal malnutrition on the bone density of the neonates, *American Journal of Clinical Nutrition* 28 (1975): 482–486.
4. L. H. Allen, Calcium bioavailability and absorption: A review, *American Journal of Clinical Nutrition* 35 (1982): 783–808; J. L. Kelsay and E. S. Prather, Mineral balances of human subjects consuming spinach in a low-fiber diet and in a diet containing fruits and vegetables, *American Journal of Clinical Nutrition* 38 (1983): 12–19.
5. S. M. Garn, M. T. Keating, and F. Falkner, Hematological status and pregnancy outcomes, *American Journal of Clinical Nutrition* 34 (1981): 115–117.
6. B. B. Peterkin, Women's diets: 1977 and 1985, *Journal of Nutrition Education* 18 (1986): 251–257.
7. C. W. Callaway, Statement on vitamin and mineral supplements, *American Journal of Clinical Nutrition* 46 (1987): 1076; D. Herber, W. Mertz, and R. E. Schucker, Food versus pills versus fortified foods, *Dairy Council Digest*, March-April 1987; A. E. Harper, "Nutrition insurance"—A skeptical view, *Nutrition Forum*, May 1987, pp. 33–37.
8. R. P. Heaney, Premenopausal prophylactic calcium supplementation (letter), *Journal of the American Medical Association* 245 (1981): 1362.
9. M. S. Sheikh and coauthors, Gastrointestinal absorption of calcium from milk and calcium salts, *New England Journal of Medicine* 317 (1987): 532–536.
10. Position of the American Dietetic Association: Nutrition for physical fitness and athletic performance for adults, *Journal of the American Dietetic Association* 87 (1987): 933–939.

11. F. T. O'Neil, M. T. Hynak-Hankinson, and J. Gorman, Research and application of current topics in sports nutrition, *Journal of the American Dietetic Association* 86 (1986): 1007–1015.

12. J. L. Greger, Food, supplements, and fortified foods: Scientific evaluations in regard to toxicology and nutrient bioavailability, *Journal of the American Dietetic Association* 87 (1987): 1369–1373.

13. B. Dawson-Hughes, F. H. Seligson, and V. A. Hughes, Effects of calcium carbonate and hydroxyapatite on zinc and iron retention in postmenopausal women, *American Journal of Clinical Nutrition* 44 (1986): 83–88.

14. R. Yip and coauthors, Does iron supplementation compromise zinc nutrition in healthy infants?, *American Journal of Clinical Nutrition* 42 (1985): 683–687; J. Albers, E. B. Dawson, and W. J. McGanity, Effect of elevated pre-natal iron supplementation on serum copper, zinc, and selenium levels (abstract), *American Journal of Clinical Nutrition* 43 (1986): 673.

15. Greger, 1987.

16. E. R. Monsen, Menstrual cycle, an address presented at the 70th Annual Meeting of the American Dietetic Association in Atlanta, Georgia, 20 October 1987.

17. K. S. Moghissi, F. N. Snyer, and T. N. Evans, A composite picture of the menstrual cycle, *American Journal of Obstetrics and Gynecology* 114 (1972): 405–415.

18. S. J. Solomon, M. S. Kurzer, and D. H. Calloway, Menstrual cycle and basal metabolic rate in women, *American Journal of Clinical Nutrition* 36 (1982): 611–616.

19. S. P. Dalvit, The effect of the menstrual cycle on patterns of food intake, *American Journal of Clinical Nutrition* 34 (1981): 1811–1815.

20. S. P. Dalvit-McPhillips, The effect of the human menstrual cycle on nutrient intake, *Physiology and Behavior* 31 (1983): 209–212.

21. Solomon, Kurzer, and Calloway, 1982.

22. *Premenstrual Syndrome*, a report by the American Council on Science and Health, July 1985.

23. B. D. Shephard, Oral contraceptives—An overview, *Journal of the Florida Medical Association* 73 (1986): 763–767.

24. Shephard, 1986.

25. J. W. Ellis, Multiphasic oral contraceptives—Efficacy and metabolic impact, *The Journal of Reproductive Medicine* 32 (1987): 28–36.

26. E. L. Marut, Oral contraceptives—Who, which, when, and why?, *Postgraduate Medicine* 82 (1987): 66–70.

27. Shephard, 1986.

28. Shephard, 1986; Marut, 1987; G. R. Huggins and P. K. Zucker, Oral contraceptives and neoplasia: 1987 update, *Fertility and Sterility* 47 (1987): 733–761.

29. The Centers for Disease Control Cancer and Steroid Hormone Study: The reduction in risk of ovarian cancer associated with oral-contraceptive use, *The New England Journal of Medicine* 316 (1987): 650–655.

30. Marut, 1987; Huggins and Zucker, 1987.

31. The Centers for Disease Control Cancer and Steroid Hormone Study: Combination oral contraceptive use and the risk of endometrial cancer, *Journal of the American Medical Association* 257 (1987): 796–800; Huggins and Zucker, 1987.

32. D. R. Miller and coauthors, Breast cancer risk in relation to early oral contraceptive use, *Obstetrics and Gynecology* 68 (1986): 863–868.

33. R. Russell-Briefel and coauthors, Cardiovascular risk status and oral contraceptive use: United States, 1976–1980, *Preventive Medicine* 15 (1986): 352–362; P. B. Moser and coauthors, Carbohydrate tolerance and serum lipid responses to type of dietary carbohydrate and oral contraceptive use in young women, *Journal of the American College of Nutrition* 5 (1986): 45–53.

34. Marut, 1987; Russell-Briefel and coauthors, 1986.

35. J. K. Williams, Oral contraceptives—The long-term perspective, *Journal of the Florida Medical Association* 73 (1986): 769–771.

36. Shephard, 1986; Williams, 1986.

37. R. Russell-Briefel and coauthors, Impaired glucose tolerance in women using oral contraceptives: United States, 1976–1980, *Journal of Chronic Diseases* 40 (1987): 3–11.

38. Williams, 1986; Moser and coauthors, 1986.

39. Ellis, 1987; Russell-Briefel and coauthors, 1987.

40. Russell-Briefel and coauthors, 1987.

41. B. L. Strom, Oral contraceptives and other risk factors for gallbladder disease, *Clinical Pharmacology and Therapeutics* 39 (1986): 335–341.

42. F. Kern, Jr. and G. T. Everson, Contraceptive steroids increase cholesterol in bile: Mechanisms of action, *Journal of Lipid Research* 28 (1987): 828–839.

43. L. B. Tyrer, Nutrition and the pill, *Journal of Reproductive Medicine* 29 (1984): 547–550.

44. K. Amatayakul and coauthors, Vitamin metabolism and the effects of multivitamin supplementation in oral contraceptive users, *Contraception* 30 (1984): 179–196.

45. S. Carpenter and L. S. Neinstein, Weight gain in adolescent and young adult oral contraceptive users, *Journal of Adolescent Health Care* 7 (1986): 342–344.

46. American Academy of Pediatrics, Committee on Drugs, The transfer of drugs and other chemicals into human breast milk, *Pediatrics* 72 (1983): 375–381; Task force on oral contraceptives of the WHO Special Programme of Research, Effects of hormonal contraceptives on milk volume and infant growth, Development and Research Training in Human Reproduction, Vol. 30, December 1984, pp. 505–522.

47. Task force on oral contraceptives of the WHO Special Programme of Research, 1984; Task force on oral contraceptives of the WHO Special Programme of Research, Long-term follow-up of children breast-fed by mothers using oral contraceptives, Development and Research Training in Human Reproduction, Vol. 34, November 1986, pp. 443–457.

48. J. Lorrain and R. Gagnon, Selection preconceptionelle du sexe, *Union Medicale du Canada* 104 (1975): 800–803; J. Stoklowski and J. Choukroun, Preconception selection of sex in man, *Israel Journal of Medical Sciences* 17 (1981): 1061–1067; and F. Papa and coauthors, Preconceptional selection of fetal sex using an ionic method: A dietary regime, *Journal de Gynecologie, Obstetrique, et Biologie de la Reproduction* 12 (1983): 415–422.

49. Lorrain and Gagnon, 1975.

50. Stoklowski and Choukroun, 1981; Papa and coauthors, 1983.

51. Z. Stein and coauthors, *Famine and Human Development: The Dutch Hunger Winter of 1944/1945* (New York: Oxford University Press, 1975).

52. C. A. Smith, The effect of wartime starvation in Holland upon pregnancy and its product, *American Journal of Obstetrics and Gynecology* 53 (1947): 599–608.

53. Smith, 1947.

54. Stein and coauthors, 1975.

55. M. Wynn and A. Wynn, The influence of nutrition on the fertility of women, *Nutrition and Health* 1 (1982): 7–13; Stein and coauthors, 1975.

56. R. E. Frisch, Fatness, menarche, and female fertility, *Perspectives in Biology and Medicine* 28 (1985): 611–633; M. E. Nelson and coauthors, Diet and bone status in amenorrheic runners, *American Journal of Clinical Nutrition* 43 (1986): 910–916.

57. Frisch, 1985; B. Goldin and coauthors, The relationship between estrogen levels and diets of Caucasian American and Oriental immigrant women, *American Journal of Clinical Nutrition* 44 (1986): 945–953.

58. Goldin and coauthors, 1986.

59. M. E. Nelson and coauthors, Diet and bone status in amenorrheic runners, *American Journal of Clinical Nutrition* 43 (1986): 910–916.

60. A. M. Frumar, D. R. Meldrum, and H. L. Judd, Hypercarotenemia in hypothalamic amenorrhea, *Fertility and Sterility* 32 (1979): 261–264; E. Kemmann, S. A. Pasquale, and R. Skaf, Amenorrhea associated with carotenemia, *Journal of the American Medical Association* 249 (1983): 926–929; P. A. Deuster and coauthors, Nutritional intakes and status of highly trained amenorrheic and eumenorrheic runners, *Fertility and Sterility* 46 (1986): 636–643.

61. Kemmann, Pasquale, and Skaf, 1983.

62. M. M. Mathews-Roth, Amenorrhea associated with carotenemia (letter), *Journal of the American Medical Association* 250 (1983): 731.

63. E. B. Dawson, W. A. Harris, and W. J. McGanity, Effect of ascorbic acid on sperm fertility (abstract), *Federation Proceedings* 42 (1983): 531; E. R. Gonzalez, Sperm swim singly after vitamin C therapy, *Journal of the American Medical Association* 249 (1983): 2747, 2751; W. A. Harris, T. E. Harden, and E. B. Dawson, Apparent effect of ascorbic acid medication on semen metal levels, *Fertility and Sterility* 32 (1979): 455–459.

64. Harris, Harden, and Dawson, 1979.

65. Dawson, Harris, and McGanity, 1983; Gonzalez, 1983.

66. M. Wynn and A. Wynn, Effects of nutrition on reproductive capability, *Nutrition and Health* 1 (1983): 165–178; Stein and coauthors, 1975.

67. C. A. Smith, Effects of maternal undernutrition upon the newborn infant in Holland (1944–1945), *Journal of Pediatrics* 30 (1947): 229–243.

68. E. Hackman and coauthors, Maternal birth weight and subsequent pregnancy outcome, *Journal of the American Medical Association* 250 (1983): 2016–2019.

69. Hackman and coauthors, 1983.

70. R. M. Pitkin, Assessment of nutritional status of mother, fetus, and newborn, *American Journal of Clinical Nutrition* 34 (1981): 658–668; R. L. Naeye, Weight gain and the outcome of pregnancy, *American Journal of Obstetrics and Gynecology* 135 (1979): 3–9.

71. J. Willis, The gender gap at the dinner table, a pamphlet available from U.S. Government Printing Office, 5600 Fishers Lane, Rockville, MD 20857, HHS Publication no. (FDA) 84-2197.

72. S. R. Johnson and coauthors, Maternal obesity and pregnancy, *Surgery, Gynecology, and Obstetrics* 164 (1987): 431–437.

73. Johnson, 1987.

74. G. L. Blackburn and G. A. Bray, Introduction, *Management of Obesity by Severe Caloric Restriction*, ed. G. L. Blackburn and G. A. Bray (Littleton, Mass.: PSG Publishing, 1985), pp. xv-xvi.

75. J. E. Haddow and coauthors, Neural tube defects after gastric bypass, *The Lancet* 1 (1986): 1330.

76. R. W. Smithells and coauthors, Further experience of vitamin supplementation for prevention of neural tube defect recurrences, *The Lancet* 1 (1983): 1027–1031; M. Tolarova, Periconceptual supplementation with vitamins and folic acid to prevent recurrence of cleft lip (letter), *The Lancet* 2 (1982): 217.

77. D. S. Richards, D. K. Miller, and G. N. Goodman, Pregnancy after gastric bypass for morbid obesity, *The Journal of Reproductive Medicine* 32 (1987): 172–175.

78. C. H. Peckham and R. E. Christianson, The relationship between prepregnancy weight and certain obstetric factors, *American Journal of Obstetrics and Gynecology* 111 (1971): 1.

79. R. E. Little and coauthors, Decreased birth weight in infants of alcoholic women who abstained during pregnancy, *Journal of Pediatrics*, 96 (1980): 974–977.

80. *Physician's Desk Reference*, 42nd ed. (Oradell, N.J.: Medical Economics Company, 1988), pp. 1705–1706.

81. After conception: Dispelling rumors about later childbearing, *Population Reports* 12 (1984): J-699–J-702.

82. L. F. Soyka and J. M. Joffe, Male mediated drug effects on offspring, *Progress in Clinical and Biological Research* 36 (1980): 49–66.

83. Soyka and Joffe, 1980. 84.

84. L. M. Hill and F. Kleinburg, Effects of drugs and chemicals on the fetus and newborn, *Mayo Clinic Proceedings* 59 (1984): 707–716.

85. Soyka and Joffe, 1980.

▶ *Focal Point 1*

Inborn Errors of Metabolism

The discussion in Chapter 1 on inheritance lays the foundation for a closer look at the ramifications of a genetic error in protein synthesis. Body functions, such as metabolic reactions and transports, that depend on proteins cannot proceed when proteins are made in an insufficient quantity or when they have an abnormal structure. If an enzyme is missing or malfunctioning in the metabolic pathway that converts compound A to compound B, then compound A accumulates and compound B becomes deficient. Both the excess of compound A and the lack of compound B can lead to a variety of physical disorders and, in many cases, death. Furthermore, high concentrations of compound A become available, and low concentrations of compound B are unavailable, for use in other metabolic pathways. These consequences, in turn, create excesses and deficiencies of other metabolites that present another array of problems. The diseases that result from these "inherited biochemical blocks in normal metabolic pathways" are known as inborn errors of metabolism.[1]

In some instances, the accumulated compound is not toxic and the deficient compound is not essential, and so individuals experience no problem. In all likelihood, they will never know about the error. However, in other cases, inborn errors have severe consequences, with many of them causing mental retardation. Without proper diagnosis and treatment, they can be lethal. As is true of most medical disorders, the earlier the diagnosis and treatment, the better the prognosis.

One goal of medical research is to detect genetic defects before they cause harm. Recent advances in medical technology allow clinicians to study the developing fetus and identify abnormal conditions during gestation. One technique, amniocentesis, analyzes amniotic fluid that has been removed by a needle or syringe puncturing the amniotic sac. This technique has proven most valuable in the identification of more than 70 different inborn errors of metabolism.[2] Analysis of the amniotic fluid and cells identifies specific enzymes and measures their concentrations, revealing abnormalities. A genetic technique called restriction enzyme analysis allows scientists to locate specific genes. Such a technique holds promise of actually correcting a genetic defect in the future. For now, prenatal diagnosis of genetic diseases allows nutritional intervention during gestation.[3]

The primary treatment for most inborn errors of metabolism is nutrition. With an understanding of the biochemical pathway involved, a clinician can manipulate the diet to correct for excesses and inadequacies. Dietary management of genetic diseases restricts dietary precursors that occur prior to the error in the metabolic pathway; administers pharmacological doses of vitamins; or replaces needed products. The goal of therapy is to:

▸ Prevent the toxic accumulation of metabolites.

▸ Replace essential nutrients that are deficient as a result of the defective metabolic pathway.

▸ Provide a diet that supports growth and development.

To meet these three requirements is a major challenge that was unattainable until earlier this century. Increased knowledge about the body's many biochemical pathways, coupled with current technology to synthesize formulas of specific nutrient compositions, have greatly enhanced the treatment of inborn errors.

Researchers are experimenting with ways to handle the toxic metabolites that accumulate in inborn errors. One solution is to administer a compound that reacts with the toxic metabolite, thus using an alternative pathway for excretion. Such alternative pathways are proving effective in the excretion of waste nitrogen in children with inborn errors of urea synthesis.[4] Another solution is to provide an antagonist that eliminates or detoxifies the accumulated metabolites. For example, the drug penicillamine is used both as a copper chelator in Wilson's disease and to increase the solubility of urinary cystine in cystinuria.[5]

This discussion focuses primarily on the most common inborn error of metabolism—phenylketonuria (PKU)—which affects approximately 200 newborns in the United States each year. The ability to detect and treat PKU has significantly improved the lives of many people and provides an example that offers hope to those suffering from other inborn errors.

PKU is only one of several inborn errors that affect amino acid metabolism. Other disorders affect not only amino acid metabolism but also carbohydrate, lipid, and vitamin metabolism. The number of possible inborn errors is limited only by the number of possible gene mutations, for genes carry the codes to make the enzymes in the body.

Consider that a small bacterial cell carries genes for at least 1000 different enzymes and that mutations are possible in all of these genes. Human cells have 1000 times as many proteins of major importance and, in theory, any of them can appear in many different mutant forms. Not only can the genes for enzymes be affected, but also those for other proteins such as the "pumps" that move nutrients into and out of cells, the carriers that transport them in the blood, and the structural proteins of cell membranes and connective tissue. Table FP1–1 provides a glimpse into the array of possible errors by identifying some of these genetic disorders, their defective pathways, associated symptoms, and treatments. The rest of this discussion provides a look at a few inborn errors that respond to nutrition therapy.

Classic Phenylketonuria

phenylketonuria (PKU): an inborn error of metabolism in which phenylalanine, an essential amino acid, cannot be converted to tyrosine. Alternative metabolites of phenylalanine (phenylketones) accumulate in the tissues, causing damage, and overflow into the urine.

Classic phenylketonuria (PKU) results from a deficiency of the enzyme phenylalanine hydroxylase. This enzyme hydroxylates the essential amino acid phenylalanine, converting it to tyrosine (see Figure FP1–1). Without phenylalanine hydroxylase, abnormally high concentrations of phenylalanine and other related compounds (phenylketones) accumulate and damage the devel-

Figure FP1–1   The Biochemical Pathway in PKU

Normally, the amino acid phenylalanine follows two pathways, one in the liver, the other in the kidney. In the liver, the enzyme phenylalanine hydroxylase adds a hydroxyl group (OH) to produce the amino acid tyrosine. Tyrosine, in turn, produces melanin, the pigmented compound found in skin and brain cells; the neurotransmitters epinephrine and norepinephrine; and the hormone thyroxine. In the kidney, enzymes convert phenylalanine to byproducts that are excreted.

In the liver:

$$\text{phenylalanine} \xrightarrow[\text{hydroxylase}]{\text{phenylalanine}} \text{tyrosine} \longrightarrow \begin{array}{l} \text{melanin} \\ \text{epinephrine} \\ \text{norepinephrine} \\ \text{thyroxine} \end{array}$$

In the kidney:

$$\text{phenylalanine} \longrightarrow \begin{array}{l} \text{phenylpyruvic acid} \\ \text{(a ketone body)} \end{array} \longrightarrow \text{other phenyl acids}$$

Individuals with PKU lack the liver enzyme phenylalanine hydroxylase, impairing conversion of phenylalanine to tyrosine. Phenylalanine accumulates in the liver and blood, reaching the kidney in abnormally high concentrations. In the kidney, an aminotransferase enzyme converts phenylalanine to the ketone body phenylpyruvic acid, which spills into the urine—thus the name phenylketonuria.

In the liver:

$$\begin{array}{l} \text{phenylalanine} \\ \text{(accumulates)} \end{array} \xrightarrow[\substack{\text{hydroxylase} \\ \text{(deficient)}}]{\text{phenylalanine}} \begin{array}{l} \text{tyrosine} \\ \text{(deficient)} \end{array}$$

In the kidney:

$$\begin{array}{l} \text{phenylalanine} \\ \text{(accumulates)} \end{array} \longrightarrow \begin{array}{l} \text{phenylpyruvic acid} \\ \text{(accumulates)} \end{array} \longrightarrow \begin{array}{l} \text{other phenyl acids} \\ \text{(accumulate)} \end{array}$$

oping nervous system. Simultaneously, the body cannot make tyrosine or other compounds (such as the hormone epinephrine) that normally derive from tyrosine. Under these conditions, tyrosine becomes an essential amino acid; that is, the body cannot make it and therefore the diet must supply it.

PKU is a hidden disease that cannot be seen at birth, yet diagnosis and treatment beginning in the first few days of life can prevent its devastating effects. For these reasons, all newborns in the United States receive a metabolic test to screen for PKU. Tests must be conducted after infants have consumed several meals containing protein. Before the 1960s, when screening became routine, children with PKU would suffer the consequences of elevated phenylalanine concentrations. At first, the only signs are a skin rash and light skin pigmentation. Between three and six months, signs of developmental delay begin to appear. The infant becomes irritable, unable to sleep restfully, and frantic. By one year, irreversible brain damage is clearly evident, and the child has already lost 40 to 50 IQ points.[6]

Table FP1–1 Inborn Errors of Metabolism

Disease name	Defect or deficiency	Result of defect or deficiency	Main effects	Therapy
Cerebrotendinous xanthomatosis (CTX)[a]	a liver enzyme	Inability to produce bile acids effectively	Accelerated hardening of the arteries Progressive neurological disorders Cataracts Deposition of cholesterol-related chemicals in the brain	Supply bile acids
Richner-Hanhart syndrome (tyrosinemia II)[b]	Tyrosine aminotransferase	High tyrosine concentrations	Eye disorders Skin disorders	Restrict tyrosine and phenylalanine
Tyrosinosis (tyrosinemia I)[c]	Fumarylacetoacetate hydrolyase	—	Failure to thrive Vomiting; diarrhea Chronic liver disease; cirrhosis Renal tubular dysfunction Vitamin D-resistant rickets Death	—
—	Ornithine transcarbamylase[d]	Inability to synthesize arginine and urea High ammonia concentrations due to altered protein metabolism	Delayed physical growth and development Extreme irritability Lethargy Muscular incoordination Seizures Vomiting Mental retardation Coma Death	Restrict protein
Hawkinsinuria[e]	—	Tyrosinemia Accumulation of toxic metabolites of tyrosine	Failure to gain weight Metabolic acidosis	—
—	Glutamate dehydrogenase[f]	High glutamate concentrations Low alpha-ketoglutarate concentrations	Neuronal degeneration	—

Disorder	Enzyme/protein	Biochemical findings	Clinical findings	Treatment
Propionic acidemia (PA)[g]	Propionyl-CoA carboxylase (PCC)—an enzyme required in branched-chain amino acid metabolism	High concentrations of ammonia High concentrations of glycine High concentrations of propionic acid High concentrations of organic acids Ketonuria	Vomiting Lethargy Ketoacidosis Seizures Osteoporosis Developmental retardation	Restrict total protein or restrict isoleucine, methionine, threonine, and valine Megadoses of biotin (in conjunction with other therapy)
Mevalonic aciduria[h]	Mevalonic kinase	Disrupts cholesterol (and other isoprenoid compounds) biosynthesis High mevalonate concentrations	Failure to grow and mature Cataracts Hypocholesterolemia	—
Wilson's disease (hepatolenticular degeneration)[i]	—	Accumulation of copper Low ceruloplasmin concentrations	Cirrhosis Neurological symptoms	Chelating agent (D-penicillamine) Oral zinc supplementation
—	Cobalamin R binding proteins	Low cobalamin concentrations	Microcytic hypochromic anemia	—
Megaloblastic anemia	Cobalamin TC II binding protein (transports cobalamin to tissues)	Normal plasma cobalamin concentrations	Megaloblastic anemia	Pharmacological doses of cobalamin

[a]New clue for prevention and treatment of hardening of the arteries, *Journal of the American Dietetic Association* 84 (1984): 567.

[b]Tyrosinemia II (abstract), *Journal of the American Dietetic Association* 86 (1986): 127.

[c]Tyrosinemia II (abstract), *Journal of the American Dietetic Association* 86 (1986): 127.

[d]Disease carriers and lowered IQ, *Science News* 117 (1980): 166; Ornithine transcarbamylase deficiency (abstract), *Journal of the American Dietetic Association* 86 (1986): 1128–1129.

[e]Hawkinsinuria: Disorder of tyrosine metabolism (abstract), *Journal of the American Dietetic Association* 80 (1982): 82–83.

[f]Glutamate metabolism in an adult-onset degenerative neurological disorder, *Journal of the American Dietetic Association* 81 (1982): 215.

[g]P. M. Queen, P. M. Fernhoff, and P. B. Acosta, Protein and essential amino acid requirements in a child with propionic acidemia, *Journal of the American Dietetic Association* 79 (1981): 562–565.

[h]An inborn error of cholesterol biosynthesis, *Nutrition Reviews* 44 (1986): 334–336.

[i]Oral zinc therapy for Wilson's disease, *Nutrition Reviews* 42 (1984): 184–186.

Table FP1-1 continued

Disease name	Defect or deficiency	Result of defect or deficiency	Main effects	Therapy
Menke's kinky hair syndrome[j]	Metallothionein synthesis or degradation (?)	Disrupts copper metabolism Reduced activity of copper metalloenzymes Low copper concentrations (blood) High copper concentrations (cells) Low ceruloplasmin concentrations	Kinky, depigmented hair Pale skin Elastin and collagen abnormalities Hypothermia Neurological disorders Skeletal demineralization Death	—
Acrodermatitis enteropathica (AE)[k]	—	Zinc malabsorption	Dermatitis Diarrhea Alopecia Depression Delayed bone maturation Growth retardation Delayed sexual development Anemia Compromised immune system	Megadoses of zinc
Homocystinuria[l]	Cystathionine synthetase	Disrupts sulfur amino acid (cysteine, cystine, methionine) metabolism; blocks transsulfuration of methionine to cysteine High methionine concentrations and related compounds High homocysteine concentrations and related compounds Low cystathionine and cystine concentrations	Dislocation of eye lenses Mental retardation Skeletal abnormalities	Restrict methionine High cystine diet Pharamacological doses of pyridoxine (cystathionine synthetase requires pyridoxal phosphate as a coenzyme)

Lysinuric protein intolerance (LPI)[m]	Disruption of dibasic amino acid (arginine, ornithine, lysine) absorption, transport, and excretion	Low arginine concentrations Low ornithine concentrations Low lysine concentrations Prevents urea cycle substrates from being renewed Low urea synthesis (with normal urea acid cycle enzymes) High ammonia concentrations after protein intake High orotic acid concentrations	Failure to thrive Vomiting Diarrhea Growth retardation Osteoporosis Low white blood cell concentrations Low blood platelet concentrations Enlarged liver and spleen Protein intolerance	Ornithine, arginine, or citrulline supplementation
Hartnup disease[n]	Disruption of monoamino-monocarboxylic acid (tryptophan, alanine, asparagine, glutamine, histidine, isoleucine, leucine, phenylalanine, serine, threonine, tryptophan, tyrosine, and valine) absorption, transport, and excretion	Low amino acid concentrations Excessive amino acid excretion Minimal biosynthesis of nicotinic acid from tryptophan	Muscular incoordination due to brain disease Pellagra and associated mental disturbances	Megadoses of nicotinic acid

[j] On the pathogenesis and clinical expression of Menkes' kinky hair syndrome, *Nutrition Reviews* 39 (1981): 391–393; Menke's disease: Are we closer to learning its cause?, *Nutrition Reviews* 42 (1984): 309–311.
[k] Zinc therapy of depressed cellular immunity in acrodermatitis enteropathica, *Nutrition Reviews* 39 (1981): 168–170.
[l] Pyridoxine-responsive homocystinuria, *Nutrition Reviews* 39 (1981): 16–18; M. A. Wallen and S. Packman, Nutrition and inborn errors of metabolism, in *Nutrition Update* vol. 2, ed. J. Weininger and G. M. Briggs (New York: John Wiley and Sons, 1985) pp. 71–89.
[m] Lysinuric protein intolerance: A rare cause of childhood osteoporosis, *Nutrition Reviews* 44 (1986): 110–113.
[n] Treatment of Hartnup disease with nicotinic acid, *Nutrition Reviews* 42 (1984): 251–253.

Table FP1–1   continued

Disease name	Defect or deficiency	Result of defect or deficiency	Main effects	Therapy
Cobalamin-responsive methylmalonic acidemias[o]	Methylmalonyl CoA mutase N[5]-methyltetrahydro-folate-homocysteine methyltransferase	Hydroxocobalamin is not converted to its active coenzymes	Protein intolerance Failure to thrive Episodic ketoacidosis Neurologic abnormalities Death (in severe, untreated cases)	Pharmacological doses of cobalamin (1 mg/day)
Galactosemia[p]	Galactose-1-phosphate uridyl transferase	Failure to convert galactose-1-phosphate to glucose-1-phosphate	Failure to thrive Jaundice; enlarged liver Renal dysfunction Cataracts Hemolytic anemia Seizures Coma; death	Eliminate galactose from the diet (feed soybean-based formulas containing sucrose or glucose, without lactose)
Phenylketonuria (PKU)[q]	Phenylalanine hydroxylase	Failure to convert phenylalanine to tyrosine	Skin rash and light pigmentation Delayed development Neurological defects Microcephaly EEG abnormalities Seizures	Restrict protein sources; supplement with a protein-containing formula with low phenylalanine content
Malignant hyperphenylalaninemia[r]	Dihydropteridine reductase	Failure to synthesize or regenerate the cofactor tetrahydrobiopterin, which is required for phenylalanine hydroxylase, tyrosine hydroxylase, and tryptophan hydroxylase Defective synthesis of neurotransmitters (dopamine, norepinephrine, serotonin)	Neurological abnormalities	Neurotransmitter replacement Tetrahydrobiopterin administration Phenylalanine restriction (not effective alone)

Disease	Enzyme defect	Metabolic findings	Symptoms	Treatment
Von Gierke's disease (glycogen storage disease type I)[s]	Glucose-6-phosphatase	Incomplete gluconeogenesis; Incomplete glycogenolysis; High concentrations of serum uric acid, cholesterol, triglycerides, and lactate	Hypoglycemia; Enlarged liver; Growth failure (due to low insulin production); Adiposity; Hemorrhagic tendency	Provide glucose between meals and during the night (continuous nocturnal intragastric infusion)
Citrullinemia[t]	Argininosuccinic acid synthetase (urea cycle enzyme that converts citrulline to argininosuccinic acid)	Elevated ammonia concentrations; Elevated citrulline concentrations	Lethargy; Rapid respiration; Tremors and seizures; Abnormal prothrombin times; Death by age 7	Feed mixture of keto acids of essential amino acids

[o]Wallen and Packman, 1985.
[p]Wallen and Packman, 1985.
[q]Wallen and Packman, 1985.
[r]Wallen and Packman, 1985.
[s]Wallen and Packman, 1985.
[t]W. L. Nyhan, Nutritional treatment of children with inborn errors of metabolism, in Textbook of Pediatric Nutrition, ed. R. M. Suskind (New York: Raven Press, 1981), pp. 563–576.

Nutritional Therapy

The effect of nutrition intervention in PKU is remarkable. In almost every case, dietary management can prevent the devastating array of symptoms described. Essentially, the diet restricts phenylalanine intake to a point that maintains blood phenylalanine concentrations within a safe range. As most dietitians can attest, this is more easily said than done.

Because phenylalanine is an essential amino acid, the diet cannot exclude it completely. If phenylalanine intake is too low, children suffer bone, skin, and blood disorders; growth and mental retardation; and death.[7] Therefore, the diet must strike a perfect balance between providing enough phenylalanine to support normal growth and health and not too much to cause harm. It is not that children with PKU require less phenylalanine than other children, but that they cannot handle excesses without detrimental effects. To ensure that blood phenylalanine concentrations remain within a safe range, children with PKU receive blood tests periodically and alterations in their diet when necessary. With a controlled phenylalanine intake, children with PKU can lead normal, happy lives.

To control phenylalanine intake requires strict dietary management that was impossible prior to 1958, when a special low-phenylalanine formula became commercially available.[8] This type of formula is now the primary source of energy and protein for children with PKU. Their diet excludes high-protein foods such as meat, fish, poultry, cheese, eggs, milk, nuts, dried beans, or peas. Also excluded are commercial breads and pastries made from regular flour, which has a high phenylalanine content. Basically, the diet allows foods that contain some phenylalanine, such as fruits, vegetables, and cereals, and those that contain none, such as sugar, jellies, and some candies. Clearly, it is impossible to create a diet of whole, natural foods, and children who depend primarily on a formula for their nourishment risk multiple trace mineral deficiencies.[9]

Infants receive a special casein hydrolysate formula with a low phenylalanine content. It does not contain all the phenylalanine an infant requires, and so parents supplement it with measured quantities of milk, rice cereal, and baby foods as the infant develops. Other formulas and products are available that provide a synthetic mixture of amino acids without phenylalanine. This allows older children to receive their entire phenylalanine quota from foods.[10]

People with PKU must also be aware of the phenylalanine content in products containing the sweetener aspartame. Aspartame is a combination of the two amino acids aspartic acid and phenylalanine, and therefore contributes phenylalanine to the diet. Sold under the trade name NutraSweet, aspartame is an ingredient in many foods and beverages such as powdered drink mixes, instant puddings, gelatin desserts, breakfast cereals, chewing gums, and the sweetener Equal. Products sweetened with aspartame bear a warning label for people with PKU. People with PKU need to consult with their physicians or dietitians before including aspartame in their diet.

Perhaps one of the hardest parts of this diet is in the children's sense of social isolation. From birth, children with PKU are on a "special diet" and cannot eat the foods that other children are eating. Some commercially available low-protein products, such as cookies, contain very little, if any, phenylalanine and allow children to share treats with others. Teachers, friends, and family members must understand that they cannot offer food to children with PKU before receiving permission from the children's parents. Until the children are old enough to know their dietary restrictions, parents must teach them to ask before eating any food. Most parents tell their children that they will become sick if they eat the wrong foods. The threat of possible brain damage and routine blood tests motivate children and their parents to adhere to the diet.[11]

No doubt, prompt nutrition intervention during the early years of central nervous system development is critical to preventing irreversible mental retardation in the young PKU child. Of less certainty is for how long the nervous system is vulnerable to the PKU defect. In the past, researchers assumed that the child with PKU could abandon the special diet after the first few years of life, once the central nervous system had completed its development. They realized that with a regular diet, phenylalanine and associated metabolite concentrations would rise, but thought perhaps these high levels would not be damaging. While the damages are less severe than at an earlier age, elevated phenylalanine concentrations in the older child do cause problems such as short attention span, poor short-term memory, and poor eye-to-hand coordination.[12] In general, children with PKU who have discontinued their controlled diet experience problems in their school performances, mood, and behavior.[13] One study reports that IQ scores of children with PKU progressively increase the longer the diets are controlled.[14] For these reasons, clinicians now encourage children to continue the low-phenylalanine diet at least through adolescence. One approach allows children over the age of ten to have one day every month or two to eat any foods they want without having to drink the special formula.[15] To reinstitute the phenylalanine-restricted diet in adolescents after several years of unrestricted diets requires intense education and reinforcement, and even then is quite often unsuccessful.[16] Reports indicate that the reinstitution of a controlled diet does improve the person's blood phenylalanine concentrations, behavior, and IQ scores.[17]

Therapy for inborn errors goes beyond nutrition, requiring psychological counseling for the people who are affected and their families. A genetic disorder is a lifelong problem that affects the entire family. All family members are at high risk for being carriers and they inevitably become involved in the care and management of the person with the inborn error. Therefore, families must learn how to handle the impact such a diagnosis has on the structure, development, and interactional processes of their family life.[18]

Maternal PKU

Before the development of routine metabolic screenings, special formulas, and restricted diets, children with PKU died young. Now that people with PKU are living longer and reaching reproductive age, researchers face a new set of PKU problems.

PKU, like all inborn errors, is a recessive disorder; that is, it only appears when a person inherits two defective genes—one from each parent. This can

carrier: an individual who possesses one dominant and one recessive gene for a recessive trait such as an inborn error of metabolism. Such a person may show no signs of the trait but can pass it on.

occur when both parents have PKU, when one has PKU and the other is a carrier, or when both are carriers. Carriers are people who inherit one defective gene and one normal gene. They may be unaware that they carry a defective gene, for their symptoms are usually mild or absent. When a person with PKU mates with a noncarrier, all of their children will be carriers. When a person with PKU mates with a carrier, their children will have a 50 percent chance of either having PKU or being a carrier. When two people with PKU mate, all of their children will have PKU. The statistical chances of two people with PKU meeting and conceiving a child would be small except for their increased contacts with each other through PKU clinics and support groups.

The risks for a PKU mother go beyond genetics. When off the diet as an adult, a woman's blood phenylalanine concentrations are high. As mentioned earlier, this causes some behavioral problems but does not cause the irreversible brain damage evident in young children. When she becomes pregnant, the fetal blood concentrations rise even higher than the mother's, and this is detrimental to fetal development.[19] A PKU mother with high phenylalanine blood concentrations is likely to give birth to an infant with mental retardation, microcephaly, congenital heart disease, and low birthweight.[20] These women frequently experience spontaneous abortions as well. These reasons, coupled with the high genetic risks of people with PKU, prompt counselors to recommend alternatives other than pregnancy, such as sterilization, therapeutic abortion, and adoption.[21]

Dietary control of maternal PKU may protect the fetus, if implemented early enough. Women who become pregnant without planning for their pregnancies expose their fetuses to high phenylalanine concentrations during a critical time of early development. A PKU woman who departed from her restricted diet as a child must resume the low-phenylalanine diet at least one to two months prior to conception and throughout her pregnancy.[22] In fact, many physicians recommend adherence to a restricted diet throughout life. To resume a low-phenylalanine diet is not easy; the special formulas are costly, inconvenient, and unpalatable to an adult who has been eating foods freely. Many women have forgotten that they were ever on a special diet as a child or may never have understood why. For these reasons, many PKU clinics recommend that females continue using the formula into adulthood. The low-phenylalanine diet for maternal PKU must also meet the energy, protein, vitamin, and mineral needs of pregnancy. Special PKU formulas for the pregnant PKU woman are now available.

A woman with PKU benefits from genetic and medical counseling. She must consider the possible consequences of pregnancy and the options of contraception to prevent pregnancy and adoption if she wants children. Dietary control does not ensure a successful outcome of pregnancy, although a low-phenylalanine diet used from before conception throughout pregnancy seems promising for women with PKU.[23]

Classic PKU is not the only inborn error to raise blood concentrations of phenylalanine. Malignant hyperphenylalaninemia has the same result, but because the error occurs elsewhere in the metabolic pathway, it does not respond to phenylalanine restriction alone.[24] In this case, treatment involves replacing missing cofactors and neurotransmitters instead of restricting the precursor in the pathway.

Other Inborn Errors

The remainder of this discussion provides a brief description of a few other inborn errors that have nutrition implications and solutions. Table FP1–1 provides additional information on several other inborn errors.

Galactosemia

Galactosemia is an inborn error of carbohydrate metabolism in which the body cannot use the monosaccharide galactose. Three enzymes are required for the conversion of galactose to glucose; in galactosemia, most commonly the enzyme galactose-1-phosphate uridyl transferase is missing or defective. When infants with galactosemia are given milk (which contains a galactose unit in each molecule of lactose), they vomit and have diarrhea. The unmetabolized galactose-1-phosphate accumulates and follows an alternative pathway to form an abnormal product that causes growth failure, liver enlargement, kidney failure, and cataracts. Infants with galactosemia experience seizures and other neurological abnormalities that lead to coma and death.[25] Early introduction of a galactose-restricted diet prevents or minimizes most of these symptoms. However, it may not prevent ovarian damage, some visual and speech problems, or other neurological abnormalities.

Dietary adjustment in galactosemia is simpler than in PKU for a couple of reasons. First, galactose is not an essential nutrient as is phenylalanine. The PKU diet is a balancing act of providing just enough phenylalanine for normal growth and development, without too much left over to be toxic; the galactosemia diet only needs to exclude galactose. Second, since galactose occurs only in lactose (the sugar in milk), only milk and milk products need to be restricted.

galactosemia: an inborn error of metabolism in which galactose cannot be metabolized normally to compounds the body can handle; an alternative metabolite accumulates in the tissues, causing damage.

Glycogen Storage Diseases

Other genetic diseases affecting carbohydrate metabolism include the glycogen storage diseases. These diseases are characterized by abnormal glycogen deposition in liver, muscle, or both.[26]

Type I, also known as von Gierke's disease, is the most common and severe of the glycogen diseases, and is caused by a deficiency of the enzyme glucose-6-phosphatase.[27] This enzyme converts glucose-6-phosphate to glucose in the gluconeogenesis pathways and glycogenolysis pathways.[28] The body's inability to handle glucose-6-phosphate results in hypoglycemia, glycogen accumulation, and their associated metabolic consequences.

Dietary management of glycogen storage disease type I involves constant provision of carbohydrate (glucose). To accomplish this, children eat frequent (at least every three hours) high-carbohydrate meals (60 to 70 percent of total kcalories) composed primarily of starch foods.[29] To maintain glucose concentrations during sleep, children receive a special glucose polymer formula by tube feeding.

Type III, or Cori's disease, is a result of a deficiency of the glycogen debranching enzyme amylo-1,6-glucosidase, which inhibits glycogen breakdown at the branches and results in short-branched glycogen. In contrast, type IV, or Andersen's disease, is due to a deficiency of the branching enzyme, which results in abnormally long glycogen chains. Type III is a fairly harmless disorder that can be managed by diet, whereas type IV leads to liver cirrhosis and death in infancy.[30]

Vitamin Disorders

Some inborn errors affect the metabolic pathways in such a way as to raise a person's vitamin requirement. The error may be in the absorption of the vitamin; the biosynthesis, transport, or accessibility of the coenzyme form of the vitamin; or the apoenzyme protein. In such a case, the person requires pharmacological doses of the particular vitamin to overcome the error and prevent its associated detrimental effects. Table FP1–1 itemizes a few of the vitamin-responsive disorders.

As scientific understanding of human genetics and biochemistry increases, more and more inborn errors are being recognized. Understanding protein structure and function makes it possible to compensate for these defects of metabolism that otherwise would destroy the quality of life. Diet cannot always be tailored to prevent the defects of inborn errors, but in many such diseases diet can make a dramatic difference in people's lives.

Focal Point 1 Notes

1. A. E. Garrod, Inborn errors of metabolism (Croonian lectures), *Lancet* 2 (1908), as cited in M. A. Wallen and S. Packman, Nutrition and inborn errors of metabolism, in *Nutrition Update*, vol. 2, ed. J. Weininger and G. M. Briggs (New York: John Wiley and Sons, 1985), pp. 71–89.
2. G. H. Lowrey, The placenta and fetal development, in *Growth and Development of Children*, 8th ed., (Chicago: Year Book Medical Publishers, 1986), pp. 53–75.
3. Wallen and Packman, 1985.
4. M. L. Batshaw and coauthors, Treatment of inborn errors of urea synthesis: Activation of alternative pathways of waste nitrogen synthesis and excretion, *New England Journal of Medicine* 306 (1982): 1387–1392.
5. Wallen and Packman, 1985.
6. Wallen and Packman, 1985.
7. P. B. Acosta and coauthors, Phenylalanine intakes of 1- to 6-year-old children with phenylketonuria undergoing therapy, *American Journal of Clinical Nutrition* 38 (1983): 694–700.
8. M. M. Hunt, H. K. Berry, and P. P. White, Phenylketonuria, adolescence, and diet, *Journal of the American Dietetic Association* 85 (1985): 1328–1334.
9. S. Stepnick-Gropper and coauthors, Trace element status of PKU children ingesting an elemental diet (abstract), *American Journal of Clinical Nutrition* 43 (1986): 676.
10. N. Reyzer, Diagnosis: PKU, *American Journal of Nursing* 78 (1978): 1895–1898.
11. S. Schild, Psychological issues in genetic counseling of phenylketonuria, in *Genetic Counseling, Psychological Dimensions*, ed. S. Kessler (New York: Academic Press, 1979), pp. 138–147.
12. Hunt, Berry, and White, 1985.
13. V. E. Schuett, E. S. Brown, and K. Michals, Reinstitution of diet therapy in PKU patients from twenty-two U.S. clinics, *American Journal of Public Health* 75 (1985): 39–42.
14. N. A. Holtzman and coauthors, Effect of age at loss of dietary control on intellectual performance and behavior of children with phenylketonuria, *New England Journal of Medicine* 314 (1986): 593–598.
15. R. Koch and E. Wenz, Phenylketonuria, in *Annual Review of Nutrition*, ed. R. E. Olson, E. Beutler, and H. P. Broquist, (Palo Alto, Calif.: Annual Reviews, Inc.), pp. 117–135.
16. S. E. Hogan, G. W. MacDonald, and J. T. R. Clarke, Experience with adolescents with phenylketonuria returned to phenylalanine-restricted diets, *Journal of the American Dietetic Association* 86 (1986): 1203–1207; Schuett, Brown, and Michals, 1985.
17. Schuett, Brown, and Michals, 1985.
18. Schild, 1979.
19. P. B. Acosta, Maternal PKU, address presented at the conference Nutrition for Pregnancy, Lactation, and Infancy, Gainesville, Florida, 13 February 1987.
20. R. R. Lenke and H. L. Levy, Maternal phenylketonuria—Results of dietary therapy, *American Journal of Obstetrics and Gynecology* 5 (1982): 548–553; H. L. Levy and S. E. Waisbren, Effects of untreated maternal phenylketonuria and hy-

perphenylalaninemia on the fetus, *New England Journal of Medicine* 309 (1983): 1269–1274.

21. Schild, 1979.
22. Lenke and Levy, 1982; Acosta, 1987.
23. E. Drogari and coauthors, Timing of strict diet in relation to fetal damage in maternal phenylketonuria, *Lancet* 2 (1987): 927–930.

24. Wallen and Packman, 1985.
25. Wallen and Packman, 1985.
26. W. C. McMurray, *Essentials of Metabolism* (New York: Harper and Row Publishers, 1977), pp. 123–165.
27. C. C. Folk and H. L. Greene, Dietary management of Type I glycogen storage disease, *Journal of the American Dietetic*

Association 84 (1984): 293–301; I. E. Daeschel and coauthors, Diet and growth of children with glycogen storage disease Types I and III, *Journal of the American Dietetic Association* 83 (1983): 135–141.
28. McMurray, 1977.
29. Folk and Greene, 1984.
30. McMurray, 1977.

Pregnancy: Nutrition for a New Life

2

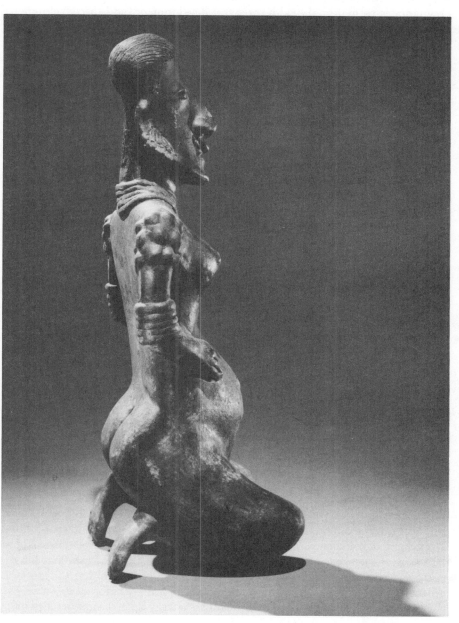

Nayarit (Pre-Columbian) pottery vessel.

Between the moment of conception and the moment of birth, innumerable events occur that determine the course and outcome of fetal development and, ultimately, the health of the newborn infant. Many of these events are beyond control—but a woman's nutrition throughout the teen and adult years, including pregnancy, is within her control, provided she has the knowledge, the means, and the motivation to attend to it. The woman who is expecting an infant and the advising health professional will be most motivated to attend to maternal nutrient needs if they understand how critical nutrition during pregnancy is to maternal health, prenatal development, and the development of the child long after birth.

Growth and Development

In the early days of pregnancy, because the zygote is so small, the nutrient-rich cells of the uterine lining provide adequate fuel and raw materials by diffusion alone. Soon, though, a specialized system is required to continue nourishing the developing embryo and fetus. To accomplish this, the placenta, an interweaving of fetal and maternal blood vessels embedded in the uterine wall, develops. The development of a healthy placenta is absolutely indispensible to fetal development, and nutrition, in turn, is crucial to placental development.

Placental Development

embryo (EM-bree-oh): the developing infant from the end of the second to the end of the eighth week after conception.

fetus (FEET-us): the developing infant from the eighth week after conception until its birth.

placenta (pla-SEN-tah): the organ inside the uterus in which the mother's and fetus's circulatory systems intertwine and in which exchange of materials between maternal and fetal blood takes place.

chorion: the outer membrane enclosing the embryo.

endometrium: defined on page 17.

The fetal portion of the placenta develops when two embryonic membranes combine, forming the chorion, which then fuses with the uterine lining (see Figure 2–1).[1] Shortly after implantation, chorionic villi develop from the chorion, establishing an internal connection with the uterus, the maternal portion of the placenta. As the villi branch and penetrate the endometrium, the placenta grows in size and complexity.

Maternal blood never leaves the mother's circulatory system. It enters the placental tissue through small artery branches of the uterus, circulates around the chorionic villi, and leaves via the uterine vein. Similarly, fetal blood never leaves the fetal vessels. It circulates through the umbilical artery and vein and their branches within the chorionic villi. Within the spongelike endometrium, exchange of materials takes place but no actual mingling of fetal and maternal blood occurs.

The placenta is a versatile, metabolically active organ. It transfers oxygen and nutrients to the fetus and returns waste products to the mother. Nutrients pass from maternal blood through the placenta into fetal blood; waste products travel from the fetal blood through the placenta into maternal blood. By exchanging oxygen, nutrients, and waste products, the placenta provides the respiratory, absorptive, and excretory functions of the embryo's lungs, gastrointestinal tract, and kidneys. Far from being passive in its transport of molecules, the placenta is a highly metabolic organ with some 60 enzymes. Much like muscles or other body tissue, it uses energy fuels to support its work.

The placenta metabolizes glucose for its own energy needs as well as actively pumping it into the fetal bloodstream. It synthesizes protein and fatty

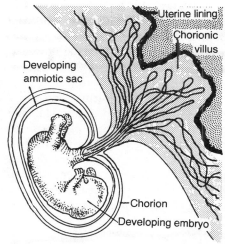

The embryonic chorion fuses with the uterine lining.

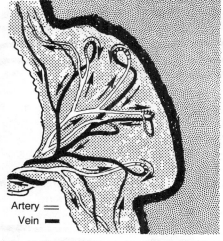

Chorionic villi (of which one is shown) develop, establishing an internal connection with the uterus.

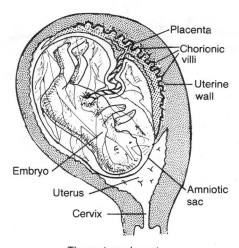

The mature placenta.

Figure 2–1 Development of the Placenta

acids from small precursors and secretes hormones and gathers up hormones from elsewhere in the body.

Of the placental hormones that are involved in maintaining a healthy pregnancy, most notable are human chorionic gonadotropin (HCG) and placental lactogen.[2] HCG increases rapidly during early pregnancy, reaching its maximum concentration in the first eight to ten weeks, and then diminishes to a low but constant concentration at the end of the third month. Most pregnancy tests are based on the detection of this hormone in urine or plasma. Early placental secretion of these hormones leads to later placental production of progesterone and estrogen. Placental synthesis of the major estrogen of pregnancy, estriol, requires a precursor from the fetal adrenal gland. Together, the placenta and fetal adrenals produce the estriol required to maintain pregnancy.

human chorionic gonadotropin (HCG): a hormone produced by the chorionic villi of the placenta that stimulates the secretion of progesterone and estrogen.

placental lactogen: a hormone produced by the placenta that stimulates the metabolism of glucose to fat.

The secretion of placental lactogen starts at low levels and increases progressively. Functioning late in pregnancy, placental lactogen stimulates growth of the mammary gland. It also inhibits insulin's action on adipose and muscle tissue. Normally insulin induces these tissues to take up amino acids, glucose, and fat, but lactogen keeps these fuels in circulation to feed the fetus and mammary gland.

Blood flow to the placenta increases dramatically during pregnancy, accounting for as much as 25 percent of the cardiac output by term.[3] The rates of maternal and fetal blood flow in turn influence the exchange of substances across the placenta. For example, the exchange of oxygen by passive diffusion improves as the flow of maternal blood increases.[4] Water, carbon dioxide, and electrolytes also cross the placenta by passive diffusion, while nutrients such as calcium, phosphorus, and magnesium cross it via active transport. Fetal accumulation of these nutrients increases throughout pregnancy, becoming greatest during the third trimester.

Glucose is the main energy source for the fetus and, as mentioned, is actively transferred from mother to fetus. The placenta also stores glycogen, reflecting the vital importance of preventing an interruption to the glucose supply. Placental glycogen stores increase early in pregnancy, but decline during later pregnancy as they give up their glucose to the rapidly growing fetus. By the third trimester, the fetus is producing its own insulin. This insulin promotes glycogen as well as protein and fat storage in the fetus for use after delivery.[5]

As mentioned, maternal nutrition is critical for placental growth. Malnutrition limits placental development and results in reduced placental blood flow. This, in turn, curtails the transfer of energy and essential nutrients to the fetus. Thus, maternal malnutrition may negatively affect the fetus in two ways—by impairing placental development and by making fewer nutrients available for transfer across the placenta.

Fetal Development

When development is proceeding, intracellular activity becomes intense. Cell division requires that every organelle of the cell be duplicated—the mitochondria, the ribosomes, the vast and intricate network of intracellular membranes, the cell membrane, the nuclear membrane, the chromosomes with their extensive DNA blueprints for enzymes, and multitudes of other intracellular bodies. To make all these new organelles requires synthesis and assembly of a multitude of different materials—DNA, RNA, protein, lipid, and more. These syntheses are carried out by enzymes that themselves have been synthesized according to instructions from the genes—a process that requires enzymes to transcribe the relevant portions of DNA to make messenger RNA for delivery to the ribosomes, transfer RNAs to line up along the messengers with their cargo of amino acids, enzymes to link those amino acids together into new proteins, and enzymes and membrane proteins to make or bring in new amino acids to make more proteins. In short, the molecular events taking place in a cell about to divide are astronomical in number. A time when so many chemical steps are proceeding is a time when many mistakes can be made, and because each cell in an early stage of development is destined to become many cells later, each mistake may ultimately have greatly amplified effects. No

cardiac output: the amount of blood discharged from the left or right ventricle of the heart per minute.

passive diffusion: the tendency of gas, liquids, or solids to move from a region of high concentration to one of lower concentration.

active transport: the energy-requiring process of concentrating a substance inside or outside a membrane by pumping it across.

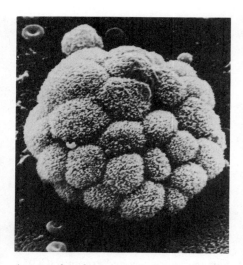

A zygote, less than one week after fertilization, is ready for implantation.

Figure 2–2 The Concept of Critical Periods

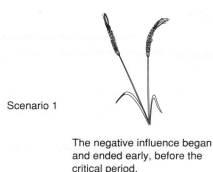

Scenario 1

The negative influence began and ended early, before the critical period.

Result: normal development

Scenario 2

The negative influence occurred during the critical period.

Result: abnormal development

Scenario 3

The negative influence began and ended late, after the critical period.

Result: normal development

wonder that times of intense developmental activity are critical periods, especially vulnerable to adverse physical and chemical influences. Figure 2-2 illustrates the concept of critical periods.

That the embryo accomplishes these developmental feats is truly amazing. The number of cells in the embryo at first doubles approximately every 24 hours. This rate slows gradually, and during the final ten weeks of pregnancy only one doubling occurs. From the ectoderm, the nervous system and skin begin to develop; from the mesoderm, the muscles and internal organ systems; and from the endoderm, the glands and linings of the digestive, respiratory, and excretory systems. At eight weeks, the 3-centimeter-long embryo has a complete central nervous system, a beating heart, a fully formed digestive system, and the beginnings of facial features. Already, an embryonic tail has formed and almost completely disappeared again, and the fingers and toes are well defined.

Each organ and tissue has its own periods of intensive developmental events, needs nourishment most during those times, and is most vulnerable to nutrient deprivation at those times. These periods of development are critical periods. In the fetus, for example, the heart and brain are well developed at 16 weeks, even though the lungs are still undeveloped 10 weeks later. Therefore, early malnutrition affects the heart and brain, later malnutrition affects the lungs.

The phase of brain growth most susceptible to malnutrition seems to be the brain's growth spurt, the period in which brain weight increases most rapidly.[6] In human beings, the brain's growth spurt begins in midpregnancy and continues into the second year of life.[7] The time of the growth spurt is a critical period in brain development, and undernutrition at this time may do irreversible damage.

The division and growth of cells of each developing organ follow a schedule unique to that organ. The development of all organs occurs by the processes of cell division, during which cells are increasing dramatically in *number* (hyperplasia), and by cell growth, when cell *size* increases (hypertrophy). These two processes may occur simultaneously, may overlap, or may occur in tandem.

critical period: a finite period during development in which certain events may occur that will have irreversible, determining effects on later developmental stages. A critical period is usually a period of cell division in a body organ.

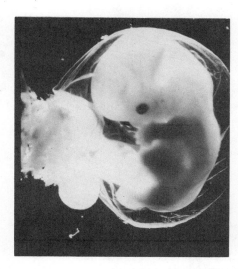

An embryo 5 to 6 weeks after fertilization; after implantation, the placenta develops and begins to provide nourishment to the developing embryo.

hyperplasia: (high-per-PLAY-zee-ah): an increase in cell number.

hypertrophy: (high-PER-tro-fee): an increase in cell size.

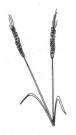

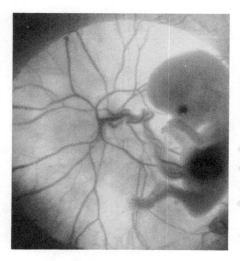

A fetus after 11 weeks of development; notice the umbilical cord and blood vessels connecting the fetus with the placenta.

Focal Point 3 discusses the effects of prenatal nutrition on fetal tooth development.

Focal Point 2 discusses the effects of alcohol consumption during pregnancy on fetal development.

Appendix A discusses nutrition assessment during pregnancy.

amniotic (am-nee-OTT-ic) **sac:** the "bag of waters" in the uterus, in which the fetus floats.

The periods during which increases in size are taking place are the times of most obvious growth. Actually, however, critical periods of cell division and differentiation may already be over. At such times, whatever nutrients and other environmental conditions are needed must be supplied if the organ is to reach its full potential. If cell division and the final cell number achieved are limited during a critical period, recovery is impossible. Early malnutrition can have irreversible effects, although they may not become fully apparent until the person reaches maturity. Here are some of the effects:

► Shortened height of people who were undernourished in their early years.[8]

► Low birthweight of infants born to mothers malnourished in early childhood.[9]

► Delayed sexual development of those undernourished during early adolescence.[10]

► Poor dental health of children whose mothers were malnourished during pregnancy.[11]

► Reduced placental cell number when malnutrition occurs around the time of conception.[12]

► Brain damage by way of central nervous system glucose deprivation caused by maternal fasting during pregnancy. Ironically, the brain damage caused by maternal fasting during pregnancy, by damaging the brain's regulatory centers, can cause later obesity in the son or daughter.[13]

► Suboptimal immune system development and lowered resistance to disease throughout life.

► Mental retardation in infants born to mothers who were iodine deficient during pregnancy.

► Diminished learning ability and attentiveness of children, even those with normal IQs, when malnutrition has occurred during pregnancy.[14]

► Irreversible physical and mental retardation of children born to mothers who drank alcohol during pregnancy (fetal alcohol syndrome).

The irreversibility of these effects is obvious when abundant, nourishing food fed after the critical time fails to remedy the growth deficit. Many growth-retarded Korean orphans adopted by U.S. families after the Korean War, for example, experienced several years of catch-up growth, but did not completely make up for the effects of early malnutrition.[15]

Recent research points strongly to the probability that malnutrition in the prenatal and early postnatal periods also affects learning ability and behavior. Much of the severe mental retardation seen in developed countries such as the United States is of unknown cause (other than profound retardation with known causes such as inherited abnormalities), but many cases are thought to be due to protein deficiency during pregnancy. Clearly, then, it is most critical to provide the best nutrition at early stages of life. The next section discusses the consequences of failing to do so.

The last seven months of pregnancy, the fetal period, bring about a tremendous increase in the size of the fetus (see Figure 2–3). Intensive periods of cell division occur in organ after organ. The amniotic sac fills with fluid to cushion the infant, as illustrated in Figure 2–4. The mother's uterus and its supporting muscles increase greatly in size; her breasts change and grow in

Figure 2–3   Stages of Embryonic and Fetal Development

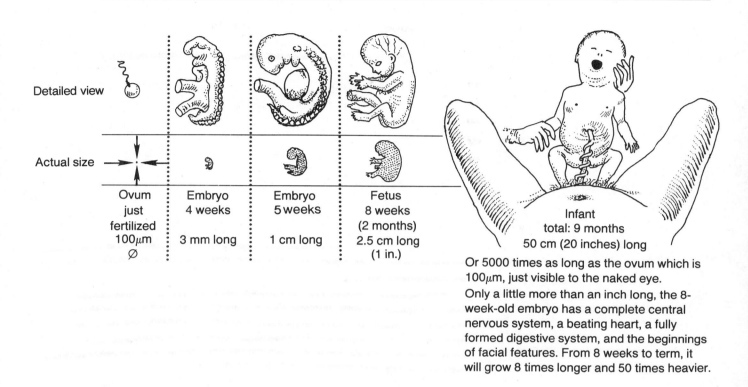

Detailed view				
Actual size →				
Ovum just fertilized 100μm ∅	Embryo 4 weeks 3 mm long	Embryo 5 weeks 1 cm long	Fetus 8 weeks (2 months) 2.5 cm long (1 in.)	Infant total: 9 months 50 cm (20 inches) long

Or 5000 times as long as the ovum which is 100μm, just visible to the naked eye.

Only a little more than an inch long, the 8-week-old embryo has a complete central nervous system, a beating heart, a fully formed digestive system, and the beginnings of facial features. From 8 weeks to term, it will grow 8 times longer and 50 times heavier.

preparation for lactation, and her blood volume increases by half to accommodate the added load of materials to be carried. The normal gain in weight of mother and child during pregnancy amounts to about 25 to 30 pounds. The gestation period, which lasts approximately 40 weeks, ends with the birth of the infant.

gestation: period of intrauterine fetal development from conception to birth.

Malnutrition during Pregnancy

Studies of nutritionally deprived animals report several significant observations. Malnourished animals bear fewer offspring per litter, the offspring are smaller, and both mother and young experience increased mortality.[16] The offspring also suffer long-term, irreversible effects, such as compromised learning ability. Such effects of malnutrition occur in people as well as animals, as mentioned, although caution is necessary in applying the results of animal studies to human beings. Animals differ from people in size, growth rates, and length of gestation; factors like these must be carefully considered in designing and interpreting animal research to examine the effects of malnutrition during pregnancy.

Occasionally, chance has designed conditions in the human environment that have provided information directly on human beings and have suggested

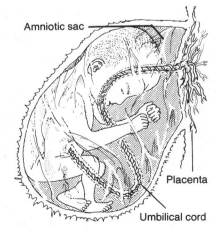

Figure 2–4   The Amniotic Sac
The amniotic sac is filled with fluid to cushion the infant.

directions for future studies using animals. Observations on live infants and autopsies of infants who have died in both affluent and poor societies have provided some evidence consistent with the theory that effects of nutrition deprivation in human beings are similar to some of those seen in animals. The following discussion attempts to sort out studies of outcome from studies of later effects. An impaired outcome may be any of the following:

► Fetal growth retardation.
► Congenital malformations, birth defects.
► Spontaneous abortion.
► Premature birth.
► Stillbirth.
► Low birthweight.
► Reduced cell number.

Of these, infant birthweight is most frequently used as a predictor of future survival and health. Malnutrition, coupled with low birthweight, is the underlying or associated cause of more than half of all the deaths of children under five years of age.[17]

low birthweight (LBW): a birthweight of 5 1/2 pounds (2500 grams) or less; used as a predictor of poor health in the newborn and as a probable indicator of poor nutrition status of the mother during and/or before pregnancy.

A low-birthweight infant who is malnourished is also likely to be unable to do its job of obtaining nourishment by sucking and to win its mother's attention by energetic, vigorous cries and other healthy behavior. It can therefore become an apathetic, neglected infant; this compounds the original malnutrition problem. Thus, for many reasons, infants of normal weight are usually more healthy than underweight infants.

About 1 in every 15 infants born in the United States is a low-birthweight infant, and about one-fourth of these infants die within the first month of life.[18] Worldwide, it is estimated that one-sixth of all live infants are of low birthweight; more than nine out of ten of these are born in the developing countries. Most of them are not preterm but are full-term infants who are small because of malnutrition.

Observations on Human Beings

Chapter 1 showed that malnutrition prior to pregnancy, as exemplified by the siege of Holland during World War II, reduced fertility and, for women who did get pregnant, increased the rate of stillbirths, neonatal deaths, and congenital malformations. Malnutrition during pregnancy has similar effects. An extreme condition that provided data on malnutrition during human pregnancy occurred during the German siege of Leningrad, which took place from 1941 to 1943.[19] Food during this time was inferior in quality and limited in quantity, at times severely limited. The infant mortality rate was unusually high. The more severe the food shortage, the greater the incidence of poor pregnancy outcomes. A substantial increase in the number of low-birthweight infants, premature births, and stillbirths occurred.

In less extreme conditions of human malnutrition, it is more difficult to observe dietary effects on prenatal development. Problems in determining dietary intake accurately and in controlling all other variables that affect development complicate the design of studies to examine the effects of diet on the outcome of pregnancy. Despite the obstacles, some relevant and interesting findings emerge.

A study conducted in the early 1940s found a correlation between the quality of the maternal diet and the condition of the infant at birth.[20] Of the mothers whose diets were classified as excellent or good, based on the RDA, 94 percent gave birth to infants whose condition was described as superior or good by pediatricians with no knowledge of the mothers' dietary intakes. In contrast, only 8 percent of women whose diets were classified as poor gave birth to infants in good or superior condition, a highly significant difference.

A more recent study examined the relationship between a single outcome variable—infant birthweight—and different environmental factors, one of which was diet quality. Diet quality was expressed as a nutrient adequacy ratio (NAR) index. This was determined by converting recorded intakes of 11 nutrients to percentages of the RDA. The percentages were then averaged to obtain the NAR index for each woman in the study. The investigators found a significant, positive correlation between the NAR index of the maternal diet and the birthweight of the infant. This study provides further evidence that poor nutrition during pregnancy impairs the outcome.[21]

More specific effects can result from individual nutrient deficiencies. The occurrence and severity of these conditions depend on many different variables, but with respect to some nutrients, the effects can be profound.

Individual Nutrient Deficiencies

The specific effects of malnutrition on pregnancy vary greatly, depending on the timing and duration of the insult, the nutrient or nutrients in question, the severity of the deficiency or excess, and the health of the mother. Single nutrient deficiencies rarely occur in human beings; if one nutrient is lacking, chances are great that one or more other nutrients are lacking as well. Nutrient deficiencies in human beings do not often occur in so orderly a manner as to be compatible with an experimental design. Thus, with regard to individual nutrients, a limited number of human studies is available. Important animal research helps to fill the gap and provides direction for studies of human beings.

Protein Studies on animals show that protein restriction during critical periods of organ development results in a reduced number of cells in the offspring at term.[22] Even after later nutrient supplementation, the liver, heart, kidney, and brain do not acquire normal numbers of cells. The effect of prenatal protein deficiency in reducing cell number in these organs is therefore irreversible.[23]

Protein deprivation in human beings during pregnancy can severely impair later development. This has been observed most frequently in the developing countries, but it is also seen in the wealthy nations when people adopt bizarre diets. In one family, for example, the mother's consuming an unbalanced

A discussion of the effects of early post-natal malnutrition in human beings appears in Chapter 4.

vegetarian diet caused her children's height and head circumference to be markedly and irreversibly diminished.[24]

Folacin   Folacin deficiency is common in pregnant women, the incidence being as high as 50 percent in some countries.[25] The poorer the folacin status at the beginning of pregnancy, the earlier deficiency symptoms appear and the more severe they become as pregnancy progresses. Folacin deficiency in early pregnancy may interfere with normal placental development.[26] A severe lack of folacin can lead to megaloblastic anemia, which, in turn, may cause miscarriage.[27] It is possible, but not yet confirmed, that miscarriage predisposes a woman to future neural tube defect births. In one study of two groups of pregnant women with histories of neural tube defect births, one group received a multivitamin supplement containing folacin, while the other group received no supplement. The incidence of neural tube defect births was five times greater in the unsupplemented women than in the supplemented women.[28] Based on results of previous studies, the researchers attributed the difference to the folacin in the multivitamin supplement.[29] A link between folacin deficiency and fetal growth retardation in human beings has also been demonstrated.[30]

Iron   Iron deficiency during critical periods of brain development in animals results in a deficit of brain iron in offspring—not the iron in the red blood cells passing through the brain, but the iron in the brain cells that facilitates cellular respiration and makes metabolism possible. This deficit persists despite adequate iron intake later.[31]

In human beings, fetal deaths, prematurity, and low birthweight correlate with low maternal hemoglobin or hematocrit concentrations.[32] These findings are disputed, however by other research.[33] For example, no significant difference in infant mortality and birthweight was found between iron-deficient women and women from the general obstetric population at a large hospital. This suggests that iron transfer across the placenta to the developing fetus is independent of maternal iron status. Furthermore, an interesting and important factor in establishing iron stores in the newborn infant relates to the attending health care professional's technique of clamping the umbilical cord.[34] When the infant is level with or below the vaginal opening for a few minutes immediately after birth, greater placental blood flow to the infant permits greater iron transfer—up to 40 milligrams of iron, or about one-sixth of the total iron content of a newborn infant.

Zinc   Biochemical changes follow rapidly on the induction of zinc deficiency. In the cases of other nutrients, a pregnant female may be able to mobilize her own stores to protect the fetus, but such is not the case with zinc. Studies on rats suggest that the mother may be unable to deliver zinc from her stores to the fetus.[35] Thus, a constant source of zinc is necessary in order to protect the fetus from the effects of deficiency. In rats, even short-term zinc deficiency during pregnancy produces a wide variety of congenital malformations.[36]

Zinc deficiency may be teratogenic for human beings as well as for animals. In one study, an association between congenital malformations in

megaloblastic anemia: the type of anemia seen in folacin or vitamin B_{12} deficiency characterized by enlarged, slightly irregular red blood cells.

neural tube defect: definition on page 36.

human beings and low maternal serum zinc concentrations has been found.[37] Another study examined the relationship between plasma zinc concentrations of adolescent women and pregnancy outcome.[38] Mothers with plasma zinc concentrations below the sample mean gave birth to infants with undescended testes and other congenital defects.

For purposes of comparisons made in this discussion, we are assuming that serum zinc concentrations and plasma zinc concentrations are comparable measures of zinc status. An important qualification to this, however, is that, as of yet, no single reliable method for assessing zinc status has appeared.[39] Interpretation of studies in which only one measure of zinc status is used must therefore proceed with caution.

Studies that examine the influence of individual nutrient deficiencies on the outcome of pregnancy serve to emphasize the varied and profound effects such deficiencies can have on fetal growth and development. Malnutrition includes overnutrition as well as undernutrition, and nutrient excesses during pregnancy may also have adverse effects. In human beings, excessive maternal energy intake corresponds to fatness of the infant.[40] Abundant animal research has examined the effects of specific nutrient excesses during pregnancy. Depending on the amount and gestational stage of administration, excess vitamin A given to pregnant animals produces many types of birth defects.[41] Recently, birth defects have been reported in human infants born to mothers treated for acne with high-dose vitamin A derivatives.[42] In human beings and animals, large doses of vitamin C during pregnancy may condition the infant such that the risk of scurvy increases at birth when the vitamin C doses cease.[43] Evidence for the conditioning effect in human beings has been questioned, however.[44]

It is apparent from these studies that critical times occur in development when deficiencies or excesses of particular nutrients may cause irreversible damage to the fetus, even with optimal nutrition at a later time. In some instances, the nutrient deficiency or excess must be severe before its effects appear. In other instances, the effects appear with only a moderate imbalance. More information is needed before all the questions are answered, but one thing is clear: optimal nutrition during pregnancy enhances the likelihood of a healthy outcome. Table 2–1 summarizes nutrient deficiency effects during pregnancy, and Table 2–4 (presented in a later section) shows the consequences of nutrient excesses.

"conditioned" scurvy: the vitamin C deficiency disease seen in newborn infants of mothers who ingested large doses of vitamin C during pregnancy; possibly induces an increased rate of vitamin C catabolism, which persists after birth.

Intervention Studies on Human Beings

The intervention studies discussed here test the effects of nutrient supplements on the progress and outcome of pregnancy. Viewed in one way, these studies might seem to be studies of nutrient adequacy, but from another point of view they are studies of *malnutrition*, for the contrasts that appear in them reveal the effects of nutrient inadequacies on pregnancy. Intervention studies do not always meet the criteria of truly rigorous experimental designs, but they do enable nutrition scientists to observe how nutrition intervention affects the health and well-being of free-living individuals. Intervention studies on pregnant women have been conducted worldwide. In the following discussion,

Table 2–1   Nutrient Deficiencies during Pregnancy

Nutrient	Deficiency Effect
Energy	Low infant birthweight[a]
Protein	Reduced infant head circumference[b]
Folacin	Miscarriage and neural tube defect[c]
Vitamin D	Low infant birthweight[d]
Calcium	Decreased infant bone density[e]
Iron	Low infant birthweight and premature birth[f]
Iodine	Cretinism (varying degrees of mental and physical retardation in infant)[g]
Zinc	Congenital malformations[h]

[a] Z. Stein and coauthors, *Famine and Human Development: The Dutch Hunger Winter of 1944/45* (New York: Oxford University Press, 1975).
[b] D. Erhard, The new vegetarians, part 1: Vegetarianism and its consequences, *Nutrition Today*, November/December 1973, pp. 4–12.
[c] R. W. Smithells and coauthors, Further experience of vitamin supplementation for prevention of neural tube defect recurrences, *Lancet* 1 (1983): 1027–1031.
[d] J. D. Maxwell and coauthors, Vitamin D supplements enhance weight gain and nutritional status in pregnant Asians, *British Journal of Obstetrics and Gynaecology* 88 (1981): 987–991.
[e] K. A. V. R. Krishnamachari and L. Iyengar, Effect of maternal malnutrition on the bone density of the neonate, *American Journal of Clinical Nutrition* 28 (1975): 482–486.
[f] S. M. Garn, M. T. Keating, and F. Falkner, Hematological status and pregnancy outcomes, *American Journal of Clinical Nutrition* 34 (1981): 115–117.
[g] P. O. D. Pharaoh, I. H. Buttfield, and B. S. Hetzel, Neurological damage to the fetus resulting from severe iodine deficiency during pregnancy, *Lancet* 1 (1971): 308–310, as cited in L. S. Hurley, Trace elements 1: Iron, copper, iodine, in *Developmental Nutrition* (Englewood Cliffs, N. J.: Prentice-Hall, 1980), pp. 183–198.
[h] S. Jameson, Effects of zinc deficiency in human reproduction, *Acta Medica Scandinavia Supplement* 593 (1976): 3–89.

pregnant women presumed to be moderately but not overtly malnourished, based on previous pregnancy outcomes and socioeconomic status, were given daily protein-energy supplements in the form of beverages or nutrient-dense foods. In the first investigation, the overall condition of the infant at birth was the outcome considered. In all the other studies, infant birthweight was the main outcome considered.

The reason why so many studies of prenatal nutrition have been undertaken is that the alarming number of low-birthweight infants worldwide demands attention. In the United States alone, the number of low-birthweight infants born in 1985 was over one-quarter of a million, or about 7 percent of total live births.[45] Worldwide, the percentage is greater.[46] In various ways, studies of prenatal nutrition test the hypothesis that prenatal dietary supplementation of moderately malnourished women can reduce the incidence of low birthweight.

Much of the research on this subject was conducted at a time when protein was considered to be *the* nutrient lacking in the diets of poor women. For this reason, protein was the nutrient most often supplemented.

As you will see, the results of these studies bring us slightly closer to unraveling the threads of uncertainty surrounding prenatal nutrition (for example, which food supplements at what point during gestation best promote fetal growth), but they also present us with new threads we have yet to untie. The results are interesting, occasionally conflicting, and often surprising.

Short-term studies   One study, conducted almost 50 years ago, showed quite clearly the impact of prenatal nutrition on pregnancy.[47] The researchers studied the prenatal diets of 400 women. They classified the women into three groups according to diet adequacy, based on specific amounts of milk, cheese, eggs, meat, vegetables, fruits, cereals, and breads eaten daily. The groups were as follows:

▶ *Poor diet:* Women consumed less than 60 grams of protein per day.

▶ *Supplemented diet:* Women with a poor diet until the fourth or fifth month were provided with additional food daily.

▶ *Good diet:* Women consumed between 60 and 80 grams of protein per day.

The women in the supplemented- and good-diet groups experienced better health throughout their pregnancies and had fewer complications. The incidence of miscarriages, stillbirths, and premature births was lower than in the poor-diet group.

In another study, a high rate of low-birthweight infants born to poor, black women was observed in New York. Because of this, researchers presumed the women to be poorly nourished and undertook a nutrient supplementation trial.[48] Based on specific criteria that identified women who were especially at risk of delivering low-birthweight infants, researchers randomly divided the women into three different treatment groups of 250 women each. They gave them:

▶ A regular prenatal vitamin-mineral supplement plus a beverage rich in protein (40 grams protein daily plus 470 kcalories)—the supplement group.

▶ A regular prenatal vitamin-mineral supplement plus a beverage with much less protein and fewer kcalories (6 grams protein and 322 kcalories)—the complement group.

▶ A regular prenatal vitamin-mineral supplement—the control group.

Contrary to the investigators' expectations, no significant differences in birthweight were seen among the three treatment groups. In fact, the supplement group bore infants with a mean birthweight *lower* than that of those born to the control group. Even more surprising was the observation that the supplement group had more premature births and, among these births, a high rate of neonatal deaths compared to the other groups. Women with a history of previous premature delivery seemed particularly susceptible to this unexpected outcome. Thus, for some women, the supplement actually seemed to have adverse effects.

The investigators used several indexes of dietary intake to assess compliance of the women in drinking the beverage. Despite this, the study is vulnerable to criticism in that some uncertainty clouded this aspect of the design.

These investigators anticipated from the start that total compliance among free-living women might be an unrealistic expectation, as well as a weak point in the study. Throughout the study, the investigators used indicators such as 24-hour dietary recalls and urine tests for a riboflavin marker in the beverages

Study 2 (cont)
no diff in smokers in supplem group

Study 3
diff esp in males

Study 4
↑ kcal, not protein that ↑ birth weight

to determine if the women substituted the beverages for food or drank them at all. They concluded that overall compliance was satisfactory.

In view of the satisfactory compliance of the women, the investigators speculate that the lower birthweights of infants born to mothers in the supplement group were due to an adverse effect of the supplement, rather than to reduced food intake. A possible explanation of the adverse effect of the supplement may be that it contained a toxic contaminant such as lead, or too much protein.

For women who were heavy smokers in the supplement group, the effect of supplements was favorable. Infants of the smoking women did not differ in birthweight from infants of comparable nonsmoking women. Women in the control group who smoked had infants with reduced birthweights. The investigators concluded that for populations of women in the United States at high risk of giving birth to low-birthweight infants, supplementation of the regular maternal diet had little effect on birthweight except in heavy smokers.

In Bogotá, Colombia, a prenatal intervention study focused on pregnant women living in a poor environment whose diets were considered deficient in protein and food energy. The women were given dietary supplements of regular foods beginning in the sixth month of pregnancy.[49] Birthweights of infants of the supplemented women were higher than birthweights of controls, and the proportion of low-birthweight infants was reduced significantly. The mean increment to the women's diet (based on two 24-hour recalls) was 136 kcalories and 20 grams of protein daily. A greater difference in infant weight was observed for thin women than for heavier women when compared to controls. In addition, the gain in birthweight for the supplemented families was seen only in male births. Unlike the New York study, this study uncovered no adverse effects of supplements. Thus, this study supports the view that additional food given to malnourished women in the third trimester of pregnancy can raise birthweight.

In Guatemala, a study was designed to examine the effects of protein supplements versus nonprotein supplements on infant birthweight across villages.[50] Comparison of the protein- and nonprotein-supplemented villages did not reveal the expected results—that protein would be more effective than food energy. The investigators then abandoned the original design in favor of comparing food energy intakes among women, regardless of the protein content of the supplements or the village in which the women lived. Ingestion by mothers of about 70 extra kcalories per day throughout pregnancy resulted in a gain of about 56 grams (2 ounces) in their infants' birthweights. This study lends support to the concept that in situations of chronic malnutrition, birthweight can be raised by sufficient food energy supplementation throughout pregnancy. In this study, it was food energy, not protein, that made the difference.

A study in Montreal, Canada, was conducted in the prenatal clinic of a large hospital serving low-income women.[51] Some of the women were referred to the Montreal Diet Dispensary, where they received dietary advice and food supplements. Mothers who were not referred to the diet dispensary served as controls. The diets of the women were presumed to be inadequate, but the women were not overtly malnourished. In this respect, the study was similar to the New York study.

The mean birthweight of the infants born to the women receiving food supplements was 40 grams (1.4 ounces) greater than that of controls. For women receiving food supplements, the frequency of low birthweight was 5.7 percent, compared with 6.8 percent in the controls. This difference was statistically significant. As in the Bogotá study, supplementation made a bigger difference in the birthweights of infants born to thin women (who had weighed less than 140 pounds when they conceived) than in the birthweights of infants born to heavier women. As in the New York study, women who had had previous low-birthweight infants gave birth to infants with lower weights than control women, but this difference was not statistically significant. The investigators concluded that prenatal supplementation of underweight and presumably underfed women can result in a modest rise in infant birthweight. At the same time, they offered the warning that for some women, nutrition supplementation can have adverse effects.

Nutrition supplementation in the Montreal study was by way of foods rather than beverage supplements. This reduces the likelihood that toxic contamination of the beverage supplement used in the New York study was responsible for the adverse effect.

A possible explanation for the lower birthweights of infants born to some of the supplemented women may be related to the timing of the intervention, which did not occur until the third trimester. Different results might have been seen with earlier intervention. In fact, in a San Francisco study, intervention was much earlier and the results dissimilar to those of the previous study.[52] Women at risk for delivering low-birthweight infants were randomly assigned to one of three dietary regimens:

- Normal diet plus a high-protein (80 grams) beverage supplement.
- Normal diet plus a low-protein (6 grams) beverage supplement.
- Normal diet plus a vitamin-mineral preparation.

The diets of all the women were generally adequate with respect to all nutrients. The diets of the women in the high-protein group were higher in protein and food energy (100 percent of the RDA) than the diets of the women in the other two groups (80 to 90 percent of the RDA). Despite these differences, mean infant birthweights were similar for all three groups, but the incidence of low-birthweight infants was half the expected rate of 6 percent.

A recent study of African women reported a significant beneficial effect of prenatal food supplementation in women who would otherwise have been in negative energy balance.[53] An energy-dense food supplement in the form of biscuits, together with vitamin-fortified tea, was consumed by about 200 women as soon as pregnancy was confirmed. Mean duration of supplementation was 24 weeks. Birthweights of infants of the supplemented women were compared with birthweights of infants born during the four years preceding intervention. Supplementation was highly effective during the wet season when food shortages and agricultural work caused negative energy balance, but was ineffective during the dry season when women were in positive energy balance. The percentage of low-birthweight infants declined significantly, from 23.7 percent to 7.5 percent, during the wet season.

Another study evaluated the effectiveness of the Women, Infants, and Children (WIC) Supplemental Feeding Program on pregnancy outcome as measured by infant birthweight.[54] Several hundred women were enrolled in this study midway through pregnancy. Women in the experimental group received vouchers for the purchase of protein-rich foods such as milk, eggs, and cheese, while women in the control group did not. The mean infant birth-weight of the supplemented women was significantly greater than that of controls. However, when entry weights of the women were controlled for, the significance of the difference disappeared, except for WIC-supplemented women who smoked.

Another WIC evaluation study of high-risk, pregnant women found the incidence of low-birthweight infants of WIC participants to be 6 percent.[55] In a group of high-risk, pregnant women who qualified for WIC but did not enter the program, the incidence of low-birthweight infants was greater than 10 percent. In addition, the greater the number of WIC food vouchers received each month, the greater the mean birthweights of the infants.

When we attempt to integrate the threads of information derived from these studies into the fabric of prenatal nutrition and fetal growth, the picture is not complete, but it is clearer, and to some researchers it looks like this.[56] Among women at risk of delivering low-birthweight infants, prenatal dietary supplementation can, in some instances, produce a slight rise (40 to 60 grams) in birthweights of infants. The degree of this rise seems to depend on the prior nutrition state of the woman. A greater rise in birthweight is seen among thin or undernourished women, compared to heavier women. It also appears that prenatal dietary supplements can offset the fetal growth retardation caused by smoking. A protein-supplemented diet may be harmful to some women, particularly those with a previous history of bearing low-birthweight infants. In addition, protein seems no more effective than nutrient-dense food in general in raising birthweight.

The studies just discussed were of short duration. All of them examined the effect of prenatal nutrition intervention on the outcome of one pregnancy, using infant birthweight as the indicator. In all cases, supplementation was initiated at some point after pregnancy was confirmed, in some cases as late as mid-pregnancy. Most of the women studied had been at least moderately malnourished for years previously. All but one of the studies confirmed that nutrient supplementation positively affected outcomes. Infants of supplemented women weighed 1 to 3 ounces more than infants of unsupplemented women and/or the incidence of low birthweights declined.

Longer-duration studies   Other researchers have tried a longer-term period of prenatal nutrition intervention and the results are more impressive.[57] Almost 200 women were involved in the Guatamalan Nutritional Supplementation study for two consecutive pregnancies and the intervening lactation period. Women received either high-kcalorie (500 kcalories or more per week) or low-kcalorie (less than 500 kcalories per week) supplements containing vitamins and minerals. Infants of women who received the high-kcalorie supplements during two consecutive pregnancies and the intervening lactation period weighed up to 10 ounces (301 grams) more than infants of women in the low-kcalorie supplement group. Infants of women who received high-kcalorie supplements while breastfeeding the first child and during the next pregnancy weighed up to 5 ounces (150 grams) more than women in the low-kcalorie supplement group. These differences are two to three times greater than those observed in previous studies. The authors speculate that it is unrealistic to expect that malnutrition that develops over long periods of time can be overcome by nutrient supplementation sustained for only a few months during pregnancy. Earlier and longer intervention periods produce greater results.

As anticipated, the results of these studies leave many more threads of doubt to untangle. When does protein supplementation have a role in prenatal diet intervention? Why is prenatal protein supplementation harmful to some women? What does this mean in terms of prenatal dietary intervention for these women? What effects will specific supplementation of a deficient nutrient have on fetal growth? These and many other questions remain to be answered. In the meantime, let us explore more knowledge.

Nutrient Needs, Diet, and Supplements in Pregnancy

A woman's nutrient needs during pregnancy are higher than at any other time in her adult life and are greater for certain nutrients than for others, as shown in Figure 2–5. A study of the figure reveals some of the key needs, and the following sections discuss them.

Food Energy and Associated B Vitamins

A recommended average food energy intake for a pregnant woman is 40 kcalories per kilogram of body weight, and energy intake should never fall below 36 kcalories per kilogram.[58] This is true for all women, even those who are overweight.

This recommendation makes the difference in food energy need one of the smallest differences in need between the nonpregnant and pregnant woman. Figure 2-5 confirms this. A daily increase of 300 kcalories (during the second and third trimesters) above the allowance for nonpregnant women is all that is recommended. This food energy is vital, however, to spare the protein needed for growth. For women of average size and moderate physical activity, 300 kcalories represents a 15 percent increase above nonpregnant food energy needs. Pregnant teenagers, underweight women, or physically active women may require more. Some research suggests that a balanced distribution of food energy from carbohydrate, fat, and protein is more important for obese pregnant women than increasing energy intake above prepregnancy intakes.[59]

The source of additional energy should be high-quality, nutrient-dense foods that will provide nutrients as well. Table 2–2 shows a suggested food pattern. For most women, appropriate food choices include nonfat milk, cottage cheese, lean meats, eggs, liver, dark-green vegetables, and whole-grain breads and cereals. For the pregnant vegan, appropriate food choices include calcium-fortified soy milk, tofu, legumes, whole-grain breads and cereals, vegetables (especially dark-green, leafy vegetables), and fruits.

Pregnant women do not always eat such nutritious foods. If a woman's diet is already meeting normal nutrient needs at the start of pregnancy, then she can easily adjust it to meet the increased demands, but if the woman has not

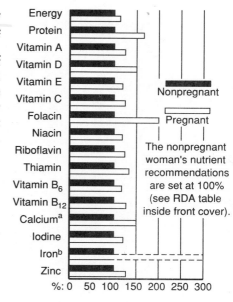

The nonpregnant woman's nutrient recommendations are set at 100% (see RDA table inside front cover).

[a]Recommended intakes of phosphorous and magnesium change similarly.

[b]The pregnant woman may need to take an iron supplement—the pregnant woman needs the RDA of 18 mg of iron, as shown here, only if her iron nutrition has been optimal prior to pregnancy—a rare case. Usually her iron needs cannot be met by ordinary diets, and she requires a supplement.

Figure 2–5 Comparison of Nutrient Needs of Nonpregnant and Pregnant Women (over 23 Years Old)
The teenage pregnant woman needs even more nutrients than shown here, as Chapter 6 discusses.

Recommended energy intake: 40 kcal/kg (18 kcal/lb). Minimum energy intake: 36 kcal/kg (17 kcal/lb).

For a 120-lb woman, this represents at least 2000 kcal and preferably 2200 kcal/day.

Table 2–2   Daily Food Guide for Pregnant Women

Food	Number of Servings	
	Nonpregnant Woman	Pregnant Woman
Protein foods		
Animal (2-oz serving)	2	2
Vegetable (at least 1 serving of legumes)	2	2
Milk and milk products	2	4
Enriched or whole-grain breads and cereals	4	4
Vitamin C-rich fruits and vegetables	1	1
Dark-green vegetables	1	1
Other fruits and vegetables	1	1

Source: California Department of Health, as cited in Nutrition and the pregnant obese woman, *Nutrition and the MD,* January 1978.

been eating well, this is definitely the time to begin. High motivation and intensive counseling and practice will help get the pregnancy on the right track (see Practical Point: Diets Tailored to Individuals). Should a pregnant woman's nutrition be poor or should she be at risk for poor nutrition status, help is available to her (see Practical Point: Maternal and Infant Assistance Programs).

Added B vitamins are needed in proportion to the added food energy intake, and normally are obtained from the same foods. Women's needs for thiamin increase early in pregnancy and then remain constant throughout; the RDA committee recommends an added 0.4 milligrams a day above the nonpregnant woman's RDA.[60] The committee also recommends 0.3 milligrams a day of riboflavin and 2 niacin equivalents above the nonpregnant woman's RDA, based on limited evidence of increased needs.[61]

Protein and Vitamin B₆

The pregnant woman's increased need for protein is more dramatic than for food energy. In addition to the 0.8 grams of protein per kilogram appropriate body weight recommended for adults, 30 more grams of protein per day are recommended during pregnancy. For example, the recommended protein intake for a woman whose appropriate weight is 120 pounds is about 45 grams; an additional 30 grams brings the total daily protein recommendation to about 75 grams—a large amount, but many women in the United States easily exceed this recommended protein intake every day, even when not pregnant. The Nationwide Food Consumption Survey of 1977 found that women between the ages of 19 and 65 had an average protein intake of 64 to 67 grams per day.[62] A more recent survey revealed that the diets of U.S. adults exceed the RDA for protein.[63] Thus, if a woman is already exceeding her RDA for protein, she may not need to add to her diet the full 30 grams of protein recommended for pregnancy. In fact, as mentioned earlier, excessive protein may affect some pregnancies adversely. The pregnant woman needs generous amounts of carbohydrate to spare the protein she eats.

Recommended protein intake: 75 g/day.

For the vegan who excludes all foods of animal origin from her diet, the increased need for high-quality protein during pregnancy demands attention. The vegan does not consume animal flesh, milk, or eggs, so the selection of protein-rich foods is limited; she faces the challenge of meeting her increased protein needs from plant foods alone. The inclusion of a variety of plant protein foods in generous quantities is imperative.

Because individual plant-protein foods contain less of certain amino acids than animal-protein foods, combining plant-protein foods that have different limiting amino acids improves dietary protein quality. This strategy of eating complementary protein foods together is known as mutual supplementation (see Figure 2-6).

The vegan can certainly improve the quality of protein consumed by practicing mutual supplementation, but need not be overly concerned about it because most plant-food diets that provide adequate energy offer a reasonable balance of amino acids in sufficient quantity.[64] A wiser use of time and concern is to obtain, prepare, and eat a wide variety of plant-protein foods and to have an adequate energy intake. The lacto-ovo vegetarian, who excludes animal flesh from the diet but eats dairy products and eggs, can continue eating these foods throughout pregnancy.

In terms of food, each of the following is equivalent to 15 grams of protein:

▸ 2 large eggs (160 kcalories).

▸ 1 cup of legumes (250 kcalories).

▸ 2 cups of nonfat milk (180 kcalories).

▸ 2 ounces of lean meat or fish (110 kcalories).

▸ 3 tablespoons of peanut butter (285 kcalories).

▸ 1/2 cup of 2 percent fat cottage cheese (100 kcalories).

Any two of these selections over and above the RDA will therefore provide the additional 30 grams of protein recommended during pregnancy. The legumes provide more energy than some of the other selections, but they are excellent sources of carbohydrate (45 grams per cup), vitamins, and minerals. To spare protein, the woman should use carbohydrate to supply 50 percent of total energy intake each day. For example, in a 2000-kcalories per day intake, this

Mixtures that provide complete protein:

▸ Legumes plus grains.

▸ Legumes plus seeds.

▸ Leafy vegetables plus grains.

▸ Leafy vegetables plus seeds.

▸ Brewer's yeast plus leafy vegetables, seeds, nuts, or whole grains.

complementary protein: two or more proteins whose amino acid assortments complement each other in such a way that the essential amino acids missing from each are supplied by the other.

mutual supplementation: the strategy, used by vegetarians, of combining two protein foods in a meal so that each food provides the essential amino acid(s) lacking in the other.

Recommended carbohydrate intake: about 50% of energy intake.

Figure 2–6   Complementary Protein Combinations for Vegetarians

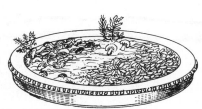

Black beans and rice, a favorite Hispanic combination.

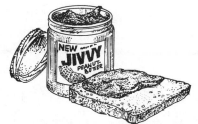

Peanut butter and wheat bread, a North American tradition.

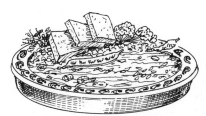

Tofu and stir-fried vegetables with rice, an Asian dish.

represents 1000 kcalories of carbohydrate, or about 250 grams. During pregnancy, 4 cups of milk per day are recommended. Four cups of milk contribute about 50 grams carbohydrate. An apple provides 10 grams carbohydrate, a large banana provides 20 grams carbohydrate, and a slice of bread provides 15 grams, so generous intakes of fruit and bread are encouraged.

Vitamin B_6 needs appear to increase in pregnancy for several reasons. For one thing, they always rise in proportion to rising dietary protein intakes. For another, all forms of the vitamin cross the placenta and are concentrated in fetal blood; furthermore, estrogen's enhanced activity during pregnancy increases the activity of an enzyme (tryptophan oxygenase) that requires a vitamin B_6 coenzyme. However, no evidence to date indicates that vitamin B_6 deficiency causes pregnancy complications or that supplements of 6 to 10 milligrams a day, which prevent biochemical changes otherwise seen, produce any therapeutic benefit. The RDA committee recommends a conservative, but protective, addition of 0.6 milligrams a day to the woman's normal 2.0 milligrams, for a total of 2.6 milligrams a day, sufficient to cover the recommended added protein intake.[65]

▸▸ PRACTICAL POINT

Diets Tailored to Individuals

No two women are alike, and no woman eats the exact diet presented in Table 2–2. One unschooled teenager driven by peer pressure might eat hamburgers, fries, and colas. A busy mother with three children and too many pressures might drink three beers in the evening and miss out on dinner. The newly converted member of a religious cult might be persuaded to give up all but a very few foods. Less extreme examples are more common; one person eats too much meat at the expense of vegetables, another drinks too much milk at the expense of iron-rich foods.

Some women's food practices are not only haphazard but irrational and rigid. Unusual beliefs, superstitions, and dietary practices have surrounded childbirth since the beginning of time. Some women, even today, regardless of age, ethnic group, or income level, may believe that over- or underconsumption of a craved food results in physical or behavioral peculiarities of the infant. For example, an unsatisfied craving for strawberries causes a strawberry-shaped birthmark. Such beliefs usually have no deleterious effect on the mother's diet nutritionally, but psychologically, they may cause stress, which can impair the outcome of pregnancy.[a]

Some women develop cravings for, or aversions to, some foods and beverages during pregnancy. These are fairly common, although not well understood. One study found that a significant number of women reduced their consumption of coffee, alcoholic beverages, and carbonated beverages

---

[a]G. M. Jonakait, M. C. Bohn, and I. B. Black, Maternal glucocorticoid hormones influence neurotransmitter phenotypic expression in embryos, *Science* 207 (1980): 551–553; I. L. Ward and J. Weisz, Maternal stress alters plasma testosterone in fetal males, *Science* 207 (1980): 328–329.

during the first half of their pregnancies.[b] Most often women attributed their reduced coffee consumption to nausea. Their reduced intakes of alcohol and carbonated beverages, however, they ascribed to concern for their infants' health or their own weight gain.

In this same study, the most common food aversions reported were to meat and poultry, a finding consistent with other reports. The most predominant food craving was for ice cream. It has often been hypothesized that food cravings may reflect physiological needs of the mother and/or fetus, although at present no evidence has proven this to be true. In other words, a woman who craves ice cream or other dairy products may not be in need of calcium, but cravings in general may reflect a nutrient-poor diet. Food aversions and cravings may arise during pregnancy due to changes in taste and smell sensitivities.

In any case, anyone providing guidance on nutrition to a pregnant woman should listen for clues about harmful dietary practices, beliefs, or superstitions. If any of these appear to be detrimental, nutritionally or otherwise, warn her that this is so. This may be easier said than done; it is extremely important not to alienate her. Our suggestions to the diet advisor are as follows.

Praise the woman for all that she is doing well during her pregnancy and, without being pushy, try to make her realize why a healthy body and mind are important to her own well-being and to that of her developing fetus. Skillful evaluation of a pregnant woman's diet is essential in determining possible risks due to alternative dietary practices. Low food energy and/or protein intakes may exist in a vegan or macrobiotic diet. A diet composed mainly of fried foods and soft drinks that offers too many kcalories in the form of fat and sugar and too few nutrients is inadequate for a pregnant woman. Such a diet lacks important vitamins, minerals, and fiber necessary to the health of mother and child. For these women, and many others, a competent nutrition counselor can make a significant difference in terms of the health and well-being of mother and child.

The advisor cannot afford to be judgmental, however. Offer support for diet and health habits that are conducive to well-being. Provide the woman with information about pregnancy in general, emphasizing the impact her own nutrition and health will have on her developing child.

Suggest small, but significant, changes she can make in her diet. The vegan who adds one serving of tofu and one serving of legumes to her diet each day does much to improve the protein adequacy of her diet. The person who replaces two soft drinks each day with two glasses of milk significantly improves the nutrient density of an otherwise high-kcalorie, low-nutrient diet. Encourage such a person to eat nutrient-dense snacks such as hard-boiled eggs, yogurt, and fresh fruits and vegetables every day and provide a list of these. As these changes gradually become part of her daily routine, the pregnant woman will feel and look better, her motivation will come from within, and the job of the health counselor will become easier.

macrobiotic diet: a diet in which ten stages of dietary restriction lead to gradual elimination of animal products, fruits, and vegetables, at which point the diet is composed only of cereals. Such a diet may be deficient in food energy, protein, iron, zinc, calcium, vitamin B_{12}, vitamin D, and other nutrients as well, depending on the level of restriction. This is dangerous, especially to pregnant women and children.

[b]E. B. Hook, Dietary cravings and aversions during pregnancy, *American Journal of Clinical Nutrition* 31 (1978): 1355–1362.

If a woman simply refuses to alter her diet, the question arises whether she should take supplements. Dietitians worth their salt will make every effort to improve food choices, but in real-life situations hard-pressed diet advisors may be forced to compromise. In the case of the vegan, for example, a dietitian might advise such a person to supplement her meals with soy-based protein powder to ensure adequate protein intake. Eating adequate amounts of a variety of whole, nutrient-dense foods is the best way to obtain needed nutrients; if such foods are just not eaten, especially in the case of pregnant women, then supplements may have to fill the gap.

Nutrients for Blood Production and Cell Growth

The nutrients required for blood production and for rapid cell proliferation in general are required in greater amounts during pregnancy. New cells are laid down at a tremendous pace as the fetus grows and develops. At the same time, the maternal red blood cell mass expands. All nutrients are important in these processes, but the needs for folacin, vitamin B_{12}, iron, and zinc are especially great, due to their key roles in DNA synthesis and the manufacture of red blood cells.

Folacin
1980 RDA: 800 μg/day.
1987 RDI: 500 μg/day.

Foods containing folacin:
▶ Green, leafy vegetables.
▶ Legumes.
▶ Liver.
▶ Orange juice and cantaloupe.
▶ Other vegetables.
▶ Whole-wheat products.

Folacin and vitamin B_{12}   The additional folacin required by the pregnant woman is due to the great increase in her blood volume, the increased urinary excretion of the vitamin, and the rapid growth of the fetus. However, folacin excess from supplements also presents a risk to pregnancy, so improvement of the diet is the better choice. The RDA for folacin doubles during pregnancy, increasing from 400 micrograms to 800 micrograms. It is possible to obtain this much folacin from food, but many diets are nevertheless inadequate in their folacin content.[66] Women who consume limited amounts of fresh fruits and vegetables should, during pregnancy, eat more of these. The physician often finds it advisable to prescribe folacin as a supplement.[67] In addition to being good sources of folacin, fruits and vegetables are low in kcalories, rich in vitamins and minerals, and high in fiber.

Recent research indicates that the determination of folate status by way of a diet history and possibly laboratory assessment may be more important than previously thought for the pregnant woman, because, it is important not only to remedy deficiencies, but also to avoid excesses. Folacin supplements taken unnecessarily, especially in combination with iron supplements (as occurs in most prenatal supplements), compromise zinc status in women with marginal zinc stores.[68] Pregnancy complications have been observed in women with high plasma folacin and low plasma zinc concentrations.[69] The folacin supplements that the pregnant women took were responsible for the high plasma folacin concentrations, and possibly for the inhibition of zinc absorption, which, in turn, caused the complications.

As you might expect, the pregnant woman also has a greater need for the B vitamin that assists folacin in the manufacture of red blood cells—vitamin B_{12}. The RDA for vitamin B_{12} for adults is 3 micrograms. During pregnancy, the RDA increases to 4 micrograms. Vitamin B_{12} is found almost exclusively in

Vitamin B_{12}
1980 RDA: 4 μg/day.
1987 RDI: 2.5 μg/day.

foods of animal origin. Meat eaters and lacto-ovo vegetarians are protected from deficiency. Vegans may need to drink vitamin B_{12}-fortified soy milk, or use nutritional yeast grown on a vitamin B_{12}-enriched diet. Some vegans have normal vitamin B_{12} status, whether or not they consume these fortified foods.[70] Researchers wonder why, since vegan diets, by definition, contain no foods from animal sources. Perhaps vegans' intestinal bacteria produce the vitamin for them.[71]

Iron   During pregnancy, the body conserves iron even more possessively than usual as a result of several changes in iron metabolism. First, menstruation, the major route of iron excretion in women, ceases. Second, absorption of iron increases up to threefold due to a rise in the level of the blood's iron-absorbing and carrier protein, transferrin. An additional adjustment is accomplished by the hormones of pregnancy, which raise the concentration of iron in the blood by increasing absorption still further and by mobilizing iron from its storage sites in the bone marrow and internal organs. Assuming that she has eaten an iron-rich diet all her life and that her iron stores are full, a woman *theoretically* needs no more iron during pregnancy than she has needed all along. Most women, however, even in the United States and Canada, have minimal iron stores due to less-than-optimal intakes over time; the demands of pregnancy deplete them to the deficiency point. Therefore, daily supplements are recommended for the pregnant woman. The exact amount should be determined by the health care professional administering prenatal care; 30 to 60 milligrams is often prescribed, on the assumption that the iron will be much more poorly absorbed than that from food.[72]

Iron-deficiency anemia is especially common in pregnancy, but the "physiological anemia" (discussed in Appendix A) of pregnancy must be considered in the diagnosis of iron-deficiency anemia. A woman may make it to the end of pregnancy without developing iron-deficiency anemia, but may bleed excessively at delivery—hence, the advisability of a prescribed iron supplement to boost her stores. At birth, an infant needs to have stored enough iron to last three to six months; this iron comes from the mother's iron stores. In order to replenish iron stores depleted by pregnancy, the National Research Council recommends continued iron supplementation for two to three months after delivery.[73]

The pregnant vegetarian again deserves special mention here. The best iron sources are meat, fish, and poultry, and, thanks to the MFP factor, iron absorption from nonmeat foods can be tripled in a meal containing MFP. Although vegetarian foods such as legumes, whole grains, dark leafy greens, and dried fruits may appear high in iron on food composition tables, the iron is not as absorbable as that of meat. The vegetarian does enjoy a compensating advantage, however. Vitamin C in fruits and vegetables can also triple absorption from iron-containing foods eaten at the same meal.

Zinc   Zinc is required for DNA and RNA synthesis and thus protein synthesis. Over 70 enzymes are now known to require zinc as a cofactor.

Small amounts of zinc must be supplied in the diet of the pregnant woman daily, as the body pool of biologically available zinc appears to be small. The zinc nutrition of many U.S. women may be marginal. A study that measured

transferrin: the blood protein responsible for the absorption and transport of iron.

Ordinarily, a hemoglobin level below 13 g/100 ml is considered low for a woman. In pregnancy, values of 12 g are not unusual, and 11 g is where the line defining "too low" is often drawn.

Food sources of iron:

▶ Liver and oysters.
▶ Red meat, fish, poultry, and other meat.
▶ Dried fruits.
▶ Legumes (dried beans and limas).
▶ Dark green vegetables.

MFP factor: a factor (identity unknown) present in **M**eat, **F**ish, and **P**oultry that enhances the absorption of nonheme iron present in the same foods or in other foods eaten at the same time.

Appendix A describes how meats and vitamin C enhance iron absorption.

Assessment of zinc status in pregnant women is discussed in Appendix A.

Zinc
1980 RDA: 20 mg/day.

the zinc content in food samples of 20 adults found an average daily zinc intake of 8.6 milligrams.[74] The RDA for zinc is 15 milligrams for adults, based on consumption of a mixed diet containing animal products.[75] The RDA for zinc for pregnant women is 20 milligrams. When dietary zinc intake of pregnant women of middle- and low-income backgrounds was examined, the average was less than two-thirds of the RDA.[76]

Zinc is most abundant in foods of high protein content, such as shellfish (especially oysters), meats, and liver. Milk, eggs, and whole grains are good sources of zinc when eaten in large quantities, but fiber and phytates in whole grains may render some of the zinc unavailable.

Nutrients for Bone Development

The nutrients involved in building the skeleton are in great demand during pregnancy. A deficiency of calcium, vitamin D, fluoride, or magnesium during pregnancy may have serious consequences for fetal bone and dental development.

Calcium
1980 RDA: 1200 mg/day.

Calcium A 50 percent increase in the intake of calcium, from 800 milligrams to 1200 milligrams, is recommended for the pregnant woman. Two-thirds of all females between 18 and 30 years of age have calcium intakes below the RDA.[77] Therefore, in order to meet the needs of the growing fetus, and because pregnancy and breastfeeding may drain women's skeletal reserves of calcium, most mothers' calcium intakes have to be boosted well above their prepregnancy levels.

Adaptive physiological changes occur during pregnancy that favor calcium retention. Intestinal absorption of calcium doubles early in pregnancy, and the mineral is stored in the mother's bones. At the same time, urinary calcium excretion decreases. During the last trimester, as the fetal bones begin to calcify, a dramatic shift of calcium across the placenta occurs and the mother's bone stores are drawn upon. Because of the adaptive mechanisms mentioned above, the consequences of a marginal calcium intake during pregnancy for maternal bone health are not entirely clear.[78]

A low calcium intake is a risk factor in the development of osteoporosis (excessive adult bone loss), which weakens bones to the point of fracturing under everyday stress. One out of four postmenopausal women will experience fractures related to osteoporosis.[79] Osteoporosis is eight times more common in women than in men.[80] This makes adequate calcium intake during pregnancy critical for a woman's health in later years.

Four cups of milk a day will supply 1.2 g calcium. The milk should be fortified with vitamin D. One cup of yogurt or 1 1/2 oz of hard cheese provides as much calcium as 1 c of milk, although these are not made from vitamin D-fortified milk.

Once again, the pregnant vegan faces a greater challenge than most. In fact, it is next to impossible for the pregnant vegan to obtain the calcium she needs without the inclusion of calcium-fortified soy milk in her diet several times a day. Other calcium food sources for the strict vegetarian include tofu (soybean curd), self-rising flour, almonds, and filberts, but no one can eat these in sufficient quantities to meet the calcium need. The vegan who does not drink calcium-fortified soy milk daily must resort to calcium supplements in order to avoid developing a deficiency for which she will pay the price in later years (see Chapter 1 for more about calcium supplements).

Vitamin D   The relationship between vitamin D and calcium is well known. Vitamin D plays a vital role in calcium absorption and utilization. Maternal vitamin D deficiency will therefore result in abnormal development of the fetal bones. The RDA for vitamin D for nonpregnant females ranges between 5 and 10 micrograms, depending on age. During pregnancy, the RDA is an additional 5 micrograms above the age-appropriate nonpregnant recommendation. Solar radiation can normally provide this amount; supplements are not normally recommended because of the risk of toxicity. The vegan's vitamin D may be obtained from daily exposure to sunlight or else must be included in the calcium-fortified soy milk.

Fluoride   Formation of the primary teeth begins within the first trimester; for this and for the bones, fluoride is needed. Because there are few food sources of fluoride, a prescription for a supplement that includes fluoride may be desirable for women in areas without fluoridated water.[81]

Magnesium   In addition to its role in building the skeleton, magnesium is also required for muscle relaxation and energy production. The RDA during pregnancy increases from 300 milligrams per day to 450 milligrams. Good food sources include nuts, legumes, cereal grains, dark-green vegetables, seafoods, chocolate, and cocoa.

Other Nutrients

The RDA for vitamin A in pregnancy is increased to 1000 RE a day (over the regular 800 RE for nonpregnant women) to permit accumulation of stores in the fetal liver without draining maternal stores.[82] As for vitamin E, a pregnant woman's RDA is raised by 2 milligrams above the nonpregnant woman's RDA of 8 milligrams a day. Vitamin E transfer across the placenta mainly occurs late in pregnancy, so in the event of a premature birth, the infant needs supplementation (see Chapter 4).

No special recommendation for vitamin K intake is made for pregnancy: normally, intestinal flora meet the need. At birth, a dose may be given to tide the infant over until internal flora are established (see Chapter 4).

Plasma vitamin C levels fall during pregnancy, due to physiological changes, increased needs, or both, and the placenta pumps vitamin C into the fetus against a concentration gradient. At term, fetal vitamin C plasma concentration is 50 percent greater than the maternal concentration. Adding 20 milligrams a day to the nonpregnant woman's RDA of 60 milligrams prevents the fall in plasma vitamin C, so this is recommended, especially for the second and third trimesters of pregnancy.[83]

The only other nutrients for which RDA are given in pregnancy are phosphorus (the recommendation matches that for calcium) and iodine (an added 25 micrograms a day are recommended, for a total of 175 micrograms). No special recommendations are made for intakes during pregnancy of the additional nutrients not in the main RDA table; it is assumed that the ranges recommended for adults will cover pregnant women as well.

Vitamin D
1980 RDA: 10–15 μg/day.

Magnesium
1980 RDA: 450 mg/day.

Vitamin A
1980 RDA: 1000 RE/day.
1987 RDI: 800 RE/day.

Vitamin C
1980 RDA: 80 mg/day.
1987 RDI: 35 mg/day (2nd trimester).
40 mg/day (3rd trimester).

Iodine
1980 RDA: 175 μg/day.

Supplements during Pregnancy

Proper food choices during pregnancy can meet most of a woman's nutrient needs. However, taking the position that diet alone cannot satisfy her requirements for iron and folacin, the National Academy of Sciences, the American College of Obstetricians and Gynecologists, and the American Dietetic Association recommend supplements of these two nutrients during pregnancy. While there is no consensus on the use of supplements, it may be prudent to recommend a supplement that contains a wide range of vitamins and minerals at physiologic levels (particularly vitamins B_6, C, D, and E, folacin, pantothenic acid, calcium, magnesium, iron, zinc, copper, and possibly selenium).[84] Such a prenatal supplement would contain:

- Vitamin B_6 (5 to 10 mg per daily dose).
- Vitamins C (80 mg per daily dose).
- Vitamin D (400 IU per daily dose).
- Vitamin E (15 IU per daily dose).
- Folacin (0.4 to 0.8 mg per daily dose).
- Elemental iron (30 to 45 mg per daily dose) of proven bioavailability.
- Zinc (15 to 20 mg per daily dose) of proven bioavailability.
- Copper (1 to 2 mg per daily dose).

It would *not* contain:

- Calcium in large amounts (greater than 250 mg).
- Calcium in the form of calcium phosphate.
- Magnesium in large amounts (greater than 100 mg).
- Artificial colorings.

Health care providers offering prenatal care commonly encourage women to take prenatal supplements that contain a variety of vitamins and minerals, including folacin and iron. In selecting which supplement to recommend, a health care provider considers both the supplement's formulation and cost. Once nutrient criteria are met, then the least expensive product is the best choice. Supplements should be reasonably priced and readily available; cost should not prohibit a woman from using them. In comparison with the costs of malnutrition during pregnancy, the cost of a supplement is relatively inexpensive.

The nutrients emphasized here have been, for obvious reasons, those most intensely involved in blood production, other cell growth, and bone growth. However, all nutrients are needed in added quantities during pregnancy, and therefore a diet of mixed whole foods is the best vehicle to supply them. The next task is to obtain the necessary nutrients within food energy allowance that will support the appropriate weight gain. Chapter 1 discussed the effects of pregravid weight on fertility and infant birthweight. The two other factors influencing infant birthweight are weight gain during pregnancy and length of gestation. These factors are discussed next.

Weight Gain and Infant Birthweight

Women who plan to become pregnant, or who are already pregnant, often express concern about the weight gain that accompanies a normal pregnancy. In a society such as ours, where body slimness is frequently equated with youth, vigor, and good looks, many prospective mothers may view the weight gain of pregnancy in a negative light. This is unfortunate. Maternal weight gain during pregnancy correlates closely with infant birthweight.[85] Infant birthweight, in turn, is a strong predictor of the health and subsequent development of the infant.

Maternal Weight Gain

The American College of Obstetrics and Gynecology recommends a pregnancy weight gain of 22 to 27 pounds.[86] Underweight women improve their chances of bearing healthy infants when they gain at least 30 pounds.[87] Adolescents need to gain more weight than older women in order to attain average or optimal infant birthweights.[88] Women who are more than 10 percent above the standard weight for height prior to pregnancy could perhaps gain less, but still should gain between 16 and 20 pounds, depending on prepregnancy weight.[89] Body composition and nutrition status are important considerations in the estimation of optimal weight gain during pregnancy for the overweight woman. For instance, some women who are 10 percent or more above the standard weight for height are well nourished, and have dense bones and substantial lean body tissue. Other women whose weight is 10 percent or more above the standard weight for height are poorly nourished, and their bodies do not contain the desirable proportions of lean and fat tissue. The first group are the ones in whom a 16-pound weight gain during pregnancy may be adequate in terms of fetal outcome. The second group, however, are probably in need of 20-pound or greater weight gains during pregnancy, in order to support the growth of healthy infants.

If a woman has gained more than the expected amount of weight early in pregnancy, she should not try to diet in the last weeks. Women have been known to gain up to 60 pounds in pregnancy without ill effects. (A *sudden* large weight gain, however, is a danger signal that may indicate the onset of pregnancy-induced hypertension, formerly called toxemia; see page 92, "Treating Medical Complications.")

Recently, some researchers have suggested that new weight-gain standards for pregnancy, based on larger, more diverse groups of women are desirable.[90] They recommend that future studies used to generate new pregnancy weight-gain charts should include adolescents, obese and underweight women, and women who are carrying more than one fetus. A new prenatal weight gain grid is shown in Appendix A.

A 22- to 27-pound weight gain for a normal-weight woman is consistent with the components of weight gain during pregnancy shown in Table 2–3. These pounds—from nutritious foods—are needed to support the growth of the placenta, uterus, blood, and breasts, as well as for an optimally healthy 7 1/2-pound infant and some maternal fat stores to provide energy for labor

The standard prenatal weight gain grid is shown in Appendix A.

Table 2–3   Weight Gain during Pregnancy

Development	Weight Gain (lb)
Infant at birth	7½
Placenta	1
Increase in mother's blood volume to supply placenta	4
Increase in size of mother's uterus and muscles to support it	2½
Increase in size of mother's breasts	3
Fluid to surround infant in amniotic sac	2
Mother's fat stores	2–8
Total	22–28

The dangers of alcohol consumption during pregnancy are discussed in Focal Point 2, Fetal Alcohol Syndrome.

and lactation.[91] There is little place in the diet for the empty kcalories of sugar, fat, and alcohol, which provide no nutrients to support the growth of these tissues and only contribute to fat accumulation. Obviously, some of the weight the pregnant woman gains is lost at delivery. In the following few weeks, much of the remaining weight is lost as blood volume returns to normal and the fluids accumulated during pregnancy are shed.

Infant Birthweight

As mentioned, maternal weight gain strongly correlates with infant birthweight. Birthweight, in turn, is a potent indicator of the infant's future health status. More is involved here, however, than birthweight alone. During the last two decades, standards of fetal growth, including physical characteristics and neurological development, have been established. These standards enable health care providers to estimate gestational age. Prior to this time, gestational age was estimated on the basis of the mother's menstrual history, consistent with clinical findings. With the development of more precise data, measurement of gestational age can be used in the classification of all newborn infants. Thus, the terms low-birthweight infant and high-birthweight infant are oversimplified.

Figure 1–1 in Chapter 1 places these newborn classification terms on a time line.

The classification of newborn infants defines infants according to birthweight, gestational age, and pattern of intrauterine growth.[92] The dividing line between term and preterm is drawn at 38 weeks; the line between term and post term is drawn at 42 weeks. A infant born between 38 and 42 weeks gestation is therefore a term infant.

large for gestational age: infants whose weight for age falls above the 90th percentile.

appropriate for gestational age: infants whose weight for age falls between the 10th and 90th percentile.

small for gestational age: infants whose weight for age falls below the 10th percentile.

Within each gestational age group, three subgroups of infants are defined by birthweight. Those above the 90th percentile are *large for gestational age*, those between the 10th and 90th percentiles are *appropriate for gestational age*, and those below the 10th percentile are *small for gestational age*. In this manner, nine groups of newborn infants are defined, based on gestational age and birthweight. When all newborns are classified at birth using this system, health care providers can easily recognize those infants who must be watched closely. They can predict the type of morbidity likely to occur, depending on the particular group into which the infant falls. Infants who are large for gestational age have different problems from those who are small for gestational age. For example, large-for-gestational-age infants are more likely to be traumatized during delivery, whereas small-for-gestational-age infants suffer more often from respiratory distress.

In summary, newborn morbidity and mortality correlate with birthweight and gestational age. For our purposes, however, "low-birthweight infant" simply refers to an infant with a birthweight below 5 1/2 pounds, unless otherwise indicated.

The distinction between preterm infants and small-for-gestational-age infants is important in terms of health and development. Preterm infants are born before their gestational development is complete. They may be small, but those who are appropriate for gestational age do catch up in growth to their full-term peers. In contrast, small-for-gestational-age infants have experienced fetal growth retardation and do not catch up as well. They reach only about the 25th percentile for height, and some fail to attain the same level of mental ability as normal-birthweight children.[93] Fetal growth retardation may also have long-term effects on development and immune function.[94] This applies both to children who are preterm and to those who are small for gestational age.

Through research, several "high-risk" groups of women have been identified who are more likely than other women to deliver low-birthweight infants. They are characterized by any or all of the following:[95]

▶ *Teenage pregnancy:* One of every four low-birthweight infants is born to a teenaged mother.

▶ *Chronic and acute conditions:* Pregnant women with diabetes, high blood pressure, pregnancy-induced hypertension, kidney or respiratory problems, or certain genetic disorders are prone to deliver low-birthweight infants.

▶ *Poor nutrition status:* Studies have shown that some infants may be born smaller than normal because of poor nutrition status of the mother.

▶ *Childbearing history:* Women who have previously delivered low-birthweight infants are more likely than others to do so again.

▶ *Cigarette, alcohol, and/or other drug consumption:* Use of any or all of these substances while pregnant has been shown to inhibit fetal growth.

The correlation between maternal weight gain and infant birthweight and the risks associated with low birthweight serve to emphasize the importance of appropriate weight gain and good nutrition during pregnancy. The pattern of maternal weight gain is even more important than total weight gain, in terms of maternal nutrition status assessment.[96] The ideal pattern is thought to be about 2 to 4 pounds during the first trimester, and about a pound per week thereafter.

The clinician who assesses a pregnant woman's nutrition status uses a set of biochemical standards specific for pregnancy. In fact, a mother's physiology changes so much during pregnancy that an observer who did not know she was pregnant might think that her lab values were abnormal. She develops an apparent anemia, she may have edema, and her carbohydrate metabolism is altered. These and other changes are normal during pregnancy, however. Should a pregnant woman's nutrition be poor or should she be at risk for poor nutrition status, help is available to her (see Practical Point: Maternal and Infant Assistance Programs).

Appendix A provides details for assessing nutrition status during pregnancy.

Maternal and Infant Assistance Programs

Pregnancy is a time of increased need. Nutrient needs increase; so do emotional and financial needs. If any of these needs are not met, the course and outcome of the pregnancy may be compromised. Frequently, low-income women may receive little, if any, prenatal care. They simply cannot afford it or are unaware of the free health services they are entitled to in their communities.

Teens, who may at first be unaware that they are pregnant, or who are trying to hide the fact that they are, may fail to seek help until late in pregnancy. Many women do not eat properly while they are pregnant because they are not aware of the importance of eating well, they do not know how to eat well, or they have too little money to purchase the food they need. Women can deal with all of these situations provided they can learn of the resources available to them.

Several options are available for anyone who may be in need of information or assistance:

- The Agriculture Extension Service provides many educational services and materials, including nutrition, food budgeting, and shopping information.
- Community hospitals and health clinics employ registered dietitians who can assist with meal planning and health care during pregnancy.
- The Women, Infants, and Children (WIC) Supplemental Feeding Program provides nutrition information and low-cost nutritious foods to low-income pregnant women and their children.
- The Food Stamp Program or other federal assistance programs may be available to some.

The health professional counseling such individuals can be invaluable in guiding them to the resources available.

Exercise

Nutrition is the main focus of this chapter and, in fact, of this entire text, but it is nevertheless only one component of optimal health. With this in mind, a few words about the importance of exercise during pregnancy are in order.

It is not unusual today to see pregnant women jogging, swimming, participating in aerobic dance classes, walking energetically, or doing other exercises with the same vigor as their nonpregnant peers. In recent years, there has been increasing interest in the effects of exercise during pregnancy: Is it harmful? Is it beneficial?

Unfortunately, the study of exercise during pregnancy is not without problems. One of the most basic problems is that many variables affect both pregnancy and exercise, making well-controlled studies difficult. Some studies on people have been conducted, but the most reliable data have been obtained from studies on animals. The animals used have four feet rather than two, as well as major metabolic differences from people, so the applicability of these results to human beings is limited.

Despite these limitations and some conflicting results, some basic conclusions seem apparent. Mild exercise during pregnancy is not associated with adverse effects on the fetus or the mother. Most studies involving the effects of strenuous exercise on the outcome of pregnancy have been conducted on women who were highly physically active prior to pregnancy, and these studies report normal fetal outcome as measured by infant birthweight and condition at birth.[97]

In view of the limited research currently available, it seems that common sense is the key to exercise during pregnancy. A woman who is not physically active prior to pregnancy should not begin a vigorous exercise program, once she is pregnant, without consulting her physician. Normally, the physician will tell her that a mild degree of exercise such as daily walking is likely to benefit her and her infant. An active, physically fit woman experiencing a normal, healthy pregnancy can more than likely continue exercising throughout her pregnancy, adjusting the intensity and duration as she goes along. Obviously, activities such as skiing, skydiving, contact sports, or games in which the pregnant woman may be hit by a ball should be replaced by safer activities—there are many from which to choose. For example, a game of tennis played by one partner on each side of the net is safer than a fast-moving doubles game of racquetball.

The American College of Obstetrics and Gynecology has developed the following safety guidelines and criteria for exercise during pregnancy. Physician consultation is recommended before starting any type of exercise program. Exercise guidelines for pregnancy include:

▶ Maternal heart rate should not exceed 140 beats per minute (faster heart rates indicate that oxygen supply is getting short and oxygen deprivation could impair fetal development).

▶ No exercise should be performed while lying on the back after the fourth month of pregnancy (the enlarged uterus obstructs the vena cava and cuts off the blood supply to the fetus).

▶ Energy intake should be adequate to meet the additional energy needs of pregnancy plus the exercise performed (an energy shortage causes protein deficiency, compromising fetal development).

▶ No exercise should be performed in hot, humid weather. Avoid overheating. Avoid saunas and hot whirlpools (the enzymes that accomplish fetal development only work within a narrow temperature range).

▶ Strenuous activities should not exceed 15 minutes in duration (longer workouts can raise body temperature to the point of inhibiting enzyme action and disrupting fetal development).

▶ The woman should drink liquids liberally before and after exercise to prevent dehydration (normal fluid and electrolyte balance is indispensable to normal fetal development).

▶ The woman should discontinue exercise at the first sign of discomfort (discomfort may be a sign of impending danger to mother or fetus).

Exercise is beneficial to all pregnant women, but is especially important for those with diabetes (see p.-ref, "Treating Medical Complications").

Potential Hazards and Problems of Pregnancy

Problems in pregnancy can arise from a variety of causes— lifestyle habits and medical problems foremost among them. These may need special attention.

Protecting Fetal Development

The potential impact of harmful practices during pregnancy cannot be overestimated. The following list itemizes the major ones.

Smoking   There is never a health advantage to smoking; during pregnancy, the disadvantages of smoking are magnified dramatically. Smoking during pregnancy harms the mother, the placenta, the embryo, the fetus, and the infant and child-to-be. Smoking increases the risk of retarded development and complications at birth. Mislocation of the placenta, premature separation of the placenta, and vaginal bleeding are 92 percent more frequent among women who smoke more than one pack of cigarettes per day than among nonsmokers (Figure 2–7 shows one such effect of smoking during pregnancy). The risk of spontaneous abortion and neonatal death increases directly with increasing levels of maternal smoking. A positive association also exists between maternal smoking and sudden infant death syndrome (SIDS).[98] This relationship is found for frequency,

Figure 2–7   Placenta Previa, an Effect of Smoking during Pregnancy
A placenta that slips down over the cerix this way may break and bleed, threatening the life of both mother and fetus.

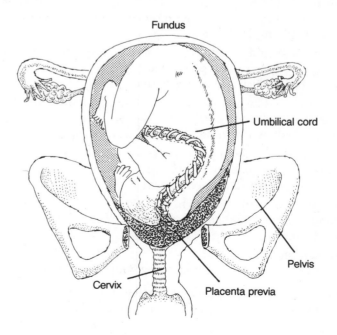

quantity, and even postnatal exposure to cigarette smoke (passive smoking). The Surgeon General's report concludes that "maternal smoking can be a direct cause of fetal or neonatal death in an otherwise normal infant."[99]

Smoking is one of the most *preventable* causes of low birthweight in the United States.[100] The more the mother smokes, the greater the reduction in birthweight. On the average, infants of mothers who smoke weigh 200 grams (7.1 ounces, or almost 1/2 pound) less than those born to nonsmoking mothers. This low birthweight reflects a small-for-gestational-age profile, not preterm birth—maternal smoking directly slows fetal growth rate.[101] Fetal growth retardation of infants born to smokers is not due to other maternal factors.

The adverse effects of smoking are not limited to the pregnancy and birth. Children of women who smoke during and after pregnancy have higher rates of morbidity and mortality up to five years of age.[102] Physical growth, mental development, and behavioral characteristics may be impaired in children at least up to the age of 11.[103]

Smoking restricts the blood supply to the growing fetus and so limits the delivery of oxygen and nutrients and removal of wastes. Tobacco smoke contains hundreds of compounds that are harmful, including nicotine and carbon monoxide. Carbon monoxide in the blood of a smoking mother may deprive the developing fetus of the oxygen necessary for optimal growth. The primary cause of most smoking-related fetal deaths is oxygen deprivation. The risks of smoking during pregnancy should be taught from junior high school through college. Any woman who smokes and is considering pregnancy or who is already pregnant should be urged to quit or at least to cut back on the number of cigarettes smoked.

Caffeine   Caffeine is a drug that crosses the placenta. The developing fetus has a limited ability to metabolize caffeine.[104] For these reasons, caffeine consumption during pregnancy should be minimal (less than 150 milligrams per day). One 6-ounce cup of coffee contains about 85 milligrams; a cup of tea or a 12-ounce cola contains about 50 milligrams.[105]

One study of pregnant women found that those who consumed more than 150 milligrams of caffeine per day were significantly more likely to experience late first- or second-trimester spontaneous abortion, compared with noncaffeine users or light users (1 to 150 milligrams per day).[106] Further studies of this same design are necessary to confirm these results. Caffeine is present not only in coffee, tea, and cola, but also in cocoa, some soft drinks, and some over-the-counter medicines. The Food and Drug Administration cautions pregnant women to avoid caffeine or to use it sparingly.

The Canadian National Guidelines on Prenatal Nutrition are more liberal in their caffeine recommendation.[107] They advise moderate caffeine consumption during pregnancy and define moderate as less than 400 milligrams per day. For persons choosing to substitute herb teas for caffeine-containing beverages, they advise moderation in the use of herb teas during pregnancy due to potential teratogenic effects.

Medications   Drugs taken during pregnancy can cause serious congenital malformations. Currently, more than 500,000 over-the-counter drugs are on the market. The public seems to be infatuated with pills, potions, and lotions. Many people routinely use antacids, aspirin, aspirin substitutes, and laxatives. A pregnant woman, however, should not take any pill, capsule, powder, or liquid medicine without consulting her health care provider. In chronic conditions such as epilepsy, which may require routine use of drugs, physician consultation may determine that dosages can be reduced or less powerful drugs substituted to minimize risk.

Illicit drugs   Women should definitely avoid the use of mind-altering drugs such as marijuana and cocaine at all times, but especially during pregnancy. In addition to effects such as interference with appetite, intellectual function, and coordination, illicit drugs such as cocaine and marijuana are harmful to the fetus. These drugs pass easily through the placenta. Tetrahydrocannabinol (THC), the psychoactive ingredient in marijuana, is stored in the fatty tissue of the fetus and is potentially damaging to the fetus.[108] Pregnancy is the most dangerous time for women to smoke marijuana.

A study of pregnant, cocaine-using women revealed a high incidence of spontaneous abortion compared with drug-free women.[109] In addition, infants exposed to cocaine during gestation had depressed interactive behavior and poor organizational responses to environmental stimuli. This study also suggests that infants exposed to cocaine are at risk for congenital malformations and perinatal mortality. Many questions remain unanswered concerning illicit drugs and narcotics and their effects during pregnancy. What is known so far, however, is that pregnancy and illicit drug use are a dangerous combination, to be avoided in all cases.

Alcohol   Alcohol consumption during pregnancy can cause irreversible brain damage and mental and physical retardation in the fetus. Fetal alcohol syndrome is the subject of Focal Point 2.

Nutrient megadoses   All of the vitamins are toxic when taken in excess. The minerals are even more so, some of them at levels not far above the RDA. This is especially significant during pregnancy. The pregnant woman who is constantly being told to eat well and take care of herself may mistakenly assume that more is better regarding vitamin-mineral supplements. This is simply not true. With the exception of iron, folacin, and, in special cases, calcium, a pregnant woman can obtain most of the vitamins and minerals she needs by eating whole foods. She should take supplements only on the advice of a registered dietitian or a physician.

Diet history forms should include questions about the use of supplements. Nutrient excesses, as well as deficiencies, can be harmful to mother and fetus. Table 2-4 presents a summary of the effects of potentially harmful substances during pregnancy.

Alleviating Maternal Discomfort

To avoid the most common nutrition-related problems encountered during pregnancy, it helps to be armed with some strategies. Most common are the conditions listed here.

Table 2–4 Effects of Potentially Harmful Substances to the Fetus[a]

Substance	Effect to Fetus
Cigarette smoke	Low birthweight; increased incidence of spontaneous abortion; CNS disturbances; increased incidence of SIDS; fetal death[b]
Caffeine	CNS stimulant; increased incidence of spontaneous abortion[c]
Medications[d]	
Salicylates (large doses)	Pulmonary hypertension and neonatal bleeding
Acetiminophen	Renal failure
Anticonvulsants	Growth retardation and mental retardation
Oral progestogens, androgens, and estrogens	Masculinization and advanced bone age
Tetracyclines	Inhibition of bone growth; discoloration of teeth
Illicit Drugs[e]	
Marijuana	Short-term irritability at birth
Heroin and methadone	Drug addiction and acute narcotic withdrawal symptoms: tremors, excessive, high-pitched crying, and disturbed sleep; low birthweight
Cocaine	Greater incidence of spontaneous abortion; uncontrolled jerking motion; paralyzation; depressed interactive behavior; poor organizational response to environmental stimuli
Phencyclidine (PCP)	Facial malformations; tremors; low birthweight
Alcohol	Fetal Alcohol Syndrome: distorted facial features, low birthweight, impaired CNS performance, cleft palate[f]
Nutrient Excesses	
Vitamin A	Microcephaly; hydrocephalus; spontaneous abortion[g]
Vitamin D	Hypercalcemia
Iodine	Congenital goiter
Heavy Metals	
Lead	Spontaneous abortion; stillbirth; low birthweight; neurobehavior deficits[h]
Mercury	CNS damage[i]

[a]Virtually any substance may be teratogenic depending on the dose, duration, time of exposure, and genetic makeup of the individual. Some viral infections such as rubella and herpes are teratogenic, as are irradiations of various types. This table presents but *some* of the vast array of substances known to be teratogenic in human beings.

[b]National Research Council, *Alternative Dietary Practices and Nutrition Abuses in Pregnancy, Summary Report* (1982): p. 17; Pregnancy and infant health, in *Smoking and Health,* a report of the Surgeon General, January 1979, available from Superintendent of Documents, U. S. Government Printing Office, Washington, D.C. 20202; T. A. Shepard, *Teratogenic Agents* 3rd ed., (Baltimore, Md.: John Hopkins University Press, 1980), pp. 73–75.

[c]W. Srisuphan and M. B. Bracken, Caffeine consumption during pregnancy and association with late spontaneous abortion, *American Journal of Obstetrics and Gynecology* 154 (1986): 14–20.

[d]W. B. Deichmann and H. W. Gerarde, *Toxicology of Drugs and Chemicals* (New York: Academic Press, 1969), p. 683; E. M. Johnson and D. M. Kochhar, *Teratogenesis and Reproductive Toxicology* (New York, N. Y.; Springer-Verlag Berlin Heidelberg, 1983), p. 217.

[e]Johnson and Kochhar, 1983, pp. 221–235; I. J. Chasnoff and coauthors, Cocaine use in pregnancy, *New England Journal of Medicine* 313 (1985): 666–669.

[f]Johnson and Kochhar, 1983, pp. 216–217.

[g]Vitamin A and teratogenesis, *Lancet* 1 (1985): 319–320.

[h]K. N. Dietrich and coauthors, Low-level fetal lead exposure effect on neurobehavioral development in early infancy, *Pediatrics* 80 (1987): 721–730.

[i]*Teratogenic Agents* 3rd ed., (Baltimore, Md.: John Hopkins University Press, 1980), pp. 212–214.

Constipation   As the hormones of pregnancy alter maternal muscle tone and the growing fetus crowds her intestinal organs, an expectant mother may complain of constipation. A high-fiber diet and a plentiful water intake will help to relieve this condition. Daily exercise may also help alleviate constipation. Laxatives should be used only on the health care provider's orders.

Heartburn   Women often complain of heartburn during pregnancy. (Heartburn is a burning sensation in the area of the lower esophagus, near the heart; hence the name.) The condition has nothing to do with the heart itself. The developing fetus puts increasing pressure on the mother's digestive tract, causing a backup of stomach acid, which creates a burning sensation. It may be especially troublesome at night, while the woman is lying down. She may find relief by sleeping with her torso slightly raised. It may also help if she shifts to smaller, more frequent meals than she has been eating. Some health care providers recommend an occasional antacid for heartburn relief.

Nausea   The nausea of "morning" (actually, any time) sickness seems unavoidable because it arises from the hormonal changes taking place early in pregnancy, but it can often be alleviated. A strategy some expectant mothers have found effective in quelling nausea is to start the day with a few bites of a soda cracker or other bland carbohydrate food, so that something is in their stomachs before getting out of bed. Some women find that drinking fluids between meals rather than with them is beneficial. The woman with nausea may want to eat small, frequent meals to avoid eating too much at one time.

Treating Medical Complications

Medical complications of pregnancy can threaten the lives of both mother and fetus. Two such complications merit discussion here due to their relationship to nutrition.

pregnancy-induced hypertension (PIH): a medical problem in pregnancy that consists of two phases. The first phase, **preeclampsia,** is characterized by increasing hypertension, edema, and protein in the urine. The presence of convulsions indicates the second phase, **eclampsia,** a major medical problem of pregnancy.

The normal edema of pregnancy responds to gravity; blood pools in the ankles. The edema of PIH is a generalized edema. This distinction helps with diagnosis.

Pregnancy-induced hypertension   A certain degree of edema is expected in late pregnancy, but in a poorly nourished woman, it may often be part of the larger cluster of symptoms known as pregnancy-induced hypertension (PIH), formerly called toxemia. PIH is a condition involving high blood pressure and renal problems that requires medical attention. It is important to keep track of maternal blood pressure throughout pregnancy and, if PIH is indicated, to initiate treatment promptly.[110] Both preexisting hypertension and PIH can cause infant death, retarded growth, lung problems, and severe birth defects.

PIH is called the "disease of theories"; its true etiology is unknown, but nutrition-related causes have been suggested for many years. The chief characteristic implicating nutrition in the etiology of PIH is its relatively high incidence in low-income mothers and pregnant teenagers. Women with PIH report consuming diets that are lower in protein and food energy than those of women without PIH. Lack of protein, food energy, and/or calcium may be involved. Adequate calcium is thought to have a direct effect in preventing high blood pressure.[111]

Epidemiological studies show that a low calcium intake during pregnancy is associated with a high incidence of PIH.[112] Excess dietary sodium has also been suggested as a cause of PIH. To avert PIH, a pregnant woman should consume ample protein-rich foods, including milk. Sodium needs increase during pregnancy, but this does not mean that foods need to be salted; sodium needs will be met simply by eating the added foods needed to meet other nutrient requirements. Sodium restriction is not advised, either, unless a medical condition makes it necessary. Even after the onset of PIH, salt intake should normally not be reduced, and diuretics (to cause sodium excretion) may be harmful. Good nutrition and rest are the basis of treatment.

Diabetes   Diabetes can make pregnancy more difficult than usual, and sometimes the onset of diabetes occurs when a woman is pregnant, a condition known as gestational diabetes. Without management of maternal diabetes, infants may suffer increased mortality and morbidity, congenital abnormalities, and other complications. Twenty to thirty percent of women who have gestational diabetes develop permanent diabetes within five years.[113] Research indicates that the incidence of permanent diabetes in women with previous gestational diabetes is twice as high in those who are 20 percent or more overweight, compared with those who are not overweight. Untreated diabetic women have a 95- to 98-percent infertility rate.[114]

gestational diabetes: the appearance of abnormal glucose tolerance during pregnancy, with subsequent return to normal postpartum.

Health care providers carefully monitor women with gestational diabetes. Persistent elevated fasting blood glucose concentrations signal a need for intervention. Health care providers evaluate a woman's potential for diabetes by checking the following risk factors associated with the condition during the first prenatal examination:

▸ Previous gestational diabetes.

▸ History of large infants (9 pounds or more).

▸ Family history of diabetes.

▸ Symptoms of diabetes and glycosuria.

▸ Obesity or excessive weight gain.

▸ Recurrent urinary tract infections.

▸ Recurrent abortions.

▸ Previous unexplained stillbirth.[115]

If the woman is at risk for gestational diabetes, a health care provider conducts a fasting or random plasma glucose test (at least two hours after eating). If the fasting level is equal to or greater than 105 milligrams per milliliter, or the random is equal to or greater than 120, she will receive a follow-up three-hour glucose tolerance test.[116] A three-hour glucose tolerance test is also administered if routine urinalysis detects glycosuria.

As added insurance against problems with diabetes, all pregnant women who have not otherwise been identified as glucose intolerant should have plasma glucose determined, following a glucose load, at 24 to 28 weeks gestation. Thereafter, at every checkup, a woman's urine should be tested for ketones. Ketonuria in conjunction with elevated blood glucose levels may be a clue to diabetes.

Women with gestational diabetes benefit from nutrition counseling. An important aspect of nutrition management is avoidance of excessive weight gain. Weight-reduction diets, however, are not recommended during pregnancy. Women with gestational diabetes should not reduce their carbohydrate intake but should include complex carbohydrates such as vegetables and whole-grain breads. They should limit their intakes of concentrated sweets. Optimum protein intake is also important. Dietary recommendations encourage three meals a day plus two snacks, each containing protein and carbohydrate and moderate fat.

Diet is the cornerstone of treatment for the person with gestational diabetes. If appropriate plasma glucose levels are not maintained, however, insulin therapy may be recommended.

In Anticipation

Pregnancy for many women is a time of adjustment to major changes. The woman who is expecting to bear an infant is a growing person in more ways than one. Physically and emotionally, her needs are changing. If it is her first infant, she senses that her lifestyle will have to change as she takes on the new responsibility of caring for a child. Ideally, she will be encouraged to develop this sense of responsibility by caring for herself during pregnancy. The expectant mother needs support in thinking of herself as a worthwhile and important person with a new and challenging task that she can and will perform well. She may still be working out her relationship with her mate, and he and she both know that the coming of a first infant will affect that relationship profoundly. There is a need for sensitive communication and understanding on both parts in this time of transition.

With all of this to worry about, can a woman relax and enjoy expecting her infant? Of course she can. With the help and guidance of health professionals, and the support of her family and friends, she can feel healthy and confident as she awaits the birth of her infant. As her uterus expands and that first little kick is felt inside, many earlier apprehensions will give way to joy and satisfaction as she realizes the special bond she has with the life inside her. She has been given the chance to nurture a new life. It is a serious and challenging task, but it is also a rewarding one. As our children grow, so do we as mothers and fathers, discovering strengths and weaknesses, abilities and emotions, and, above all, an appreciation for life that we may have never known before.

Chapter 2 Notes

1. G. H. Lowrey, The placenta and fetal development, in *Growth and Development of Children*, 8th ed. (Chicago: Year Book Medical Publishers, 1986), pp. 53–75.

2. H. N. Munro, Placental factors conditioning fetal nutrition and development, *American Journal of Clinical Nutrition* 34 (1981): 756–759.

3. H. N. Munro, S. J. Pilistine, and M. E. Fant, The placenta in nutrition, *Annual Review of Nutrition* 3 (1983): 97–124.

4. R. B. Wilkening and coauthors, Placental transfer as a function of uterine blood flow, *American Journal of Physiology* 242 (1982): H429—H436, as cited in H. N. Munro, S. J. Pilistine, and M. E. Fant, The placenta in nutrition, *Annual Review of Nutrition* 3 (1983): 97–124.

5. Lowrey, 1986.

6. M. Winick and P. Rosso, The effect of severe early malnutrition on cellular growth of human brain, *Pediatric Research* 3 (1969): 181–184.

7. L. S. Hurley, Malnutrition, brain growth, and learning, in *Developmental Nutrition* (Englewood Cliffs, N.J.: Prentice-Hall, 1980), pp. 94–109.

8. K. Satyanarayana and coauthors, Effect of nutritional deprivation in early childhood on later growth—a community study without intervention, *American Journal of Clinical Nutrition* 34 (1981): 1636–1637.

9. J. M. Tanner, Growth before birth, in *Fetus into Man: Physical Growth from Concep-*

tion to Maturity (Cambridge, Mass.: Harvard University Press, 1978), pp. 37–51.

10. Satyanarayana, 1981.

11. Tanner, 1978.

12. P. Rosso, Placental growth, development, and function in relation to maternal nutrition, *Federation Proceedings* 39 (1980): 250–254.

13. G. P. Ravelli, Z. A. Stein, and M. W. Susser, Obesity in young men after famine exposure in utero and early infancy, *New England Journal of Medicine* 295 (1976): 349–353, as cited in J. Kirtland and M. I. Gurr, Adipose tissue cellularity: A review part 2, The relationship between cellularity and obesity, *International Journal of Obesity* 3 (1979): 15–55.

14. C. G. Neumann and E. F. P. Jelliffe, Effects of infant feeding, in *Adverse Effects of Foods*, ed. E. F. P. Jelliffe and D. B. Jelliffe (New York: Plenum Press, 1982), pp. 529–574.

15. N. M. Lien, K. K. Meyer, and M. Winick, Early malnutrition and "late" adoption: A study of the effects on the development of Korean orphans adopted into American families, *American Journal of Clinical Nutrition* 30 (1977): 1734–1739.

16. F. J. Zeman, Effect of protein deficiency during gestation on postnatal cellular development in the young rat, *Journal of Nutrition* 100 (1970): 530–538.

17. A. Petros-Barvazian and M. Behar, Low birthweight: What should be done to deal with this global problem? *WHO Chronicle* 32 (June 1978): 231–232; *New Trends and Approaches in the Delivery of Maternal and Child Care in Health Services* (sixth report of the WHO Expert Committee on Maternal and Child Health), as cited in *Journal of the American Dietetic Association* 71 (1977): 357.

18. National Institute of Child Health and Human Development, *Facts about Premature Birth*, HHS Publication no. (NIH) 461-338-841-25324 (Washington, D.C.: Government Printing Office, 1985).

19. A. N. Antonov, Children born during the siege of Leningrad in 1942, *Journal of Pediatrics* 30 (1947): 250–259.

20. B. S. Burke and coauthors, The influence of nutrition during pregnancy upon the condition of the infant at birth, *Journal of Nutrition* 26 (1943): 569–583.

21. C. Phillipps and N. E. Johnson, The impact of quality of diet and other factors on birth weight of infants, *American Journal of Clinical Nutrition* 30 (1977): 215–225.

22. Zeman, 1970.

23. F. J. Zeman, R. E. Shrader, and L. H. Allen, Persistent effects of maternal protein deficiency in postnatal rats, *Nutrition Reports International* 7 (1973): 421–436.

24. D. Erhard, The new vegetarians, part 1: Vegetarianism and its consequences, *Nutrition Today*, November/December 1973, pp. 4–12.

25. M. S. Rodriguez, A conspectus of research on folacin requirements of man, *Journal of Nutrition* 108 (1978): 1983–2103.

26. G. R. Wadsworth, Some historical aspects of knowledge about folate deficiency, *Nutrition* 27 (1973): 17–22.

27. *Facts about Premature Birth*, 1985; B. M. Hibbard, Folates and the fetus, *South African Medical Journal* 49 (1975): 1223–1226.

28. R. W. Smithells and coauthors, Further experience of vitamin supplementation for prevention of neural tube defect recurrences, *Lancet* 1 (1983): 1027–1031.

29. K. M. Laurence and coauthors, Double-blind randomised controlled trial of folate treatment before conception to prevent recurrence of neural tube defects, *British Medical Journal* 282 (1981): 1509–1511, as cited in M. Tolarova, Periconceptional supplementation with vitamins and folic acid to prevent recurrence of cleft lip (letter), *Lancet* 2 (1982): 217.

30. N. Baumslag, T. Edelstein, and J. Metz, Reduction of incidence of prematurity by folic acid supplementation in pregnancy, *British Medical Journal* 1 (1970): 16–17.

31. P. R. Dallman, M. A. Siims, and E. C. Manies, Brain iron: Persistent deficiency following short-term iron deprivation in the young rat, *British Journal of Haematology* 31 (1975): 209.

32. S. M. Garn, M. T. Keating, and F. Falkner, Hematological status and pregnancy outcomes, *American Journal of Clinical Nutrition* 34 (1981): 115–117.

33. J. A. Pritchard, The effects, if any, of maternal iron deficiency on pregnancy and lactation, Report of the Eighty-second Ross Conference on Pediatric Research, *Iron Nutrition Revisited—Infancy, Childhood, Adolescence* (Columbus, Ohio: Ross Laboratories, 1981) pp. 89–94

34. A. C. Yao and J. Lind, Effect of gravity on placental transfusion, *Lancet* 2 (1969): 505–508.

35. L. S. Hurley and coauthors, The movement of zinc in maternal and fetal rat tissues in teratogenic zinc deficiency, *Teratology* 1 (1968): 216.

36. L. S. Hurley, J. Gowan, and H. Swenerton, Teratogenic effects of short-term and transitory zinc deficiency in rats, *Teratology* 4 (1971): 199–204.

37. S. Jameson, Effects of zinc deficiency in human reproduction, *Acta Medica Scandinavia Supplement* 593 (1976): 3–89.

38. F. F. Cherry and coauthors, Plasma zinc in hypertension/toxemia and other reproductive variables in adolescent pregnancy, *American Journal of Clinical Nutrition* 34 (1981): 2367–2375.

39. J. C. King, Assessment of techniques for determining human zinc requirements, *Journal of the American Dietetic Association* 86 (1986): 1523–1528.

40. J. N. Udall and coauthors, Interaction of maternal and neonatal obesity, *Pediatrics* 62 (1978): 17–21.

41. L. S. Hurley, Fat-soluble vitamins, *Developmental Nutrition* (Englewood Cliffs, N.J.: Prentice-Hall, 1980), pp. 125–142.

42. Vitamin A and teratogenesis, *Lancet* 1 (1985): 319–320.

43. E. P. Norkus and P. Rosso, Changes in ascorbic acid metabolism of the offspring following high maternal intake of this vitamin in the pregnant guinea pig, *Annals of the New York Academy of Sciences* 258 (1975): 401–409.

44. M. Levine, New concepts in the biology and biochemistry of ascorbic acid, *New England Journal of Medicine* 314 (1986): 892–902.

45. National Center for Health Statistics, personal communication, 3700 West Highway, Hyattsville, Maryland.

46. Petros-Barvazian and Behar, 1978.

47. J. H. Ebbs, F. F. Tisdall, and W. A. Scott, The influence of prenatal diet on the mother and child, *Journal of Nutrition* 22 (1941): 515–526.

48. D. Rush, Z. Stein, and M. Susser, *Diet in Pregnancy: A Randomized Controlled Trial of Prenatal Nutritional Supplementation* (New York: Alan Liss, 1979).

49. J. O. Mora and coauthors, Nutritional supplementation and the outcome of pregnancy. I. Birthweight, *American Journal of Clinical Nutrition* 32 (1979): 455–462.

50. J. P. Habicht and coauthors, Relation of maternal supplementary feeding during pregnancy to birth weight and other sociobiological factors, in *Current Concepts in Nutrition*, vol. 3, ed. M. Winick, (New York: John Wiley and Sons, 1974), pp. 127–146.

51. D. Rush, Nutrition services during pregnancy and birthweight: A retrospective

matched-pair analysis, *Canadian Medical Association Journal* 125 (1981): 574–576.

52. S. O. Adams, G. D. Barr, and R. L. Huenemann, Effect of nutritional supplementation in pregnancy, *Journal of the American Dietetic Association* 72 (1978): 144–147.

53. A. M. Prentice and coauthors, Increased birthweight after prenatal dietary supplementation of rural African women, *American Journal of Clinical Nutrition* 46 (1987): 912–925.

54. J. Metcoff and coauthors, Effect of food supplementation (WIC) during pregnancy on birth weight, *American Journal of Clinical Nutrition* 41 (1985): 933–947.

55. E. T. Kennedy and coauthors, Evaluation of the effect of WIC supplemental feeding on birthweight, *Journal of the American Dietetic Association* 80 (1982): 220–226.

56. M. Susser, Prenatal nutrition, birthweight, and psychological development: An overview of experiments, quasi-experiments, and natural experiments in the past decade, *American Journal of Clinical Nutrition* Supplement 34 (1981): 784–803.

57. J. Villar and J. Rivera, Nutritional supplementation during two consecutive pregnancies and the interim lactation period: Effect on birth weight, *Pediatrics* 81 (1988): 51–57.

58. Food and Nutrition Board, Committee on Dietary Allowances, *Recommended Dietary Allowances*, 9th ed. (Washington, D.C.: National Academy of Sciences, 1980), p. 26.

59. J. C. King, Obesity in pregnancy, in *Dietary Treatment and Prevention of Obesity*, ed. R. T. Frankle and coeditors, (London: John Libbey, 1985), pp. 185–191.

60. Food and Nutrition Board, 1980, p. 85.

61. Food and Nutrition Board, 1980, pp. 89, 94.

62. H. Tippett, Nationwide food consumption survey results, *Family Economics Review*, Spring 1980, pp. 3–22.

63. B. H. Dennis and coauthors, Nutrient intakes among selected North American populations in the Lipid Research Clinics prevalence study: Composition of energy intake, *American Journal of Clinical Nutrition* 41 (1985): 312–329.

64. K. Akers, *A Vegetarian Sourcebook* (New York: Putnam, 1983).

65. Food and Nutrition Board, 1980, pp. 100–101.

66. R. M. Pitkin, Assessment of nutritional status of mother, fetus, and newborn, *American Journal of Clinical Nutrition* Supplement 34 (1981): 658–668

67. L. B. Bailey, C. S. Mahan, and D. Dimperio, Folacin and iron status in low-income pregnant adolescents and mature women, *American Journal of Clinical Nutrition* 33 (1980): 1997–2001; V. Herbert, The vitamin craze, *Archives of Internal Medicine* 140 (1980): 173–176.

68. K. Simmer and coauthors, Are iron-folate supplements harmful? *American Journal of Clinical Nutrition* 45 (1987): 122–125.

69. M. D. Mukherjee and coauthors, Maternal zinc, iron, folic acid, and protein nutriture and outcome of human pregnancy, *American Journal of Clinical Nutrition* 40 (1984): 496–507.

70. T. A. B. Sanders, F. R. Ellis, and J. W. T. Dickerson, Haematological studies on vegans, *British Journal of Nutrition* 40 (1978): 9–15, as cited in A. M. Immerman, Vitamin B_{12} status on a vegetarian diet: A critical review, *World Review of Nutrition and Dietetics* 37 (1981): 38–54.

71. M. J. Albert, V. I. Mathan, and S. J. Baker, Vitamin B_{12} synthesis by human small intestinal bacteria, *Nature* 283 (1980): 781–782.

72. Food and Nutrition Board, 1980, p. 138.

73. Food and Nutrition Board, 1980, p. 138.

74. J. M. Holden, W. R. Wolf, and W. Mertz, Zinc and copper in self-selected diets, *Journal of the American Dietetic Association* 75 (1979): 23–28.

75. Food and Nutrition Board, 1980, p. 146.

76. K. M. Hambidge and coauthors, Zinc nutritional status during pregnancy: A longitudinal study, *American Journal of Clinical Nutrition* 37 (1983): 429–442.

77. M. D. Carroll, S. Abraham, and C. M. Dresser, *Dietary Intake Source Data: United States, 1976–1980*, Vital and Health Statistics, series 11, no. 231, HHS Publication no. (PHS) 83–1681, National Center for Health Statistics, Public Health Service (Washington, D.C., U.S. Government Printing Office, March 1983).

78. Food and Nutrition Board, 1980, p. 130.

79. The American Society for Bone and Mineral Research, *Osteoporosis*, Kelseyville, Calif., 1982.

80. National Institute of Arthritis, Diabetes, and Digestive and Kidney Diseases, *Osteoporosis: Cause, Treatment, Prevention*, NIH Publication no. 83-2226, April 1983.

81. F. B. Glenn, W. D. Glenn, and R. C. Duncan, Fluoride tablet supplementation during pregnancy for caries immunity: A study of the offspring produced, *American Journal of Obstetrics and Gynecology* 143 (1982): 560–564.

82. Food and Nutrition Board, 1980, p. 58.

83. Food and Nutrition Board, 1980, pp. 76–77.

84. V. Newman, R. B. Lyon, and P. O. Anderson, Evaluation of prenatal vitamin-mineral supplements, *Clinical Pharmacy* 6 (1987): 770–777.

85. A. Gormican, J. Valentine, and E. Satter, Relationships of maternal weight gain, prepregnancy weight, and infant birthweight, *Journal of the American Dietetic Association* 77 (1980): 662–667.

86. Committee on Nutrition: *Nutrition in Maternal Health Care* (Chicago: American College of Obstetricians and Gynecologists, 1974).

87. R. L. Naeye, Weight gain and the outcome of pregnancy, *American Journal of Obstetrics and Gynecology* 135 (1979): 3–9.

88. A. R. Frisancho, J. Matos, and P. Flegel, Maternal nutritional status and adolescent pregnancy outcome, *American Journal of Clinical Nutrition* 38 (1983): 739–746.

89. Naeye, 1979.

90. P. Rosso, A new chart to monitor weight gain during pregnancy, *American Journal of Clinical Nutrition* 41 (1985): 644–652.

91. F. E. Hyten and I. Leitch, in *The Physiology of Human Pregnancy* (Oxford: Blackwell Scientific Publications, 1971).

92. F. C. Battaglia and L. O. Lubchenco, A practical classification of newborn infants by birthweight and gestational age, *Journal of Pediatrics* 71 (1967): 159.

93. Tanner, 1978, p. 46.

94. R. Fancourt and coauthors, Follow-up study of small-for-date babies, *British Medical Journal* 1 (1976): 1435–1437; C. Neumann, E. R. Stiehm, and M. Swenseid, Longitudinal study of immune function in intrauterine growth retarded infants (abstract), as cited in *Federation Proceedings* 39 (1980): 888.

95. *Facts about Premature Birth*, 1985.

96. Pitkin, 1981.

97. F. K. Lotgering, R. D. Gilbert, and L. D. Longo, The interactions of exercise and pregnancy: A review, *American Journal of Obstetrics and Gynecology* 149 (1984): 560–568.

98. Pregnancy and infant health, in *Smoking and Health*, a report of the Surgeon General, January 1979, available from Superintendent of Documents, U.S. Government Printing Office, Washington, DC 20402.

99. Surgeon General, 1979.

100. Committee on Nutrition of the Mother and Preschool Child, Food and Nutrition Board, Commission on Life Sciences, Na-

tional Research Council, *Alternative Dietary Practices and Nutrition Abuses in Pregnancy, Summary Report* (Washington, D.C.: National Academy Press, 1982), p. 16.

101. Surgeon General, 1979.

102. National Research Council, 1982.

103. Surgeon General, 1979.

104. National Institute of Nutrition in Canada, Caffeine: A perspective on current concerns, *Nutrition Today*, July/August 1987, pp. 36–38.

105. National Institute of Nutrition in Canada, 1987.

106. W. Srisuphan and M. B. Bracken, Caffeine consumption during pregnancy and association with late spontaneous abortion, *American Journal of Obstetrics and Gynecology* 154 (1986): 14–20.

107. Department of Health and Welfare, Federal-Provincial Subcommittee on Nutrition, Canada's National Guidelines on Prenatal Nutrition, *Nutrition Today*, July/August 1987, pp. 34–35.

108. J. C. Gampel, Marijuana and health, in *Drug Use in Society: Proceedings of Marijuana and Health Conference* (Washington, D.C.: Council on Marijuana and Health, 1984), pp. 1–9.

109. I. J. Chasnoff, Cocaine use in pregnancy, *New England Journal of Medicine* 313 (1985): 666–669.

110. Blood pressure of 140/90 mm mercury during the second half of pregnancy in a woman who has not previously exhibited hypertension indicates PIH. So does a rise in systolic blood pressure of 30 mm or in diastolic blood pressure of 15 mm on at least two occasions more than six hours apart. R. J. Worley, Pathophysiology of pregnancy-induced hypertension, *Clinical Obstetrics and Gynecology* 27 (1984): 821–835.

111. J. M. Belizan and J. Villar, The relationship between calcium intake and edema-, proteinuria-, and hypertension-gestosis: An hypothesis, *American Journal of Clinical Nutrition* 33 (1980): 2202–2210.

112. H. M. Linkswiler and coauthors, Protein-induced hypercalciuria, *Federal Proceedings* 40 (1981): 2429–2433.

113. Management of gestational diabetes, *Nutrition and the M.D.*, February 1982, pp. 2–3.

114. M. Wynn and A. Wynn, Effects of nutrition on reproductive capability, *Nutrition and Health* 1 (1983): 165–178.

115. I. L. Spratt, Session V: Report of Workshop Chairmen, Summary and Recommendations, *Diabetes Care* 3 (1980): 499–501; C. P. Weiner and M. W. Varner, Nutritional considerations in diabetic pregnancy, *Clinical Nutrition* 3 (1984): 5.

116. Spratt, 1980.

▶ *Focal Point 2*

Fetal Alcohol Syndrome

Every pregnant woman wants her child to be "normal"—to be free of mental or physical defects. When asked if she wants a boy or a girl, a pregnant woman will oftentimes reply that it does not really matter as long as the child is healthy.

Some women bear children who are not perfectly healthy, however, and often this is beyond their control. Much of an infant's development is genetically determined, and so some errors are inherited. One such disorder, PKU, is highlighted in Focal Point 1. For such a defect, prevention is impossible, but the disorder can be controlled with proper treatment. The subject of this discussion is fetal alcohol syndrome (FAS), a defect for which the reverse is true. FAS can only be prevented; no treatment is possible. In this situation, the expectant mother can take control; she can actively reject beverages that can harm her child.

fetal alcohol syndrome (FAS): the cluster of symptoms seen in an infant or child whose mother consumed excess alcohol during her pregnancy; includes mental impairment, growth retardation, and facial malformations.

Fetal Alcohol Syndrome

The many mental and physical characteristics that FAS children have in common define the syndrome. The one characteristic that all mothers of FAS infants have in common is alcohol consumption during pregnancy.

FAS is not always recognized by physicians; therefore its incidence can only be estimated. The actual numbers may be higher than we realize. The incidence of FAS in the United States is estimated to range from 0.4 to 2.6 per 1000 live births.[1] The lower rates are seen in rural areas where the alcoholism rate is low, and the higher rates in metropolitan areas where alcoholism is more prevalent.

Effects of FAS

fetal alcohol effects (FAE): effects of maternal alcohol consumption on the fetus, not severe enough to be diagnosed FAS, but still detectable.

Alcohol damages the fetus in several ways. It retards growth, impairs development of the central nervous system, and causes facial malformations. Abnormalities in these three areas are used as the minimum criteria for diagnosing FAS. Some infants suffer the consequences of alcohol consumption yet do not meet all these criteria for diagnosis. The term fetal alcohol effects (FAE) is used in such cases. The exact criteria for FAS are as follows:[2]

1. *Prenatal and/or postnatal growth retardation with weight, length, and/or head circumference below the tenth percentile on growth charts.*

It is easy to see that the infant with FAS is much smaller than others, even at birth. The head circumference is smaller than would be expected, even for a small infant. Infants with FAS experience little postnatal catch-up growth, even with adequate nutrition and care.[3] With proper nutrition, most other infants born with a low weight or height experience a period of catch-up growth that takes them closer to the average. FAS children are frequently evaluated as having failure to thrive syndrome, and remain growth deficient until puberty. With the onset of the adolescent growth spurt, these children approach normal weight for height values.[4]

failure to thrive syndrome: failure of a child to develop mentally and physically.

2. *Central nervous system involvement with neurologic abnormality, developmental delay, or intellectual impairment.* Signs may include:

▸ Low IQ.

▸ Poor coordination.

▸ Extreme nervousness.

▸ Irritability.

▸ Hyperactivity.

▸ Fine motor problems.

▸ Delayed gross motor development.

FAS is the third most common cause of mental retardation in this country.[5] In addition to their mental disabilities, FAS children often have behavioral problems. They are irritable and fussy as infants and difficult to control as children.

3. *Characteristic facial disfigurations.*

The most obvious symptoms of FAS are the abnormal facial features, as illustrated in the photograph. These facial abnormalities reflect inadequate development of the brain, as well as of parts of the face, and they are permanent. The child does not outgrow them.

This is an important point. The FAS child's physical features are different from those of normal children, but these features alone are not a handicap. What is a handicap is that the brain's capabilities mirror the facial structure. The more severe the facial characteristics, the more severe the mental function impairment. Alcohol is responsible for both.

Another effect of alcohol is that many FAS infants are too weak to suck effectively. Sucking is an infant's natural response to hunger. Sucking develops facial muscles and enables the infant to obtain nutrients from either a bottle of formula or a mother's breast. An infant who does not suck vigorously may appear apathetic to feeding. This serious feeding problem can easily lead to malnutrition, which further limits the growth of the infant, who is destined never to reach full potential.

In addition to the effects seen in the FAS child, alcohol prevents the birth of some children. Spontaneous abortions occur more frequently in women who drink more than two alcoholic beverages daily than in women who do not drink.[6]

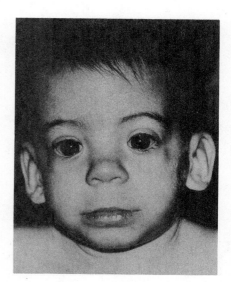

Characteristic facial abnormalities of FAS include low nasal bridge, short eyelid opening, underdeveloped groove in center of the upper lip below the nose, thin reddish upper lip, small midface, short nose, and small head circumference.

How FAS Arises: Alcohol Metabolism

When a person drinks an alcoholic beverage, the alcohol moves rapidly from the digestive system into the blood. The alcohol-laden blood then enters the

Focal Point 6 discusses alcohol metabolism in more detail.

liver, which can detoxify it. There is a limit, however, to the amount of alcohol the liver can process in a given time. The potential for fetal damage arises when the liver receives more alcohol than it can handle. Alcohol that is not detoxified on the first pass through the liver enters the general circulation; once in the bloodstream, it circulates to all parts of the body.

In a pregnant woman, alcohol freely crosses the placenta to the fetus. Fetal blood-alcohol concentrations rise until they reach an equilibrium with maternal blood-alcohol concentrations.[7] This might not seem to be a problem if the mother is functioning well (is not drunk), but while blood levels are the same for the mother and unborn child, the fetus's body is significantly smaller and its detoxification system is less developed. Blood-alcohol concentrations tend to fall more slowly in the fetus than in the mother, and alcohol can be detected in fetal blood after it has totally disappeared from maternal blood. As Dr. C. F. Enloe, past editor of *Nutrition Today*, has observed: After she [the mother] has become drunk she usually has a hangover. That will pass away in a few hours. For the fetus, the hangover may last a lifetime.[8]

How Much Is Too Much?

The Surgeon General has issued a statement that pregnant women should drink absolutely no alcohol. Dr. Enloe agrees. So far, no "safe" level of alcohol consumption during pregnancy has been established, and there is no evidence of benefits to mother or fetus. Thus, such advice is in the best interest of both mother and fetus.

Dr. Enloe creates the following hypothetical situation. Suppose a pregnant woman drinks *one* martini on an empty stomach. The alcohol will be rapidly absorbed and will quite likely be more than the liver can readily detoxify. Excess alcohol will circulate through the body to the uterus, cross the placenta, and enter the fetal bloodstream. If vital cells are being developed at that moment, the exposure to alcohol may irreversibly damage those cells.

The American Council on Science and Health (ACSH) takes a more liberal stand that many health care providers do not support. Its position statement recommends that women be cautious about alcohol use during pregnancy, and advises a daily limit of two 12-ounce beers, two 4-ounce glasses of wine, or two drinks with 1 1/2 ounces of 80-proof liquor.[9] It maintains that the health risks associated with this level of alcohol consumption are low or nonexistent. While it is true that no risks have been observed at a low level of drinking, absence of risk cannot be conclusively established.[10]

The ACSH issued this statement after a review of current scientific evidence examining the relationship between alcohol consumption and reproductive effects. While it is clear that excessive alcohol consumption is hazardous to the fetus, it is not clear at what level, if any, it is safe. The ACSH recommendation allows the many women who drink in this country to continue limited, occasional drinking during pregnancy without feelings of guilt.

The ACSH supports the pregnant woman who has a margarita on a Saturday night, sips a glass of champagne on her birthday, or drinks a beer at a ball game. She should not endure the nine months of her pregnancy, they say, with feelings of fear or guilt. Such stress may, indeed, be more damaging to the unborn child than an occasional alcoholic beverage.

The percentage of alcohol in distilled liquor is stated as proof: 100-proof liquor is 50% alcohol; 90 proof is 45% , and so forth. A drink is a dose of any alcoholic beverage that delivers 1/2 oz of pure ethanol:

► 3 to 4 oz wine.
► 10 oz wine cooler.
► 12 oz beer.
► 1 oz hard liquor (whiskey, gin, rum, vodka).

No doubt it is important to distinguish between heavy drinking, which almost invariably affects the unborn child, and moderate drinking, which in some cases does not. The difference between Dr. Enloe's "no-drinks" position and the ACSH's "occasional-drinks" position is one of philosophy. There is undeniably a risk associated with *any* drinking during pregnancy; the ACSH position simply states that that risk is small enough to be negligible.

Indeed, in comparison with other risks in pregnancy, *moderate* drinking does not stand out as a *great* danger. Many other factors affect the outcome of pregnancy. The mother's socioeconomic level, age, emotional stability, diet, drug use, smoking habits, genetic makeup, and prenatal care all play at least as great a role as an alcoholic beverage or two. However, the effects of alcohol during pregnancy may be intensified by nicotine, caffeine, or other drugs. In studies of both women and animals, the extent of fetal damage seems to correlate directly with the quantity of alcohol the mother consumes.[11]

Now it remains to define moderate drinking. A pregnant woman need not be an alcoholic in order to give birth to a baby with FAS characteristics. She only needs to drink in excess of the liver's capacity to detoxify. Reports from mothers of FAS children reveal they consumed an average of five or more drinks daily throughout their pregnancies. Does this mean that four drinks or less per day are safe? Probably not, for researchers cannot be sure they are obtaining accurate measures of alcohol consumption. Many women are reluctant to admit they drank during their pregnancies. Mothers of deformed infants often feel guilty and responsible for their children's defects. It is not surprising that they are not willing to be interviewed or to let it be known that they have understated their alcohol intakes.

Most FAS studies speak only of average intake. Little is known about the effects of periodic binge drinking. How does a drinking binge at a critical time compare with the same amount of alcohol consumed over a longer period of time? Most likely it depends on the frequency of binges, the quantity consumed, and fetal development at the time.

In conclusion, it is impossible to say whether small amounts of alcohol are safe during pregnancy. The risk associated with occasional drinking is less than that associated with heavy drinking, but why take any risk? The mother who chooses to drink during pregnancy, even moderately, is at greater risk than the mother who abstains completely.

There seems to be a gap between people's understanding of the effects of alcohol on an unborn child and their estimation of how many drinks constitutes a "moderate" level of safe drinking. One study reported that 90 percent of those surveyed were aware of the risks of drinking during pregnancy, but thought that an average of three drinks daily was safe.[12] We believe it was wise for the Surgeon General to have taken such a conservative position after all.

When Is the Damage Done?

There is no time when drinking excessively is safe. The type and extent of abnormality observed in an FAS infant seems to depend on the developmental events that are occurring at the time the fetus is exposed to alcohol.

In experiments on laboratory animals, the effects of alcohol on fetal development are most marked when the female takes alcohol during the earliest period—that of organ formation. Effects also appear when a dose of alcohol elevates the female's blood-alcohol level immediately prior to conception; the amount of alcohol in the female's blood is critical. Male alcohol ingestion may also affect fertility and fetal development. Animal studies have found decreased litter size, birthweight, survival, and learning ability in the offspring of males consuming alcohol prior to conception.[13] One human study found an association between paternal alcohol intake one month prior to conception (defined as an average of two or more drinks daily or at least five drinks on one occasion) and decreased infant birthweight.[14] This relationship was independent of parents' smoking or maternal use of alcohol, caffeine, or other drugs.

Different dangers are associated with each trimester of pregnancy.[15] In the first trimester, developing organs such as the brain, heart, and kidneys may be malformed. During the second trimester, the risk of spontaneous abortion increases. During the third trimester, when the fetus is fully formed and rapidly growing, body and brain growth may be retarded.

Maternal Malnutrition

One of the health hazards associated with alcohol abuse is malnutrition. Alcohol depresses appetite because it produces euphoria, so that heavy drinkers usually eat poorly, if at all. Alcohol also attacks the digestive tract lining, causing pain and malabsorption of nutrients.

Many women who abuse alcohol can easily drink 100 grams of ethanol a day. This amount is roughly equivalent to eight beers, a pint of whiskey, or a bottle of wine. Alcohol provides 7.1 kcalories per gram, so the daily kcaloric intake from alcohol alone can be over 700 kcalories. The woman who derives so many kcalories from a source that has no nutritive value finds it difficult to obtain, from the additional kcalories she can consume, the many essential nutrients she needs to maintain her health and support the fetus's growth.

Not only do alcohol abusers suffer malnutrition from lack of food, but even if they eat well, the direct effects of alcohol take their toll. Alcohol hinders the absorption, alters the metabolism, and increases the excretion of many nutrients, so that malnutrition can occur even in a well-fed drinker. Many nutrient deficiencies are associated with alcohol abuse. For example, folacin deficiency is common in people with a history of alcoholism. During pregnancy, the need for this vitamin is doubled. Women with poor nutrition status and such high nutrient needs put themselves in a precarious situation when they drink alcohol.

Thus, an alcohol-abusing pregnant woman harms her unborn child not only by consuming alcohol but also by not consuming food. This combination enhances the likelihood of malnutrition and a poorly developed infant. However, it is important to realize that malnutrition is not the cause of FAS. It is true that mothers of FAS children often have unbalanced diets and nutrient deficiencies. It is also true that malnutrition may augment the clinical signs seen in these children, but it is the *alcohol* that is the determining factor. An adequate diet will not prevent FAS if alcohol is abused during the pregnancy; without alcohol, the pattern of FAS is not seen.

Ethanol is the alcohol in beer, wine, and liquor. For purposes of comparison, 100 g of ethanol is more than 3 oz (1 oz is equivalent to 28 g). An ounce of 100-proof whiskey (1 "drink") is 50% alcohol, so it requires 6 or 7 drinks to imbibe 3 oz of pure alcohol.

Counseling and Prevention

The health care provider who realizes a pregnant woman drinks heavily and has no intention of quitting faces a difficult challenge. Drinking is more important to this woman than the theoretical possibility of harming an infant she has never touched and does not yet love. The task is to provide her with the information that alcohol causes birth defects, and make it clear that the connection is well established. She should understand that the only way to be sure of excluding the possibility of this kind of retardation is to abstain from drinking altogether throughout the pregnancy. The decision to abstain or not is hers, however, not the health care provider's. The responsibility of the health care provider ends when the woman has been given the information. Pushing the woman to make the decision will alienate her. She will thereafter be less inclined to confide in those trying to help her. This will also limit opportunities to guide her in other nutrition choices.

If she does decide to quit drinking, at least during the pregnancy, she deserves a pat on the back. Let her know she has made a wise decision and that the sooner she abstains, the less risk for her unborn child.

At the other extreme is the anxious woman who is usually quite careful of her health but who had a cocktail with friends during the first month of her pregnancy, before she even knew she was pregnant. Now she fears her infant will be born with mental and physical defects. In such a situation, the chances are very small that harm will have been done. The woman should be reassured that such small quantities of alcohol often does not harm the developing infant. Many drinkers, even heavy drinkers, bear normal babies. Furthermore, and even more important, the episode is in the past, and nothing can be done to change it. The choices she makes now affect the present and the future, not the past.

A pregnancy can be a long, suspenseful experience, especially if parents fear an imperfect outcome. The health care provider should minimize the things that cannot be changed and emphasize what can be done now and in the future to ensure the best possible outcome.

The one happy note in this FAS story is that, of the leading causes of mental retardation, it is the only one that is totally preventable. Every female, indeed every person, should know the potential dangers of alcohol use during pregnancy. Proper health care instructions and education should begin *before* conception. FAS information should be included in all classes that discuss birth control, sexual intercourse, or pregnancy.[16] The message should be clear: FAS can be prevented by maternal avoidance of alcohol.

Focal Point 2 Notes

1. F. L. Iber, Fetal alcohol syndrome, *Nutrition Today*, September/October 1980, pp. 4–11.
2. H. L. Rosett and L. Weiner, Alcohol and pregnancy: A clinical perspective, *Annual Review of Medicine* 36 (1985): 73–80.
3. M. Lee and J. Leichter, Alcohol and the fetus, in *Adverse Effects of Foods*, ed. E. F. P. Jelliffe and D. B. Jelliffe (New York: Plenum Press, 1982), pp. 245–251.
4. A. P. Streissguth, S. K. Clarren, and K. L. Jones, Natural history of the fetal alcohol syndrome: A 10–year follow-up of eleven patients, *Lancet* (1985): 85–91.
5. A report by the American Council on Science and Health, *Alcohol Use during Pregnancy*, 1981.
6. Iber, 1980.
7. C. F. Enloe, How alcohol affects the developing fetus, *Nutrition Today*, September/October 1980, pp. 12–15.
8. Enloe, 1980.
9. A report by the American Council on Science and Health, *Alcohol Use during Pregnancy*, 1981.

10. H. L. Rosett and L. Weiner, Alcohol and pregnancy: A clinical perspective, *Annual Review of Medicine* 36 (1985): 73–80.

11. W. S. Beagle, Fetal alcohol syndrome: A review, *Journal of the American Dietetic Association* 79 (1981): 274–276.

12. R. E. Little and coauthors, Public awareness and knowledge about the risks of drinking during pregnancy in Multnomah County, Oregon, *American Journal of Public Health* 71 (1981): 312–314.

13. L. F. Soyka and J. M. Joffe, Male mediated drug effects on offspring, *Progress in Clinical and Biological Research* 36 (1980): 49–66.

14. R. E. Little and C. F. Sing, Father's drinking and infant birth weight, *Teratology* 36 (1987): 59–65.

15. Rosett and Weiner, 1985.

16. An excellent ten-minute film entitled *Born Drunk: The Fetal Alcohol Syndrome* is available from ABC Wide World of Learning, Inc., 1330 Avenue of the Americas, New York, NY 10019, (212) 887–5000.

Postpartum:
Breastfeeding and Formula Feeding

3

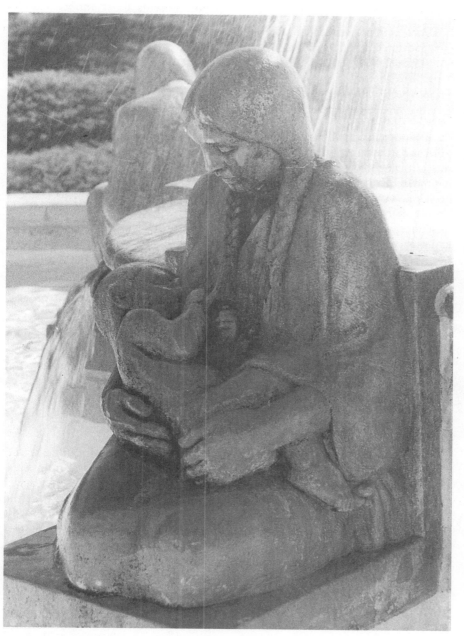

Detail from *Fountain of the Seasons* by Christian Petersen.

Childbirth marks the end of pregnancy and the beginning of a new set of parental responsibilities, decisions, and behaviors. Many of these focus on care of the newborn. Newborns arrive without an instruction manual, and people become parents without any formal training. Parents must gather information from a variety of sources to determine what to do and how and when to do it. Translating this information into action requires making many adjustments and learning a number of new behaviors. This chapter describes the responsibility of feeding an infant—the factors that influence the decision of what to feed the infant and the behaviors parents must adopt to do so successfully.

Infant Feeding: Breast Milk or Formula?

An infant grows most rapidly during the first four to six months of life. Breast milk and infant formula are the only recommended sources of nutrients during this critical time. In many countries around the world, a woman breastfeeds her newborn without considering the alternatives or consciously making a decision. In other parts of the world, a woman feeds her newborn formula simply because she knows so little about breastfeeding. She may have misconceptions or feel uncomfortable about a process she has never seen or experienced. In both settings, mothers might benefit from knowledge about both alternatives before deciding what best meets their own needs and the needs of their infants.

Appendix F provides a list of nutrition resources.

To learn about infant feeding practices, a pregnant woman can read one of the many books available. Other good sources of information are health care providers and mothers who have successfully breastfed and formula fed their infants. In addition to these resources, a woman examines her personal values and those of the society in which she lives. Each contributes to the decision-making process. The following discussion examines factors influencing the decision whether to breastfeed or formula feed an infant.

Societal Support

Prior to the eighteenth century, substitutes for breast milk were nonexistent. Human milk was the only source of nourishment for a newborn infant. If a mother could not or did not want to breastfeed her infant, she hired a wet nurse. Deplorable sanitary conditions, as well as strange beliefs held at the time, precluded even the thought of using cow's milk to feed an infant.

wet nurse: a woman who breastfeeds another woman's infant.

Around the mid-1700s, women adopted the practice of feeding infants a mixture of bread and flour soaked in water once the first tooth had erupted. In 1874, an author first wrote of the usefulness of cow's milk when breast milk was unavailable.[1] A major problem at the time was the lack of an appropriate feeding instrument for the infant. (Cow's milk was first fed, logically, by way of a cow's horn.) By the end of the eighteenth century, the advantages of glass bottles and the need for cleanliness were recognized.

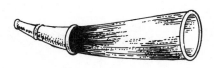

Cow's horn

Formula feeding gained popularity as the "modern," efficient, and practical way to feed an infant at the turn of this century. For the infants of women who were unable to breastfeed or who had died in childbirth, formulas offered an alternative. Formula feeding coincided with the rise in hospital births and the associated practice of separating mothers from infants after delivery. Other twentieth-century phenomena also influenced the shift from breast to formula. One obvious accomplishment of this time was the development of the technology required to analyze breast milk and to create a formula that was similar. Systems to purify water supplies and to control pathogenic organisms allowed formula feeding to develop as a safe method of nourishing infants. Simultaneous trends were seen in the advertising and fashion industries as they grew bolder in glamorizing women's bodies to a point of distorting the natural function of breasts. To view the breasts primarily as sex objects is to forget that their primary function is to provide milk to a suckling infant.

Breastfeeding steadily declined until less than one in five U.S. mothers of newborns was engaging in it. During the 1970s, the trend reversed until, by the 1980s, three out of every five new mothers were choosing to breastfeed.[2] About half of these women are still breastfeeding at three months and only one-fourth of those still breastfeeding at three months continue through the first year.[3] Statistics for Canada are somewhat lower and follow a similar trend. As might be expected, the incidence of breastfeeding progressively declines throughout the first year of the infant's life. In developing countries, the initial incidence of breastfeeding is much higher than in developed countries and the decline over the first year is much smaller.[4]

The medical profession, recognizing the nutritional and immunological benefits, endorses breastfeeding as the preferred method of infant feeding. Society now embraces the old practice of breastfeeding once again as an integral part of motherhood and child care. The increasing incidence of breastfeeding in recent years coincides with the decreasing incidence of formula feeding *during the early months of infancy*. Formula feeding is also on the increase, however, due to the trend toward diminished use of cow's milk *during the later months of infancy*. Specifically, for infants three to five months old, the use of formulas has increased 20 percent since 1971.[5]

Although lactation is an automatic physiological process, breastfeeding is a learned behavior. This learning is most successful in a supportive cultural environment. In societies where few women breastfeed, appropriate breastfeeding etiquette remains undefined. A woman faces conflict, confusion, and frustration. Must she retreat to a private place to nurse? What if she cannot find such a place in a public setting? A hungry infant is impatient, and a mother must act quickly. With abundant role models, a consensus defines accepted behaviors, thus offering a nursing mother guidance and confidence. Many public buildings now offer "baby rooms" with tables for changing diapers and comfortable chairs for nursing. These rooms are open to both mothers and fathers, in response to current parenting needs.

Another need of parents in today's society is to coordinate work and family. All mothers are working women—many of them with jobs outside of the home. A social system that provides extended, paid maternity leaves, nursing breaks on the job, and at-the-job-site child care promotes breastfeeding as a realistic option for infant feeding.

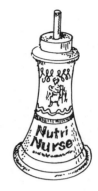

18th century German pewter nursing bottle

"There is a reason behind all these things in nature." Aristotle

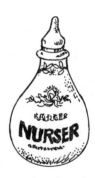

19th century American glass nurser

lactation (lack-TAY-shun): maternal secretion of milk for a suckling offspring.

Differences between Breast Milk and Formula

Breast milk is the ideal infant food. With the possible exception of vitamin D and fluoride (whose concentrations in breast milk are extremely low), breast milk is tailor-made to meet the nutrient needs of a newborn.[6] The breast milk of a healthy, well-nourished mother contains most essential nutrients in the appropriate quantities and proportions to support optimal growth and development. In addition, the nutrients are of high bioavailability and digestibility (Chapter 4 describes each nutrient in detail). For example, breast milk iron, although low in quantity, is available in a highly absorbable form.[7] Chemists working for formula manufacturers attempt to copy human milk as closely as possible.

The well-nourished mother can therefore feel confident that the quality of milk she gives her infant is the best available. There is a limit to the supply per feeding for the breastfed infant, but most mothers can produce more than adequate quantities by feeding frequently if necessary. On the other hand, the differences in nutrients delivered by breast milk and formula are not great enough to cause the formula-feeding mother any anxiety. The mother who feeds her infant formula, of course, can feel confident that the quantity of milk she gives her infant is adequate, even at a single feeding. She can see the bottle being emptied and can replenish it as needed. The supply is limited only by finances.

No matter how close they get, formula manufacturers cannot duplicate human milk exactly. Breast milk confers immunological protection that formula cannot provide. Milks of each species contain natural factors that are highly individual and characteristic of the species. These factors protect infants from infections, as is evident in the higher hospitalization rates of formula-fed infants the first 18 months of life.[8]

This does not necessarily mean that feeding human milk is the only way to protect infants from illnesses. Formulas prepared under sanitary conditions minimize exposure to pathological organisms. In developed countries, preventive medical care (such as vaccinations) and public health measures (such as purified water) help to protect infants from infections. Safety and sanitation can be achieved with either mode of feeding by the informed mother whose water supply is reliable.

In countries where poor sanitation is prevalent, breastfeeding takes priority over feeding formula. Failure to breastfeed an infant who lives in a house without piped water and a toilet incurs twice the risk of perinatal mortality as for a breastfed infant living in a house with good sanitation.[9]

Chapter 4's discussion on feeding the infant provides more details on colostrum and immune resistance.

Medical Considerations

Some medical situations weigh on the question whether breastfeeding is the appropriate choice. If a woman has a communicable disease that could threaten the infant's health so that they have to be separated, then, of course, she cannot breastfeed. Similarly, a physician may advise a woman with a chronic disease against breastfeeding if it would be a drain on her energy and a strain on her emotional health.

Formula feeding is preferred, and can even be lifesaving, in some medical circumstances. The woman who has a positive antibody test for AIDS is advised to formula feed her infant. The AIDS virus can be transmitted through breast milk and infect the infant.

Infants with specific metabolic disorders, such as PKU, must receive special formulas, such as Lofenelac. In these cases, not only must the infant receive formula instead of or in addition to breast milk, but the formula must meet exact specifications (see page 131, "Special Formulas"). Some circumstances, such as lactose intolerance and protein allergies, may appear to warrant formula feeding in preference to breastfeeding. Yet infants with these conditions often do better with mother's milk than with formulas.

If a woman must take medication that is known to harm the infant and that will be secreted in breast milk, she must opt for formula feeding, at least temporarily. Many prescription drugs do not reach nursing infants in sufficient quantities to affect them adversely. Some, however, do. Table 3–1 presents a list of drugs that are contraindicated during breastfeeding and shows their effects on infants and lactation. In addition, drugs containing radioactivity (such as iodine 131) require temporary cessation of breastfeeding. The length of cessation depends on the specific drug. To maintain lactation during times of cessation, the mother should express her milk and discard it. If a woman must take a medication that is regarded as generally safe, she can minimize any effects by taking the drug while or immediately after the infant nurses. This will provide the lowest amount of drug in the breast milk at the next feeding.[10]

Considerations for Preterm Infants

Preterm infants have special needs, which are discussed in Chapter 4. Researchers have compared three sources of nutrients to meet these needs: breast milk from mothers of preterm infants, breast milk from mothers of term infants, and formula designed for preterm infants. They find that preterm milk and special formulas support infant growth better than full-term milk, even though preterm infants tolerate full-term milk well.[11]

A preterm mother's milk supports more rapid infant growth better than the milk of a full-term mother because its composition is more suited to a preterm infant's needs. Formula designed for preterm infants also offers a growth advantage over feeding with mature human milk. The breast milk of preterm mothers differs in some nutrient concentrations and in milk volume from that of term mothers.[12] During early lactation, preterm milk contains higher concentrations of protein and is lower in volume than term milk. Controversy surrounds the question of whether the higher protein concentrations are real or merely a reflection of milk volume.[13] The low milk volume is advantageous because preterm infants are unable to consume large quantities of milk per feeding, and the higher protein concentration allows for better growth. Some researchers argue that the differences are real and reflect a premature stage of lactation.[14] The physical and hormonal activities of the reproductive cycle and of mammary gland development have been prematurely halted. The composition of preterm milk closely resembles colostrum, the

Table 3–1 Drugs That Are Contraindicated during Breastfeeding

Drug	Registered name	Indications	Reported Sign or Symptom in Infant or Effect on Lactation
Amethopterin methotrexate[a]			Possible immune suppression; unknown effect on growth or association with carcinogenesis
Bromocriptine mesylate	Parlodel	Amenorrhea, female infertility, suppress lactation, Parkinson's disease	Suppresses lactation
Cimetidine hydrochloride[b]	Tagamet	Ulcers	May suppress gastric acidity in infant, inhibit drug metabolism, and cause central nervous system stimulation
Clemastine fumarate	Tavist	Allergies	Drowsiness, irritability, refusal to feed, high-pitched cry, neck stiffness
Cyclophosphamide[a]	Cytoxan	Malignancies	Possible immune suppression; unknown effect on growth or association with carcinogenesis
Ergotamine tartrate	Cafergot	Migraine headaches	Vomiting, diarrhea, convulsions (doses used in migraine medications)
Gold salts	Myochrysine	Rheumatoid arthritis	Rash, inflammation of kidney and liver
Methimazole	Tapazole	Hyperthyroidism	Potential for interfering with thyroid function
Phenindione			Hemorrhage
Thiouracil			Decreased thyroid function; does not apply to propylthiouracil

[a] Data not available for other cytotoxic agents.
[b] Drug is concentrated in breast milk.

Sources: Adapted from American Academy of Pediatrics, Committee on Drugs, The transfer of drugs and other chemicals into human breastmilk, *Pediatrics* 72 (1983): 375–384; and *Physician's Desk Reference* 42nd ed. (Oradell, N.J.: Medical Economics Company, 1988).

earliest secretion of lactation. In either case, most authorities agree that preterm milk best meets the specific needs of a preterm infant.

In many instances, mixtures of nutrients specifically designed for preterm infants are added to the mother's expressed breast milk and fed to the infant from a bottle. Based on theoretical estimates of the requirements of preterm infants, preterm milk may be an inadequate source of some nutrients. Specifically, the calcium and phosphorus in preterm milk may be insufficient. The combination of preterm human milk fortified with a preterm supplement supports growth at a rate that approximates the rate that would have occurred in utero.[15]

A mother can provide her preterm infant with her milk even if she is unable to actually breastfeed. That is, if her infant is isolated in an incubator in the intensive care unit, she can express her milk for the infant to receive by bottle.

A description of expressing breast milk is given on page 125.

Alcohol, Other Drugs, and Environmental Contaminants

Drug addicts, including alcohol abusers, are capable of consuming such high doses that their infants can become addicts by way of breast milk; in these cases, formula feeding is preferred. Moderate consumption of alcohol is compatible with breastfeeding (one cocktail, or one glass of wine, or one beer per day). However, indiscriminate or excessive drinking while breastfeeding may cause drowsiness, weakness, and slowed growth in infants.[16]

A woman may hesitate to breastfeed because she has learned that environmental contaminants can find their way into breast milk and she fears their potential harm to her infant. As adaptable and nutritious as human breast milk is, it does not contain a magic filter for contaminants. Substances, such as pesticides and toxic wastes, may at times be present in breast milk. Whether they are present depends on what the mother has ingested, the quantity consumed, and the interval between ingestion and breastfeeding.

Contaminants are often widespread in the environment; consumed by people in the foods they eat and the air they breathe; stored in the body's fat tissues; and slowly degraded and excreted.[17] Long-term exposure to contaminants leads to a gradual accumulation in the body's fat, including breast milk fat. Lactation is a means of excreting contaminants.

Prior to the 1972 federal restrictions on the use of the pesticide DDT, several studies reported DDT in the milk of mothers at concentrations greater than the federal government allows in dairy milk meant for human consumption.[18] This may be partly explained by the difference in the DDT excretion rate between women and cows. Lactating women excrete most of their DDT intake, while cows excrete very little.[19] Fortunately, studies did not find that breastfed infants of mothers excreting DDT were less healthy than formula-fed infants.

DDT is dichlorodiphenyl trichloroethane.

Other toxic wastes of concern are the PCBs, found in rivers and waterways polluted by industry. PCBs are organic chemicals used in such products as paint and caulking compounds. According to the Committee on Environmental Hazards of the American Academy of Pediatrics, only women who have eaten large amounts of fish caught in PCB-contaminated rivers, such as the Saint Lawrence Seaway, or who have been directly exposed to PCBs in their occupations need fear breast milk contamination.[20] A woman with concerns

PCBs are polychlorinated biphenyls.

about her exposure to toxic substances can obtain information from her local health department.

Effects on the Mother's Body

Breastfeeding may offer medical benefits to the mother as well as to the infant. Evidence suggests that lactation protects women from later breast cancer.[21] Whether the physical and hormonal events of breastfeeding are protective or the imbalances that lead to unsuccessful lactation also predispose a woman to breast cancer is unclear. Of course, in either case, the fear of contracting a life-threatening disease is an unsound basis for deciding to breastfeed.

Some women fear that breastfeeding will cause their breasts to sag. The breasts do swell and become heavy and large immediately after the infant is born, but they eventually shrink back to their prepregnant size, even when they are producing enough milk to nourish a thriving infant. With proper support, diet, and exercise, breasts return to their former shape and size after weaning, at the latest. Breasts change their shape as the body ages, but breastfeeding does not accelerate this process.

Breastfeeding can actually aid in restoring a woman's body to its nonpregnant state. The infant's suckling stimulates the nerves controlling the muscles of the uterus, causing them to contract. The contractions expel any tissue remaining after the birth, and return the uterus to its normal size. Milk production also requires energy, which can help a lactating mother lose weight more quickly. Breastfeeding facilitates the mobilization of fat stored during pregnancy. A woman who chooses nutrient-dense foods during lactation will experience a gradual weight loss, even though her energy intake is greater than normal. Breastfeeding does not, however, promote rapid, easy, weight loss and should not be expected to do so. Disappointment arising from such false expectations may lead some women to stop nursing their infants earlier than they had originally intended.[22]

Some women find the delayed onset of ovulation, and the consequent delay of menstruation during lactation, a pleasant bonus. (They should not, however, count on it for contraception, as explained in the upcoming section, Postpartum Amenorrhea.) The onset of menstruation does not interfere with lactation.

Bonding

bonding: a process that occurs immediately after birth in which a mother forms an affectionate attachment to her infant.

Some breastfeeding proponents argue that breastfeeding encourages bonding. The affection of a mother for her infant depends more on the time spent in close physical contact than on the method of feeding. There is evidence, however, to suggest that mothers allowed early extended contact with their newborns are more likely to breastfeed and to continue to do so for a longer duration than mothers denied contact. This is not to say that breastfeeding mothers bond better than mothers who feed their infants formulas, but that early, prolonged contact facilitates both bonding and breastfeeding.

Controversy surrounds the question whether early and extended mother-child contact is crucial to bonding.[23] The notion that a bond develops during a sensitive period just after birth that has a profound effect on the parent-child relationship is based on observations of farm animals. In animals, the bond between a mother and her offspring forms within the first few minutes of life. If the two are separated during this crucial time, the mother later rejects the offspring. She refuses to nurse and exhibits physically hostile behaviors toward the newborn. A brief initial contact, even if followed by a separation, is sufficient to establish the relationship. A variety of visual, auditory, and olfactory cues establishes the maternal acceptance of the offspring. Most likely, postpartum hormonal conditions influence maternal acceptance.

In human beings, mothering behaviors are more complex than can be explained by cues and hormones alone. The actual birth in human beings is preceded by months of maternal thought and anticipation. Many women begin the bonding process during pregnancy. They pat their bellies when they feel a kick, attend childbirth classes, read books, seek advice from friends, and decorate the baby's room. A woman enters motherhood with memories of her own relationship with her mother. She has learned her culture's patterns of mother-child interaction. Whether the infant was planned or wanted also affects the mother's maternal behaviors, as does her relationship with the father.

The notion that events at the time of birth can influence the bonding process has altered birth practices in this country. Earlier this century, mother and newborn were separated at birth and cared for in the maternity and nursery wards, respectively. More recently, there has been a trend toward allowing mother and newborn to lie together in a warm and quiet room, often joined by father. Health care providers encourage breastfeeding mothers to nurse their infants immediately after delivery.

Such family-centered birth experiences may indeed promote loving relationships, but the theory is difficult to prove. As is often the case in research involving human beings, designing a methodologically sound and ethical study is close to impossible.[24] In this instance, the results would require subjective interpretations of significance. If one mother picks up her infant more often than another, who is to determine the significance and effects of that behavior?

Convenience

In a society that embraces microwave ovens and frozen foods, convenience plays a large part in the many decisions parents make about feeding themselves and their children. The lifestyles, attitudes, and habits of each individual dictate what is defined as convenient.

The natural way to nourish infants since the beginning of time, breastfeeding is a simple, yet elegant, procedure. Once a woman learns the correct technique, she becomes confident and finds the experience enjoyable. In a few short weeks, the mother and infant adjust to the feeding process and the milk supply is established. Many women find that breastfeeding is as easy as breathing. It can be done anywhere, anytime, as long as mother and infant are together. Breast milk is sterile and always at the appropriate temperature. The breastfeeding mother is free of sterilizing bottles and mixing formulas.

Breastfeeding may not be convenient, however, for a mother whose schedule does not permit her to be with her infant easily at feeding times. A woman who works outside the home may find it less troublesome to feed her infant formula. Hot cycles on a dishwasher make bottle sterilization easy, and measuring, mixing, and pouring formula is easier than preparing any other meal. Ready-to-pour formulas that do not need mixing, although more expensive, are available for busy mothers who can afford them. Another advantage of formulas is that they allow the father and other family members an opportunity to enjoy feeding the infant.

A working mother need not give up breastfeeding. She can breastfeed exclusively until she returns to work. Then, depending on her schedule and location, she can continue to breastfeed some feedings and supplement with formula or expressed breast milk for others. Breastfeeding manuals provide a multitude of hints and suggestions to help her work out the details.

Making the Decision

The decision whether to breastfeed is best made by the parents with the advice of their health care providers. However, quite likely, many friends, relatives, and strangers will voice their opinions. Some will consider breastfeeding old-fashioned and formula feeding more convenient. Others believe the breast best and formulas unnatural. After listening to these people, a woman will ultimately need to rely on well-informed sources for advice and information. She can also obtain help from registered dietitians, instructors at natural childbirth classes, and nurses in the maternity wing of the hospital.

Some women are convinced that breastfeeding offers the best nourishment to their newborns. They are sure within themselves that the suckling of an infant at their breast is a most rewarding experience. Breastfeeding is compatible with their views on mothering and easily fits into their work and home arrangements.

Some women are uncomfortable with breastfeeding; they may attempt to breastfeed, but find they are too nervous or too distracted to successfully nurse an infant. Other women find breastfeeding just does not work with their lifestyles and schedules. These mothers have valid reasons for making their choices, and their feelings need to be honored. Bearing and nurturing an infant involves much more than merely pouring in nutrients.

Many health care providers and dietitians believe breastfeeding is sufficiently important to warrant that every effort be made to do so, even if only for a short time. Of those women who do breastfeed, 25 to 50 percent discontinue within the first month, and 50 to 70 percent discontinue by four months.[25] This duration is long enough to allow the infant to receive immunological protection and other special advantages of breastfeeding during the most critical first few weeks or months. The mother can then shift to formula, knowing she has given her infant those benefits.

If this discussion appears biased in favor of breastfeeding, it is not an accident. Breastfeeding offers many benefits to both mother and infant, and every pregnant woman should seriously consider it. Still, as mentioned earlier, there are many valid reasons for not breastfeeding, and formula-fed infants grow and develop into healthy children. After all, the primary goal is to provide optimal nourishment in a relaxed and loving environment.

The responsibilities and decisions continue once a mother decides how she will feed her infant. If she decides to breastfeed, she will need to learn how to eat to promote optimal milk production. If she decides to feed formula, she will need to learn how to select the appropriate formula and prepare it. Each of these options is discussed in the following sections.

Lactation and Breastfeeding

While much attention is focused on nutrition for pregnant women, infants, and children, nutrition for lactating women is often neglected, but the lactating mother has unique nutrient needs and concerns. Her care and feeding deserve special attention. First, a description of the physiology of lactation sets the foundation for understanding the special nutrient needs of a new mother. Then, a discussion of the behavior of breastfeeding builds on that (see Practical Point: How to Breastfeed, at the end of this section).

Physiology of Lactation

Lactation is the natural extension of pregnancy—of the mother's body nourishing the infant. The mammary glands secrete milk for this purpose.

Figure 3–1 illustrates breast development from puberty to lactation. The mammary glands, stimulated by estrogen during puberty, develop a system of ducts, lobes, and alveoli. This system remains fairly inactive until pregnancy. During pregnancy, hormones stimulate a proliferative stage of mammary gland activity. Estrogen promotes growth and branching of the duct system, while progesterone stimulates development of the alveoli. During pregnancy, the elevated concentrations of these hormones support mammary gland development, while inhibiting the actual secretion of milk. These two hormones return to their basal concentrations within a few days postpartum, thus allowing milk production to begin.[26]

mammary glands: glands of the female breast that secrete milk.

ducts: narrow tubular vessels that drain the lobes of the mammary gland into the tip of the nipple.

lobes: segments of the mammary gland.

alveoli (al-VEE-oh-lie): the milk-producing cells of the mammary gland; the singular is **alveolus**.

Figure 3–1   Breast Development from Puberty to Lactation
During puberty, a system of ducts, lobes, and alveoli develops and remains inactive until pregnancy. During pregnancy, growth proliferates, with ductal branching and lobular-alveolar development proceeding at a spectacular rate, yet in an orderly fashion.

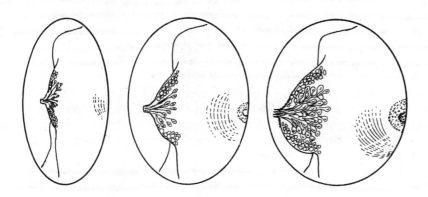

Figure 3–2   Prolactin and Oxytocin Activity

(1) An infant suckling at the breast stimulates the pituitary to release prolactin and oxytocin. Each of these hormones act on the mammary glands, (2) prolactin encourages milk production and (3) oxytocin stimulates milk ejection. Each of the hormones also act on the reproductive organs, (2) prolactin inhibits ovulation and (3) oxytocin promotes uterus contractions.

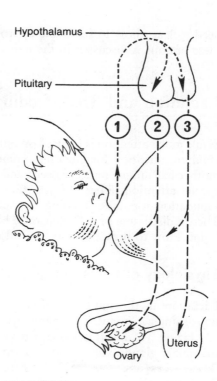

prolactin (pro-LAK-tin): a hormone secreted from the anterior pituitary gland that acts on the mammary glands to initiate and sustain milk production.
pro = promote
lacto = milk

oxytocin (OK-si-TOE-sin): a hormone secreted from the posterior pituitary gland that stimulates the uterus to contract and the mammary glands to eject milk.
oxy = quick
tocin = childbirth

prolactin-inhibiting hormone: a hormone secreted from the hypothalamus that acts on the anterior pituitary gland to regulate the release of prolactin.

myoepithelial cells: contractile cells of the mammary glands.

let-down reflex: the reflex that forces milk to the front of the breast when the infant begins to nurse.

As illustrated in Figure 3–2, the hormones prolactin and oxytocin finely coordinate lactation. Prolactin is responsible for milk production. Throughout pregnancy, the blood concentration of prolactin increases.[27] With the delivery, its concentration rises substantially in preparation for infant feeding.

High prolactin concentrations signal the release of prolactin-inhibiting hormone, which ensures that prolactin concentrations and milk production do not exceed the need. This is an example of hormone regulation by negative feedback—prolactin is turned off by its own high concentrations.

In contrast, the slow, steady rise in estrogen production during the final trimester of pregnancy requires prolactin-inhibiting hormone to remain inactive, allowing prolactin concentrations to rise in preparation for lactation. Another message to turn off prolactin-inhibiting hormone comes from infant suckling. The suckling on the breast signals a demand for milk production (which requires prolactin) and a demand for prolactin-inhibiting hormone to turn off (which elicits the release of prolactin). The consequence of these hormonal interactions is that prolactin concentrations remain high and milk manufacture continues as long as the infant is nursing. The infant's demand for milk causes the mammary glands to supply milk.

In breastfeeding mothers, concentrations of prolactin are extremely high for the first three months but then decline to near-normal levels, even with continued milk production.[28] In nonbreastfeeding mothers, prolactin concentrations decline to prepregnant levels within the first two to three weeks postpartum.

The hormone oxytocin causes the myoepithelial cells surrounding the alveoli to contract, thus initiating milk ejection into the ducts, known as the let-down reflex. (The mother feels this as a contraction of the breast, followed by flow of milk and relief of pressure.) After the birth, the elevated progester-one concentrations of pregnancy (which turn off oxytocin) decline, allowing oxytocin's release. Oxytocin also responds to the stretching of the cervix during childbirth, causing two organs to react: the uterus to contract and the mammary glands to eject milk.

An infant's suckling also elicits oxytocin to eject milk from the mammary glands. At first, the stimulus for let-down is the infant's suckling. Later, when the reflex is well established, the sound of the infant's crying may be enough to trigger it. An efficient let-down reflex is essential to successful lactation. Emotional upset, pain, and fatigue may inhibit the let-down reflex. By relaxing and eating well, the nursing mother promotes easy let-down of milk and greatly enhances her chances of successful lactation.

From early to late in a nursing session, the character of milk changes. The milk released first, known as the foremilk, provides most of the nutrients the infant receives. The draught reflex, which occurs later during a nursing session, draws milk from the hindmost milk-producing glands of the breast after the foremilk has been released. The mother feels this as a tingly sensation within the breast. Hindmilk has a higher fat content than foremilk, leading research-ers to speculate that its appearance late in a breastfeeding session permits the infant to satisfy its sucking need and receive sufficient nutrients from the foremilk before achieving satiety.

foremilk: the milk released early in a nurs-ing session, the milk at the front of the breast; low in fat, high in nutrients.

draught reflex (DRAFT reflex): the reflex that moves the hindmilk toward the nip-ple after the infant has drawn off the foremilk.

To stop lactating, a woman may be given an injection of estrogen or a large dose of vitamin B_6. Such measures hasten the end of lactation, but are not necessary. Without the stimulation of suckling, milk production will eventually stop.

hindmilk: the milk released late in a nurs-ing session, higher in fat than foremilk.

Postpartum Amenorrhea

Women who breastfeed their infants experience prolonged postpartum amen-orrhea. An infant's suckling serves the dual purpose of not only promoting milk production, but also of causing lactational anovulation; both of these effects are mediated by the hormone prolactin. As mentioned earlier, prolactin inhibits the release of the hormones responsible for ovulation. This is beneficial because it allows time for the replenishment of maternal nutrient reserves.

postpartum amenorrhea: the normal tem-porary absence of menstrual periods im-mediately following childbirth.

lactational anovulation: the normal sup-pression of ovulation during lactation.

Physically, the new mother's body is still undergoing major changes. Hormones are shifting from a state of pregnancy to one of lactation or nonpregnancy. Some nutrient stores may be low or depleted, and energy levels are low. A new mother rarely sleeps more than four hours at a time. Even with optimal nourishment and adequate rest, she will not be back to "100 percent" for at least a year. Repeated pregnancies at intervals of less than one year deplete nutrient reserves. Whether contraception is passive or active, it seems best to avoid pregnancy until the mother has had time to readjust to nonpregnancy, restore nutrient banks, and recharge her energy. The reproduc-tive system needs a rest before being called into active duty again.

Chapter 1 discusses preparation for preg-nancy and contraception.

The uterus returns to its normal size about six weeks after delivery. Menstruation usually occurs four to eight weeks postpartum in nonlactating women. Women need not be concerned if menstruation is delayed for three or four months, since variation is quite normal. The duration of postpartum amenorrhea is as individual as the women themselves. Absent menstrual periods, however, do not protect a woman from pregnancy. An ovum may be

The effect of nutrition on fertility is discussed in Chapter 1.

released at any time, so to avoid pregnancy a couple must use some form of contraception.

Maternal nutrition status plays a role in altering plasma prolactin concentration and, therefore, in postpartum amenorrhea and anovulation. When diets of undernourished lactating women are supplemented to provide the needed energy, protein, vitamins, and minerals to support lactation, plasma prolactin concentrations decline.[29] The duration of postpartum amenorrhea is shortened.[30] Thus, the length of postpartum amenorrhea depends on both lactation and nutrition. Prolonged lactation and poor nutrition lengthen the period of postpartum amenorrhea and consequently reduce fertility.

The endocrine events preceding the first menstruation postpartum are rarely like those of an ordinary interpregnancy cycle. Many women do not ovulate before that first menstruation; menstruation results from the degeneration of an ovarian follicle. When ovulation does precede the first menstruation, it is often followed by an incomplete luteal phase of the cycle. These conditions are unlikely to support a pregnancy even if the ovum is fertilized. Fewer than 20 percent of postpartum women have a normal ovulatory cycle prior to their first menstruation.[31] Given a 25 percent probability of conception in a normal menstrual cycle, it is estimated that only 5 percent of lactating women who engage in unprotected intercourse before their first menstruation are likely to conceive. Indeed, the incidence of conception during lactational amenorrhea in developing countries is less than 10 percent. Such statistics, seen in populations, bespeak the effectiveness of lactation as a contraceptive influence, but do not make it acceptable as a contraceptive method for an individual.

Unfortunately, a simple or reliable procedure to detect the onset of fertility has yet to be developed. Many biological factors influence the variability in duration of postpartum infertility. Hormonal responses to the frequency and vigor of sucking are thought to be responsible for much of the variation. Women who frequently nurse their infants have elevated plasma prolactin concentrations. The number of feeding periods as well as the total time at the breast also raise plasma prolactin. As mothers begin to supplement their infants' diets and nurse for shorter periods less often, prolactin levels decline and ovarian activity resumes. Most lactating women will start to menstruate and ovulate prior to weaning.

Maternal Nutrient Needs

During lactation, as during pregnancy, the mother requires sufficient nutrient intakes and stores to support the infant's growth and her own health. If she does not eat well throughout pregnancy and lactation, her health may be compromised, in some instances, to a greater extent than that of her child. In addition, lactation is likely to falter or fail. Ideally, a woman will have consumed high-quality foods throughout pregnancy, and will continue to eat them after she has given birth.

The pattern of nutrient needs for a lactating mother is unique. Depending on the specific nutrient, her need may be less than, equal to, or greater than during pregnancy. Figure 3–3 repeats Figure 2–5 of Chapter 2, adding the nutrient needs of lactating women. Table 3–2 offers a daily food guide to meet these nutrient needs.

Table 3–2   Daily Food Guide for Lactating Women

Food	Number of Servings
Protein foods	
Animal (2-oz serving)	2
Vegetable (at least 1 serving of legumes)	2
Milk and milk products	5
Enriched or whole-grain breads and cereals	4
Vitamin C-rich fruits and vegetables	1
Dark-green vegetables	1
Other fruits and vegetables	1

Source: California Department of Health, as cited in Nutrition and the pregnant obese woman, *Nutrition and the MD,* January 1978.

Energy intake and exercise   Energy from maternal diet and tissue reserves provides for both lactation and maternal health and activities. A nursing mother produces approximately 30 ounces of milk in a day.[32] At 20 kcalories per ounce, this quantity represents 600 kcalories per day. Additional kcalories are required to compensate for the less-than-100 percent efficiency of the mammary glands in converting maternal energy into milk energy. Thus, the food energy requirement for a lactating woman is about 750 kcalories a day above her nonpregnant need.[33] To meet these energy needs, the RDA recommends that a lactating woman consume an additional 500 kcalories from foods each day. The fat reserves accumulated during pregnancy provide the balance of the energy required for milk production. The addition of only 500 of the estimated 750 required kcalories allows for gradual weight loss. Many postpartum women want to lose weight rapidly and disregard advice to consume recommended energy intakes. Women with energy intakes below the RDA can successfully breastfeed their infants while losing weight.[34] However, when a woman's energy intake is too low, her milk volume decreases. Such restrictions are detrimental in the early weeks of lactation when milk production is still getting established.

On the energy output side, the lactating mother can and should exercise regularly as before she gave birth. Exercise at the same level as was maintained during pregnancy does not compromise lactation. For the woman who was sedentary during pregnancy, the postpartum period is a good time to begin regular walks or workouts.

Maternal diet has a different influence on each of the nutrients found in breast milk. First and most important is water.

Water   Water is the major nutrient in breast milk. Total milk volume varies with infant age, but not with maternal fluid intake, as might be expected.[35] The mother can therefore become dehydrated while lactating. To prevent dehydration, two quarts of fluid a day are recommended for the lactating mother. A beneficial habit she may want to adopt is to drink a glass of milk, water, or juice each time she nurses.

Carbohydrate   Maternal diet has a different influence on each of the energy nutrients found in breast milk. For carbohydrate, maternal nutrition has no effect on the lactose concentration in breast milk.[36]

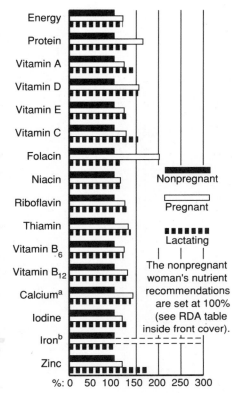

[a]Recommended intakes of phosphorous and magnesium change similarly.
[b]The pregnant woman may need to take an iron supplement, as dicussed in Chapter 2.

Figure 3–3   Comparison of Nutrient Needs of Nonpregnant, Pregnant, and Lactating Women

Protein Maternal nutrition may have no effect on breast milk's protein contents, either. Protein supplementation has been reported to increase milk volume and both increase and decrease the protein concentrations in breast milk. In general, the protein concentration of breast milk in malnourished women is similar to that of well-nourished women. Studies reporting otherwise may have used analytical methods that measured nonprotein nitrogen. Nonprotein nitrogen accounts for 25 percent of the nitrogen in breast milk; if used as an indicator of protein per se, it makes breast milk's protein concentration appear spuriously high.[37] The protein RDA is 20 grams per day above nonpregnant requirements, well within most women's intakes; the average protein intakes of many women exceed their RDA.[38]

Lipid Maternal dietary intake alters the fatty-acid composition of breast milk, but not the total fat concentration or milk volume.[39] Consequently, the omega-3 fatty acid docosahexaenoic acid (DHA) concentrations of breast milk increase with maternal consumption of fish oil rich in DHA.[40] This, in turn, raises the infant's consumption of DHA, which may support brain development, considering that DHA is one of the most abundant structural lipids in the brain. DHA does accumulate in the brain as it develops after birth. In addition to the DHA found in human milk, infants can synthesize DHA from linolenic acid. Cholesterol concentrations in breast milk are unaffected by maternal fat and cholesterol consumption.

Vitamins Breast milk volume does not change with maternal dietary excesses and deficiencies of the fat-soluble vitamins, but its composition may change, depending on the vitamin. The vitamin A concentration in the milk is maintained at the expense of the mother's stores, and therefore vitamin A deficiency is rare in breastfed infants, as long as maternal stores last. However, megadoses of vitamin A can increase the concentration of the vitamin in breast milk to a level that threatens to be toxic. Vitamin D in breast milk is minimal even with adequate maternal dietary intake. Vitamin E in breast milk varies directly with maternal intake and stores. Breast milk vitamin K concentrations and the infant's intestinal flora activity are minimal.

Like the fat-soluble vitamins, water-soluble vitamins in breast milk reflect maternal intake to varying extents. Marginal deficiencies and daily fluctuations have little, if any, influence on breast milk composition, but severely vitamin-deficient mothers produce vitamin-deficient breast milk. For example, lactating women who consume a strict vegetarian diet produce vitamin B_{12}-deficient milk. Milk concentrations of vitamin C rise with maternal intakes up to 90 milligrams per day. Daily vitamin C intakes greater than 90 milligrams per day do not further raise the vitamin C concentrations in breast milk.[41] The RDA for most of the vitamins during lactation are greater than during pregnancy; the RDA for vitamin D and vitamin B_{12} remain at their pregnancy level during lactation; the RDA for vitamin B_6 and folacin during lactation are lower than during pregnancy.[42]

Minerals The calcium, phosphorus, and magnesium RDAs are the same during lactation as during pregnancy. The calcium concentration in human milk remains fairly constant even when maternal calcium intakes are low.[43] However, a low calcium intake promotes mobilization of calcium from maternal bone stores. Thus, dietary intake is more critical in preventing maternal bone demineralization than in producing calcium-rich milk. A lactating woman whose daily diet lacks calcium-rich foods may find herself with weakened bones later in life.

As with calcium, the phosphorus and magnesium contents of breast milk remain fairly constant, regardless of maternal dietary intake. In general, maternal dietary intake of minerals does not influence the total minerals in milk, although specific amounts of individual minerals may vary with the stage of lactation.[44]

Breast milk iron concentration remains fairly constant whether the mother takes an iron supplement or suffers iron-deficiency anemia. Even when maternal stores and dietary intake are inadequate, the iron that is available reaches the breast milk. (The mother's body is designed to deliver iron to the infant, no matter the cost to her health.)

Supplements for Lactating Women

Postpartum maternal iron stores are often depleted. During gestation, the fetus takes enough iron to meet its own needs for the first four to six months after birth.[45] In addition, blood losses may have occurred at delivery. That is why the recommendation is made that the woman should continue taking iron supplements during lactation, after the infant's birth. The intent is not to enhance the iron content of her breast milk, but to replenish her depleted maternal iron stores. When iron stores become depleted, the symptoms of iron-deficiency anemia (such as weakness, fatigue, and headaches), become evident. A new mother trying to care for her infant cannot do so optimally if she is tired and weak. Her compromised emotional and physical health will eventually deplete her milk supply.

The health care provider may recommend supplements that contain the full range of vitamins and minerals. However, for most lactating women, iron supplements are all that are necessary, and as always, foods are a better choice for the delivery of nutrients.

The lactating mother needs to pay special attention to her own nutrition at the same time as she is adjusting to the presence of a new, needy, and time-consuming individual in her life. The support of her family and companions can help her succeed at this. In fact, the support of a lactating mother is important enough to warrant a section of its own.

Care of the Lactating Mother

Life is hectic, to say the least, for any new mother, whether she is breastfeeding or formula feeding. The breastfed infant demands frequent feedings in the early weeks, stimulating milk production. The nursing mother may at first feel as if she is doing little else. Finding time to prepare meals for herself and other family members is often difficult in the beginning.

Nutrition plays a significant role in successful lactation, affecting both the physical and mental well-being of the mother. Thus, it is important that she eat well. In order to do so, she needs help and support. She cannot expect, nor should she be expected, to prepare family meals, breastfeed her infant, attend to other responsibilities, and get the rest she so urgently needs, without help from family members and friends. Her main priorities at first are to feed and care for herself and her newborn infant.

Family members can help by shopping and preparing food. Meals may be quick and simple for a while, but they can still be nutritious. Casseroles, salads, and soups are easy to prepare. They also provide many nutrients, especially when foods such as instant, nonfat dry milk, vegetable broth, nuts, seeds, cheese, eggs, and nutritional yeast are added to them. Table 3–3 lists quick and nutritious food suggestions.

Rest is vital to successful lactation and an important feature of the road to recovery. Giving birth to an infant is an exhausting and stressful experience. Friends and family members can help by caring for the infant for a few hours while mother rests or spends some time away from home. Mothers can benefit by napping when the infant naps.

Once postpartum bleeding has stopped and the mother is feeling stronger, exercise and fresh air are excellent "medicines" to improve her strength, well-being, and self-esteem. Exercise classes, including free babysitting, are offered throughout the country today. If the mother can afford this luxury, these classes provide an excellent opportunity to do something just for herself, with the added bonus of a break from the infant and the social stimulation of other new mothers' company.

Nursing women are frequently the recipients of unsolicited, "friendly" advice on how to care for themselves and their newborns, including what they should or should not eat during lactation. Aside from creating unnecessary confusion for the mothers, this advice is often incorrect. Each mother and

Table 3–3 Quick and Nutritious Food Suggestions

Foods that derive a large proportion of their kcalories from sugar, fat, salt, or alcohol are not included here since they are not nutrient dense. This list includes only those foods that require minimal preparation. Don't forget about leftovers from previously prepared meals. Last night's dinner may make a quick, nutritious snack, lunch, or even breakfast.

Nonfat milk and cereal
Cheese and crackers
Cottage cheese and fruit
Yogurt shake (yogurt, juice, and a banana)
Sardines or tuna fish on crackers
Green pepper stuffed with tuna
Deviled eggs
Peanut butter on bread or crackers
Nuts and raisins or other dried fruit
Fruit and cheese
Raw vegetables and clam, onion, or other dip
Fruit and yogurt

infant combination is unique, and what is true for one nursing mother may not be for another. For example, one mother may find that when she eats garlic, her infant becomes irritable, while another mother has no such experience. Infant reactions to substances in mother's milk are matters that require individual detective work.

In addition to the support friends and family members offer by helping, a new mother (and her infant) benefit from accurate information on breastfeeding (see Practical Point: How to Breastfeed for a summary of instructions). When women receive early and repeated postpartum breastfeeding information and support, they breastfeed their infants longer than other breastfeeding women.[46]

In conclusion, successful lactation requires the support of all those who care. This, plus adequate nutrition, rest, exercise, and fresh air will do much to support lactation and enhance the well-being of mother and infant.

▶▶ PRACTICAL POINT

How to Breastfeed

Most healthy women who want to breastfeed can do so. The mother-to-be may find it reassuring to learn that 95 percent of all women who try are successful. The size and shape of a woman's breasts do not affect her ability to breastfeed an infant.

Newborn infants readily adapt to breastfeeding. In fact, fetuses evince sucking behaviors before birth. Newborns are prepared to suckle immediately after birth and demonstrate a rooting reflex that orients them toward a nipple. Nursing the infant immediately after birth facilitates successful lactation.

Beginning at the first feeding, the mother needs to learn how to relax and position herself so that she and the infant will be comfortable. The position must also allow the infant to nurse without obstructing breathing. The mother squeezes the areola, the colored halo around the nipple, between two fingers, slipping enough of it into the infant's mouth to promote good pumping action (see Figure 3–4). If the infant is to successfully milk the mammary glands, the nipple must rest well back on the infant's tongue. The infant's lips and gums pump the areola, thus releasing milk from the mammary glands into the ducts that lie beneath the areola. The sucking and swallowing reflexes work together. The infant's tongue and jaw suck milk from the breast and the swallow follows. To break the suction, the mother can slip a finger between the infant's mouth and her breast.

The let-down reflex forces milk to the front of the breast when the infant begins to nurse, allowing it to flow. Let-down has to occur for the infant to obtain milk easily, and the mother needs to relax for let-down to occur. This means that at a time when the stress response might be more natural, she must will the relaxation response. Willed relaxation first requires that a person assume a comfortable position in a noninterrupting environment and then maintain a passive attitude toward intervening thoughts. It may take several feeding sessions for the mother to learn how to respond to cries of hunger before she can achieve let-down promptly and fully.

rooting reflex: a reflex that causes an infant to turn toward whichever cheek is touched, in search of a nipple.

areola (ah-REE-oh-la): the colored portion of the mammary gland that surrounds the nipple.

stress response: the body's response to a physical or psychological threat, mediated by nerves and hormones.

relaxation response: the opposite of the stress response; the normal state of the body.

Figure 3—4   Infant's Grasp on Mother's Breast
The mother squeezes the areola, slipping enough of it into the infant's mouth to promote good pumping action. The infant's lips and gums pump the areola, releasing milk from the mammary glands into the milk ducts that lie beneath the areola.

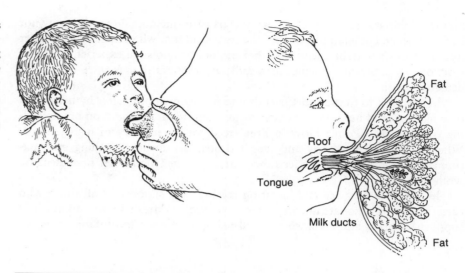

The infant sucks half the milk from the breast within the first two minutes, and 80 to 90 percent of it within four minutes. However, sucking on one breast is encouraged for 8 to 12 minutes. The sucking itself, as well as the complete removal of milk from the breast, stimulates lactation. After ten minutes or so, the mother offers the other breast to finish satisfying the infant's hunger. Nursing sessions start on alternate breasts to ensure that each breast is emptied regularly. This pattern maintains the same supply and demand for each breast, and thus prevents either breast from overfilling. At regular intervals, the mother holds the infant upright to expel any swallowed air, and then offers another chance to nurse.

Approximately six feedings a day, when the infant cries with hunger, promote optimal milk production and infant growth. The mother encourages the infant to nurse the full 15 to 20 minutes per feeding. Some infants fall asleep in less time and may need to be aroused to continue feeding. Feeding intervals vary with each infant, but should be at least two hours apart. If they are less than two hours apart, the mother may begin to feel like a human pacifier, and her milk supply, at first unable to meet the demand, may come to exceed it. If a feeding interval exceeds four hours, the mother may need to express some milk to relieve pressure and maintain the demand. Figure 3—5 illustrates methods of expressing milk. Until lactation is well established, the infant should be encouraged to feed regularly and not allowed to sleep through a feeding.

What if a mother is breastfeeding twins? As far as milk supply is concerned, a woman need have no problem breastfeeding twins. The more milk the infants drink, the more milk the breasts produce. Most mothers of twins agree that the problem lies in finding time to feed two—whether by breast or by bottle. Each infant has a unique "hunger clock," and every mother has to work out her own system. Breastfeeding twins is no more difficult than any other task involving twins.

If an infant seems thirsty after a long feed, or prior to the next scheduled feeding, a parent can offer a bottle of water. Sweetened water or supplemental

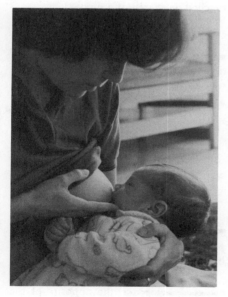

A mother breastfeeds her infant while sitting in a relaxed, comfortable position.

Figure 3–5 Methods of Expressing Milk

Milk Expression by Hand

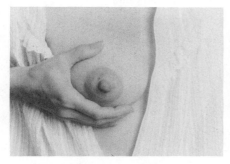

1. The hand is placed on the breast near the chest wall, with the thumb on top and the fingers cupped around and under the breasts. The hands gently move toward the nipple.

2. With the thumb and forefinger about an inch back from the nipple, the woman presses gently inward toward the chest wall and squeezes the thumb and finger together. This "push back and squeeze" motion is continued until no more milk comes out. Then the fingers are rotated to another position and the procedure is repeated.

Manual Breast Pump

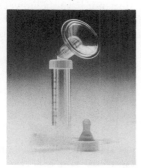

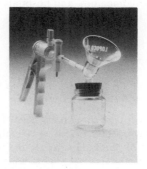

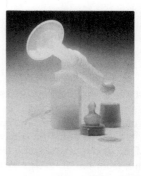

The most popular manual (non-electrical) pump is the piston or cylinder pump. Two cylinders fit together, and breast milk is pumped with a piston-type motion into the outer cylinder. The outer cylinder can be used as a baby bottle. The cylinder pump is easy to use and clean. It is small, lightweight, and transportable.

The Loyd-B® pump has a trigger-shaped handle that initiates the suction. Its pumping action, which can be regulated from gentle to strong, makes it one of the most effective of the manual pumps. Although somewhat bulky, the Loyd-B® comes apart and is small enough to transport easily. It is available with two breast shields—one plastic, one glass. The plastic shield fits a regular baby bottle so mother can pump directly into a bottle if desired.

Medela makes a pump that can be operated manually or used in conjunction with Medela's electric pump. The system is designed around the suck, release, relax cycle of the baby's nursing pattern.

Figure 3–5   Continued

Electric Pump

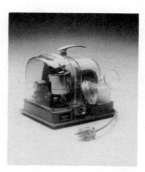

Battery-Powered Pump

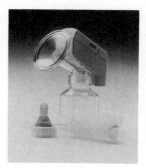

An electric pump is the easiest way to express breast milk. Of all pumps, it is most effective at emptying the breast to stimulate milk production. Electric pumps range in price from $100 to $1,000. The larger, more expensive models can be rented from some large pharmacies, medical supply companies, and hospitals.

The battery-operated pump is the newest addition to the growing line of breast pumps. Two AA batteries supply the power for this small, light-weight, easily cleaned pump. A six-stage suction adjustor allows for individual control, so the pump can be operated with one hand. While this pump does not have the power of the electric pump, the convenience and cost make it worth investigating.

Techniques for Pumping Breast Milk

Learning how to effectively express breast milk will take time, regardless of the method selected. Practice improves efficiency. Effectiveness of pumping may vary due to let-down, stress, and time available for pumping.

One of the best ways to learn the mechanics of pumping is to use the pump on one breast at the same time the baby is nursing from the other. It's easier to master the technique of pumping when milk is flowing, than to try to master it without the milk ejection reflex.

1. Massaging the breasts just before pumping helps to increase the quantity of milk collected and to decrease the time needed for collection. To massage the breasts, a woman makes small circular motions with her fingertips starting near the chest wall, and moving toward the areola.

2. She then uses the palms of both her hands to apply gentle but firm pressure starting from the outside edge of the breast working toward the nipple. She massages around each breast several times before attempting to express milk.

3. After massaging the breasts, she moistens the edges of the pump flange with expressed milk or water to lubricate it and to make a better seal with the skin. The nipple should slide along the inside of the top edge of the pump flange to help stimulate the milk ejection reflex and initiate the flow of milk.

4. The flange is held just tightly enough against the breast to make a good seal, making sure the edge of the flange does not block milk flow from the nipple. Initiate the pumping according to the pump manufacturer's instructions. Continue to pump until one minute after the flow stops. Break the seal by pressing a finger against the breast where it meets the flange. Repeat the pumping process with the other breast.

Source: Mead Johnson Nutritional Division, Mead Johnson and Company, Evansville, Ind. 47721.

formula feedings in the first two weeks are ill advised. Sweetened water provides energy, which should come to the infant only from a nutrient-dense source. The full extent of the infant's demand should be communicated to the mother's body by way of sucking, so that the milk supply will increase to meet it.

A mother might want to know if she can skip an occasional feeding, substituting a bottle of formula. To avoid suppressing lactation, the mother will need to express her milk; that way, the breast receives the message to continue producing milk. This may not be necessary once lactation is well established.

A mother who wants to skip one or two feedings daily—for example, if she works outside the home—can substitute formula for those feedings and continue to breastfeed at other feedings. Or the infant can be fed, in a bottle, the breast milk she has expressed and frozen on previous occasions. Breast milk can be kept refrigerated for up to 24 hours or frozen for up to six weeks.

If the mother feels that she is spending immense amounts of time breastfeeding, she should remind herself that the parent who is feeding formula is also spending time sterilizing bottles, preparing formula, and feeding an infant. Breastfeeding will be less time consuming after the first few weeks. The mother is encouraged to remember the advantages and to enjoy this time with her infant while it lasts.

Most problems associated with breastfeeding can be resolved. Many new mothers experience sore nipples during the initial days of breastfeeding. Sore nipples need to be treated kindly, but nursing can continue. Air and sunlight between feedings help to heal them. Before let-down, the infant must suck hard on the nipple to receive milk. For this reason, a mother will want to nurse on the less-sore breast first. Then, when the milk lets down and is freely flowing, she can switch to the sore nipple. When the fast-flowing, early milk from that sore breast is gone, she can switch back and satisfy the infant's hunger and sucking need.

Engorgement is common before lactation is established, when the schedule is changed as in weaning, or when a feeding is missed. The breasts become so full and hard that the infant cannot grasp the nipple and mother is most uncomfortable. A gentle massage or warming the breasts (with a heating pad or in a shower) helps to initiate let-down and to release some of the accumulated milk. The best solutions are to pump out some of the milk; to use a nipple shield that will help the infant grasp the nipple; and to allow the infant to nurse. The breasts will, in time, get smaller and softer, while still producing ample milk.

engorgement: overfilling of the breasts with milk so that they become swollen and hard.

A mother can also manage to nurse with an inverted nipple. An inverted nipple folds inward toward the breast when the areola is pressed between two fingers. Pushing the areola toward the chest wall—manually or with a shield—everts the nipple, making it available for infant sucking.

An undrained duct can make a hard, uncomfortable lump in the breast. By massaging the lump while the infant is nursing, the mother can move the milk toward the nipple, where it will join the main supply.

Infection of a breast, known as mastitis, is best managed by *continuing to breastfeed*. By drawing off the milk, the infant helps to relieve pressure in the infected area. The infant is safe because the infection is between the milk-producing glands, not inside them.

mastitis: inflammation of the breast, most common in women during lactation.

Most importantly, if the infant is irritable and wakeful, the mother may fear that her milk supply is inadequate. The infant's normal small bowel movements may suggest to her that the infant is underfed, but the health care provider can reassure her that breast milk contains little indigestible material and therefore little waste. The stress of worrying, itself, can inhibit lactation. All infants cry. The mother's ability to relax and set her fears aside will better support lactation than will anxiety about inadequate milk production. However, if she wants to wean the infant to formula, that is an acceptable alternative. Breastfeeding, even for a few days, provides the infant with protective factors from colostrum, which contribute to the infant's health and development.

To wean an infant, the mother gradually introduces small amounts of formula or milk and solid foods to the infant while she continues to breastfeed. (The type of food or milk and the age of weaning is discussed in the next chapter.) As the infant consumes more solid foods and formula or milk, breast milk consumption will descrease. Because the breasts need time to adjust their supply to the diminishing demand for milk, the key to a comfortable weaning is to wean *gradually*. The less breast milk an infant drinks, the less the mother produces until finally weaning is complete—that is, the infant is eating solid foods, drinking milk or formula, and not receiving any breast milk.

The mother should allow several weeks for complete weaning. The first step is to replace any one breast feeding with formula or milk and solid foods. After a few days, a second breast feeding is replaced in the same way. This process continues until all breast feedings have been replaced. Such a gradual schedule will allow the breasts to adjust with little discomfort until they are no longer producing milk.

Formula Feeding

Appendix D provides a table comparing the composition of infant formulas available in the United States.

A woman who breastfeeds for the better part of one year can wean her infant to cow's milk, bypassing the need for infant formula. However, a woman who decides to feed her infant formula from birth, to wean to formula after a short time, or to substitute formula for breastfeeding on occasion must select an appropriate infant formula and learn to prepare it. A variety of infant formulas are available, and the selection must be made carefully. Once other foods begin to supply nutrients in significant quantities, then cow's milk can partially replace the formula. However, the continued use of iron-fortified formula throughout the first year of life helps ensure an adequate iron intake. The following discussion offers help with the question: What type of formula is appropriate? (See Practical Point: How to Feed Formula at the end of this section.)

Standard Formulas

Formula makers duplicate human milk as closely as they reasonably can. Not all human milk is the same, though. Breast milk composition varies from one woman to another, from one feeding to another, with the duration of each feeding, and with the duration of lactation. Nevertheless, national and international standards have been established for the nutrient contents of infant formulas. The standard developed by the American Academy of Pediatrics (AAP) reflects "human milk taken from well-nourished mothers during the first or second month of lactation, when the infant's growth rate is high."[47] Manufacturers in the United States use this standard to develop their formulas. The Infant Formula Act of 1980 requires that formulas meet nutrient standards based on the AAP recommendations. Formulas meeting the standard have similar nutrient compositions; small differences are sometimes confusing but usually unimportant.

Throughout the years, infant formula composition and labeling have reflected the knowledge of the time regarding the nutrient needs of infants. In 1941, labeling regulations pertained only to vitamins A, D, C, and thiamin, plus the minerals calcium, phosphorus, and iron. The remaining vitamins and minerals were considered adequate because the formulas of the time contained enough milk to provide them. In 1967, as knowledge about the nutrient needs of infants expanded, the AAP proposed minimum, and in some cases maximum, amounts for vitamins and minerals in formulas. As of 1986, labeling regulations specify how nutrient contents and preparation must be listed on labels. The progression of nutrient labeling recommendations for infant formulas is shown in Table 3–4.

To prepare a standard infant formula, manufacturers start with a nonfat cow's milk base or a mixture of nonfat cow's milk and added whey (if they are creating a whey-predominant formula, for reasons described later). They replace the poorly absorbed butterfat of cow's milk with vegetable oils. They then add lactose, vitamins, and minerals so that the energy content and nutrient distribution closely resemble those of human milk. All standard infant formulas in the United States contain lactose as the principal carbohydrate. Fat is the major source of energy, as well as of essential fatty acids, in infant formulas and human milk. Infant formulas provide 20 kcalories per ounce, as does human milk.

Chapter 4 discusses the differences in fat and its absorption between human milk and cow's milk.

The proteins of human milk are whey and casein, in a ratio of 80 to 20.[48] In contrast, the whey-to-casein ratio of cow's milk is 20 to 80. Some infant formulas maintain the whey-to-casein ratio of 20 to 80 (casein-predominant formulas), while others add whey, changing the ratio to 60 to 40 (whey-predominant formulas). Full-term infants grow equally well on either formula. Preterm infants require whey-predominant formulas, which contain an amino acid profile better suited to their metabolic capacities.[49]

whey: the prinicpal protein in human milk, found in the liquid that remains after milk has been coagulated.

casein: the principal protein in cow's milk, found in coagulated milk curds. *caseus* = cheese

In 1984, formula makers began to add the amino acid taurine to infant formulas.[50] Analysis of human milk reveals that it is a rich source of taurine. Infants receiving taurine-free formulas do not show clinical signs of taurine deficiency, nor are there any known risks associated with its addition. Infants consuming taurine-supplemented formulas have plasma concentrations similar to those of breastfed infants. Most infant formulas are now supplemented with taurine at a concentration approximating that of human milk.

The role of taurine in infant growth is discussed in Chapter 4.

Further recommendations of the AAP include recognition of interrelationships among nutrients such as vitamin E and linoleic acid, calcium and phosphorus, and vitamin B_6 and protein. For example, the calcium-to-phosphorus ratio must be between 1 to 1 and 2 to 1.

Table 3–4 Labeling Standards and AAP Recommendations for Formulas

1941[a]	1967	1976	1983 Recommendations (per 100 kcal)
Protein	Protein	Protein	1.8–4.5 g
Fat	Fat	Fat	3.3–6.0 g[c]
Carbohydrate	Carbohydrate	Carbohydrate	—
Ash			
Vitamin A	Vitamin A	Vitamin A	75–225 µg
Vitamin D	Vitamin D	Vitamin D	1.0–2.5 µg
	Vitamin E	Vitamin E	0.5 mg tocopherol equivalent
		Vitamin K	4 µg
Vitamin C	Vitamin C	Vitamin C	8 mg
Thiamin	Thiamin	Thiamin	40 µg
	Riboflavin	Riboflavin	60 µg
	Niacin	Niacin	250 µg
	Vitamin B_6	Vitamin B_6	35 µg[d]
	Folacin	Folacin	4 µg
	Pantothenic acid	Pantothenic acid	300 µg
	Vitamin B_{12}	Vitamin B_{12}	0.15 µg
		Biotin	1.5 µg
		Choline	7.0 mg
		Inositol	4.0 mg
Calcium	Calcium	Calcium	60 mg[e]
Phosphorus	Phosphorus	Phosphorus	30 mg[e]
	Magnesium	Magnesium	6 mg
		Sodium	20 mg (6 mEq[f])
		Potassium	80 mg (14 mEq[f])
		Chloride	55 mg (11 mEq[f])
Iron	Iron	Iron	0.15 mg
	Iodine	Iodine	5 µg
	Copper	Copper	60 µg
		Zinc	0.5 mg
		Manganese	5.0 µg
		Chromium[b]	—
		Cobalt[b]	—
		Molybdenum[b]	—
		Selenium[b]	—
		Fluoride[b]	—

[a] FDA Regulations—1941 Infant Formula Labeling Requirements, from the Federal Register, 1941.
[b] These trace minerals require further study; recommendations have not been made.
[c] The AAP recommends 300 mg of the essential fatty acid linoleic acid.
[d] The vitamin B_6 recommendation provides 15 µg/g protein in formula.
[e] The recommended calcium-to-phosphorus ratio is 1:1–2:1.
[f] A milliequivalent (mEq) describes the concentration of electrolytes in a solution.

Source: Adapted from H. P. Sarett, The modern infant formula, in *Infant and Child Feeding*, ed. J. T. Bond (New York: Academic Press, 1981), pp. 99–121; American Academy of Pediatrics, Committee on Nutrition, Recommended ranges of nutrients in formulas, in *Pediatric Nutrition Handbook*, 2nd ed., ed. G. B. Forbes, (Elk Grove Village, Ill.: American Academy of Pediatrics, 1985), pp. 356–357.

The AAP also makes recommendations specific to iron. All formulas must contain bioavailable iron in amounts approximately equal to that of human milk, which averages about 0.3 milligrams per liter. Formulas fortified with iron contain 6 to 12 milligrams per liter. Both iron-fortified and non-fortified formulas are available. However, it is recommended that all formula-fed infants receive iron-fortified formulas by four months. Table 3–5 compares nutrient composition of human milk, cow's milk, and an infant formula.

Special Formulas

Standard infant formulas are inappropriate for some infants. Special formulas are available, designed to meet the dietary needs of infants with specific conditions such as milk intolerance, prematurity, or congenital abnormalities.

Milk intolerance   Special soy-protein formulas are available for infants who are unable to tolerate the standard milk-based formulas. Originally developed for infants with milk allergy or lactose intolerance, these formulas are prepared using soy for the protein source, and corn syrup and sucrose instead of lactose. Soy formulas solve the problem of feeding an infant with any of several conditions: a temporary lactase deficiency due to diarrhea, a congenital lactase deficiency, or galactosemia. They are also useful as an alternative to milk-based formulas for vegetarian families. However, soy formulas are often used in situations for which they are inappropriate, such as when an infant fed a standard formula is colicky or regurgitates often. The infant's digestive tract adapts enzymatically to the milk it is fed: if not fed cow's milk, it will not produce the enzymes necessary to digest the ingredients that are found in cow's milk. The inappropriate use of soy formulas throughout infancy may make the later transition to cow's milk more difficult than if milk-based formula had been used.

> Soy-based formulas include Prosobee, Nursoy, Isomil, Isomil SF, and Soyalac.

Some infants with milk allergy are also allergic to soy protein. Infants with multiple food allergies, chronic diarrhea, or lactose intolerance may require a hydrolysate formula. In a hydrolysate formula, the casein is hydrolyzed to amino acids and peptides to permit easier absorption. Some of these formulas also replace the long-chain triglycerides with medium-chain triglycerides for infants with impaired fat absorption. Hydrolysate formulas are expensive and taste unappealing, but for the infant unable to tolerate milk- or soy-based formulas, they are indispensable.

> Casein hydrolysate formulas include Nutramigen and Pregestimil.

Preterm infants   Preterm infants, especially very-low-birthweight infants (less than 1500 grams), often have limited digestive abilities. For this reason, formulas designed for preterm infants contain a mixture of lactose and glucose polymers, and a blend of medium-chain triglycerides and unsaturated long-chain triglycerides.[51] Preterm infants also have greater nutrient needs than full-term infants. For this reason, formulas for preterm infants generally have higher protein, mineral, and vitamin concentrations than standard formulas. They also have a kcaloric density of 24 kcalories per ounce, slightly greater than that of regular infant formulas.

The whey-to-casein ratio in formulas for preterm infants is adjusted to 60 to 40, to make it approach that in human milk. Whey protein is preferred

Table 3–5   Human Milk, Cow's Milk, and Infant Formula Compared

Characteristic	Human Milk	Cow's Milk	Formula[a]
Carbohydrate (g/100 ml)	7.2	5.0	7.0–7.2
Energy (kcal/100 ml)	74	67	68
Fat (g/100 ml)	2.7–4.6	3.5	3.6–3.7
Linoleic acid (% of total fatty acids)	10–15	4	13–23
Minerals			
Calcium (mg/l)	340	1200	510–550
Calcium-to-phosphorus ratio	2.4	1.3	1.2–1.3
Iron (mg/l)	0.2–1.0	0.5	12 or 1.5[b]
Phosphorus (mg/l)	140	955	390–460
Potassium (mEq/l)[c]	13	35	18–20
Sodium (mEq/l)[c]	7	25	11–12
Protein (g/100 ml)	1.1	3.5	1.5–1.6
Renal solute load (mOsm/l)[d]	74	220	105–108
Vitamins (per 100 ml)			
Folacin (μg)	2–5	0.3	5–11
Niacin (mg)	0.15–0.18	0.09	0.7–1.3
Pantothenic acid (mg)	0.18–0.23	0.4	0.30–0.32
Riboflavin (μg)	36–37	175	63–100
Thiamin (μg)	14–16	44	53–65
Vitamin A (IU)	190–250	103 or 190[d]	169–250
Vitamin B_6 (μg)	10–11	64	40
Vitamin B_{12} (μg)	0.03–0.05	0.4	0.15–0.21
Vitamin C (mg)	4.3–5.2	1.1	5.5
Vitamin D (IU)	2.2	1.3 or 38[e]	40–42

[a]These numbers represent two formulas, Similac and Enfamil.
[b]These formulas are available unfortified or with iron fortification.
[c]Milliequivalents per liter of formula. A milliequivalent is the amount of a substance that contains the same number of charges as 1 mg of hydrogen—a useful measure, because the number of charges present is an index of the osmotic pressure the solution will exert.
[d]The ability of solutes to cause osmosis is measured in terms of *osmols;* the osmol is a measure of the total number of particles. A *milliosmol* equals 1/1000 of an osmol. Renal solute load is measured in milliosmols per liter of solution (mOsm/l).
[e]The higher value represents fortified milk, which should contain 2000 IU vitamin A and 400 IU vitamin D per quart (1900 and 375 IU/l, respectively).

Source: Adapted from K. Brostrøm, Human milk and infant formulas: Nutritional and immunological characteristics, in *Textbook of Pediatric Nutrition,* ed. R. M. Suskind (New York: Raven Press, 1981); *Milk-based and Soy-based Formulations Used for Feeding Newborns in the Hospital,* an information sheet (January 1979) available from Ross Laboratories, Columbus, OH 43216. Data on vitamins for all milks are adapted from S. J. Fomon, Milks and milk-based formulas, in *Infant Nutrition* (Philadelphia: Saunders, 1967), pp. 195–224.

because it is higher in cystine than in casein protein. Preterm infants may lack the hepatic enzyme cystathionase needed to convert methionine to cystine.[52] Soy formulas are not recommended for preterm infants.

Congenital disorders   Other formulas are available for infants with inborn errors of metabolism who cannot metabolize specific amino acids. These formulas purposely lack one or more nutrients and are called *incomplete* formulas. For this reason, they are not appropriate for other infants. Figure 3–6 illustrates the process of choosing a formula, and the accompanying

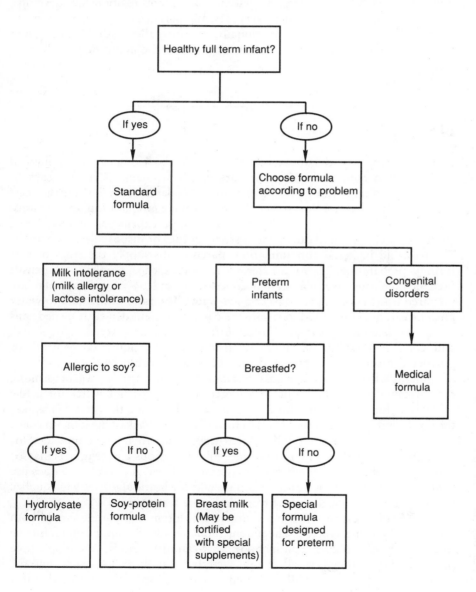

Figure 3–6   Choosing a Formula

Practical Point: How to Feed Formula provides directions for the feeding process itself.

Infants born in technologically advanced countries are fortunate to have a diverse array of formulas available to them. Not too long ago, death was the inevitable outcome for infants without access to breast milk. Recent changes in government regulations of formula manufacturing ensure protection for formula-fed infants. Mothers feeding their infants formula can feel confident that modern infant formulas offer a safe, nutritionally sound alternative to breast milk.

The initial care of a healthy newborn involves such simple tasks as the parents' providing clean diapers, warm clothing, a place to sleep, nourishment, and love. With each interaction, the parent and infant relationship develops. During each of several feedings every day, the parent has the opportunity to nurture the infant physically, emotionally, and mentally. With each day, their relationship continues to grow and change, just as the infant does.

▶▶ PRACTICAL POINT

How to Feed Formula

Formulas in the United States and Canada are available in a variety of physical forms. Liquid concentrate formulas are relatively inexpensive and easy to prepare by mixing with equal parts water. Powdered formulas are the least expensive and lightest for travel. Labels provide preparation instructions. Ready-to-feed formulas are the easiest and most expensive; premixed and sterile formula is poured directly into sterile bottles or disposable bottle liners.

To avoid bacterial contamination, parents must apply the rules of safe formula preparation. They must sterilize all bottles, caps, nipples, and utensils used in preparing formula. Liquid concentrate and powdered formulas are prepared using cooled, previously boiled water. The ratio of formula to water must be carefully measured to ensure the correct nutrient density. Opened cans of liquid concentrate and ready-to-feed formulas must be covered, refrigerated, and consumed within 48 hours or thrown away. Liquid concentrate or powdered formula, once prepared, should be used within 24 hours.

Infants will drink cold formula, but most prefer it warm. To warm formula, the caretaker places the bottle in a larger container of hot water for a few minutes. Before offering the bottle of formula to the infant, the caretaker shakes the bottle and sprinkles a few drops of formula on the back of the hand to check that the temperature is not too hot. Microwave ovens are not recommended for heating formulas; they tend to heat unevenly. The drops a parent feels may be warm, while the sip an infant takes may cause a burn. A parent who does use a microwave oven to heat formula should shake the bottle vigorously to equalize the temperature throughout the formula before testing it.

Close contact during feeding is important. Infant and parent should both be comfortable and relaxed. The parent should cradle the infant on an incline so that its head is higher than its body, so it can drink easily. The nipple hole should be large enough to allow one swallow of milk to flow each time the infant sucks; if it is too small, it should be enlarged with a sterile needle; if it

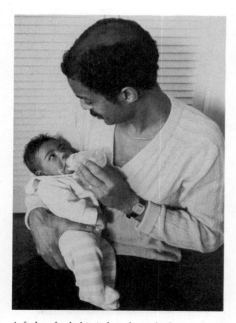

A father feeds his infant formula from a bottle.

is too large, it should be replaced. The parent tilts the bottle so that the nipple is full of formula, not air, while the infant is sucking.

Now and then, the parent should hold the infant upright and give a gentle pat on the back to help eliminate any bubbles of air. Infants generally feed for about 15 minutes and should not be forced to finish the bottle. Like making children clean their plates, this promotes obesity. Formula left in a bottle after feeding should be discarded.

The feeding schedule can vary, but is best if adjusted to the infant's expressed hunger needs at first, within reason. Some infants need to feed more frequently than others. Most infants enjoy bottles; the sucking provides stimulation and satisfaction, as well as nutrients. Infants cannot be allowed to sleep with bottles, however, because of the potential damage to developing teeth. A bedtime bottle may be the most wanted, but it must be firmly denied.

Nursing bottle syndrome is discussed in Focal Point 3.

Chapter 3 Notes

1. M. Underwood, as cited in T. E. Cone, History of infant and child feeding: From the earliest years through the development of scientific concepts, in *Infant and Child Feeding*, ed. J. T. Bond and coeditors (New York: Academic Press, 1981), pp. 3–34.
2. G. A. Martinez, Trends in breastfeeding in the United States, in *Report of the Surgeon General's Workshop on Breastfeeding and Human Lactation*, HHS Publication no. (HRS-D-MC) 84–2 (Washington, D.C.: Government Printing Office, 1984).
3. United Nations Children's Fund (UNICEF), *The State of the World's Children* (Oxford University Press, New York: 1988), pp. 61–67.
4. United Nations Children's Fund (UNICEF), 1988.
5. S. Fomon, Reflections on infant feeding in the 1970s and 1980s, *American Journal of Clinical Nutrition* 46 (1987): 171–182.
6. American Academy of Pediatrics, Committee on Nutrition, Vitamin and mineral supplement needs of normal children in the United States, in *Pediatric Nutrition Handbook*, 2nd ed., ed. G. B. Forbes (Elk Grove Village, Ill.: American Academy of Pediatrics, 1985), pp. 37–48.
7. J. A. McMillan, S. A. Landaw, and F. A. Oski, Iron sufficiency in breast-fed infants and the availability of iron from human milk, *Pediatrics* 58 (1976): 686–691.
8. Y. Chen, S. Yu, and W. Li, Artificial feeding and hospitalization in the first 18 months of life, *Pediatrics* 81 (1988): 58–62.
9. J. P. Habicht, J. DaVanzo, and W. P. Butz, Mother's milk and sewage: Their interactive effects on infant mortality, *Pediatrics* 81 (1988): 456–461.
10. W.A. Bowes, The effect of medications on the lactating mother and her infant, *Clinical Obstetrics and Gynecology* 23 (1980): 1073–1080.
11. S. J. Gross, Growth and biochemical response of preterm infants fed human milk or modified infant formula, *New England Journal of Medicine* 308 (1983): 237–241.
12. D. M. Anderson and coauthors, Length of gestation and nutritional composition of human milk, *American Journal of Clinical Nutrition* 37 (1983): 810–814; J. A. Lemons and coauthors, Differences in the composition of preterm and term human milk during early lactation, *Pediatric Research* 16 (1982): 113–117.
13. Anderson, 1983.
14. Lemons, 1982.
15. M. S. Brady and coauthors, Formulas and human milk for premature infants: A review and update, *Journal of the American Dietetic Association* 81 (1982): 547–552.
16. American Academy of Pediatrics, Committee on Drugs, The transfer of drugs and other chemicals into human breastmilk, *Pediatrics* 72 (1983): 375–384.
17. W. J. Rogan, A. Bagniewska, and T. Damstra, Pollutants in breast milk, *New England Journal of Medicine* 302 (1980): 1450–1453.
18. Rogan, Bagniewska, and Damstra, 1980.
19. J. A. Knowles, Drugs in milk, *Ross Timesaver* 21 (1972): 28–32.
20. Committee on Environmental Hazards, American Academy of Pediatrics, PCB in breastmilk, *Pediatrics* 62 (1978): 407.
21. T. Byers and coauthors, Lactation and breast cancer: Evidence for a negative association in premenopausal women, *American Journal of Epidemiology* 121 (1985): 664–674.
22. A. M. Ferris and coauthors, Biological and sociocultural determinants of successful lactation among women in eastern Connecticut, *Journal of the American Dietetic Association* 87 (1987): 316–321.
23. B. J. Myers, Mother-infant bonding: The status of this critical-period hypothesis, *Developmental Review* 4 (1984): 240–274.
24. Myers, 1984.
25. S. E. Saunders and J. Carroll, Post-partum breast feeding support: Impact on duration, *Journal of the American Dietetic Association* 88 (1988): 213–215.
26. R. A. Lawrence, Human lactation as a physiologic process, in *Report of the Surgeon General's Workshop on Breastfeeding and Human Lactation*, HHS Publication no. (HRS-D-MC) 84–2 (Washington, D.C.: Government Printing Office, 1984).
27. A. S. McNeilly, Effects of lactation on fertility, *British Medical Bulletin* 35 (1979): 151–154.
28. Lawrence, 1984.
29. P. G. Lunn and coauthors, The effect of improved nutrition onn plasma prolactin concentrations and postpartum infertility in lactating Gambian women, *American Journal of Clinical Nutrition* 39 (1984): 227–235.
30. H. Delgado, Nutrition. lactation, and postpartum amenorrhea, *American Journal of Clinical Nutrition* 31 (1978): 322–327.

31. R.V. Short, Breast feeding, *Scientific American* 2540 (1984): 35–41.
32. N. F. Butte and coauthors, Effect of maternal diet and body composition on lactational performance, *American Journal of Clinical Nutrition* 39 (1984): 296–306.
33. Food and Nutrition Board, Committee on Dietary Allowances, *Recommended Dietary Allowances*, 9th ed. (Washington, D.C.: National Academy of Sciences, 1980), p. 27.
34. Butte and coauthors, 1984.
35. Committee on Nutrition, American Academy of Pediatrics, nutrition and lactation, *Pediatrics* 68 (1981): 435–443.
36. B. Lonnerdal, Critical review: Effects of maternal dietary intake on human milk composition, *Journal of Nutrition* 116 (1986): 499–513.
37. Lonnerdal, 1986.
38. B. B. Peterkin, Women's diets: 1977–1985, *Journal of Nutrition Education* 18 (1986): 251–257.
39. Lonnerdal, 1986.
40. W. S. Harris, W. E. Connor, and S. Lindsey, Will dietary w-3 fatty acids change the composition of human milk?, *American Journal of Clinical Nutrition* 40 (1984): 780–785.
41. L. O. Byerley and A. Kirksey, Effects of different levels of vitamin C intake on the vitamin C concentration in human milk and the vitamin C intakes of breast-fed infants, *American Journal of Clinical Nutrition* 81 (1985): 665–671.
42. Food and Nutrition Board, 1980, pp. 55–124.
43. Food and Nutrition Board, 1980, p. 130; L. H. Allen, Calcium bioavailability and absorption: A review, *American Journal of Clinical Nutrition* 35 (1982): 783–808.
44. D. B. Jelliffe, Unique properties of human milk, *Journal of Reproductive Medicine* 14 (1975): 133.
45. Committee on Nutrition, 1981.
46. Saunders and Carroll, 1988.
47. K. Brøstrom, Human milk and infant formulas: Nutritional and immunological characteristics, in *Textbook of Pediatric Nutrition*, ed. R. M. Suskind (New York: Raven Press, 1981), pp. 41–64.
48. K. Brostrøm, 1981, p. 43.
49. D. Wink, Getting through the maze of infant formulas, *American Journal of Nursing* 4 (1985): 388–392.
50. T. A. Picone, Taurine update: Metabolism and function, *Nutrition Today*, August 1987, pp. 16–20.
51. M. S. Brady and coauthors, Specialized formulas and feedings for infants with malabsorption or formula intolerance, *Journal of the American Dietetic Association* 2 (1986): 191–200.
52. O. G. Brooke, Nutritional requirements of low and very low birthweight infants, in *Annual Review of Nutrition*, ed. R. E. Olson, E. Beutler, and H. P. Broquist (Palo Alto, Calif.: Annual Reviews, 1987), pp. 91–116.

▶ *Focal Point 3*

Dental Health

Teeth begin to develop in the fetus before birth, erupt during the first year, and serve their owners thereafter for a lifetime. It seems appropriate to present the relationships between nutrition and oral health early in this book, because the care parents deliver early in their children's lives can make a lifelong difference to their children's dental health.* As one authority put it, "The best time to start practicing good oral hygiene was yesterday. The next best time is today."**

The mouth is the normal passageway for all foods and beverages entering the body. Its parts work to prepare foods for their journey through the digestive system. The tongue senses the flavors that encourage or discourage food consumption. The teeth break large pieces of food into smaller ones, and saliva blends with these pieces to ease swallowing. The teeth also contribute to diction and facial appearance, and the gums support the teeth.

Nutrition and diet are important to dental and periodontal health. Conversely, oral health is important to nutrition. Due to both dental and periodontal disease, almost half of U.S. adults over age 65 have no teeth at all.[1] *wow!* Tooth loss and alveolar bone resorption change the contour of the jaw, impairing chewing ability and the fit of dentures. The loss of a tooth can reduce chewing efficiency, thereby creating difficulty in making food ready for swallowing. Dentures, even when they are comfortable, well-designed, and well-maintained, are less effective than natural teeth.

As surprising as it may sound, tooth loss can even be fatal. Circumstantial evidence points to toothlessness as a cause of death: a large majority of adult choking victims are denture wearers, and choking correlates with absence of *choking ↑ c̄ dentures* teeth. Missing teeth or improperly fitting dentures reduce chewing efficiency, and this results in the attempt to swallow dangerously large pieces of food.[2]

People with advanced gum disease, tooth loss, and ill-fitting dentures tend to select soft foods over fibrous, sometimes more nutritious foods. Foods such as corn on the cob, apples, and hard rolls that are difficult to chew are swallowed mostly unchewed, or avoided altogether. If they are replaced by creamed corn, applesauce, and rice, then nutrition status may not be greatly affected, but when food groups are avoided and variety is limited, nutrient deficiencies follow.

Since this discussion is about the connections of nutrition with oral health, it speaks little about dental care and oral hygiene, merely acknowledging their high priority. This discussion is intended to answer the questions:

saliva: the secretion of the salivary glands.

periodontal health: health of the tissues surrounding and supporting the teeth.

alveolar (al-VEE-oh-lar) bone: the part of the jawbone that forms the sockets of the teeth.

*This discussion is adapted from S. R. Rolfes and E. N. Whitney, Say cheese and smile: The nutrition and oral health picture, *Nutrition Clinics* (George F. Sickley Company, Philadelphia: December 1987).
**H. Hopkins, editorial director of *FDA Consumer*.

▶ How does nutrition before birth affect tooth development?

▶ How do nutrition, food, and eating patterns throughout life affect the health of the teeth and gums?

It concludes with a set of recommendations for the person interested in applying the answers.

Tooth Development

primary teeth: the first set of 20 teeth that are eventually replaced with permanent teeth; also called **deciduous** or **baby** teeth.

permanent teeth: the final set of 32 teeth that replace the primary teeth.

dentin: the main tissue of a tooth surrounding the pulp.
dens = tooth

enamel: the hard, white, dense substance made up mainly of calcium and phosphorus that covers the crown of the teeth. Enamel is the hardest substance in the human body.

caries (KARE-eez): gradual decay and disintegration of a tooth.
carius = rottenness

odontoblasts: cells from which dentin is formed.

ameloblasts: cells from which tooth enamel is formed.

Primary tooth development in human beings begins between two and three months in utero. By the last trimester of gestation, permanent teeth are forming. Of the ultimate 52 primary and permanent teeth that human beings form, 32 have begun to develop during gestation.[3] Maternal nutrition during pregnancy therefore profoundly influences the development of the teeth. Maternal nutrients must supply the preeruptive teeth with the building materials needed to develop in the proper sequence.

Like other tissues, the tissues in the mouth develop in stages. When nutrition insults occur during critical stages of their growth, the damage that results is irreversible. For example, defects in dentin or enamel formation cannot be corrected at any time after the critical stage.

To a great extent, heredity determines the potential arrangement of teeth, their eruption time, the tooth pattern and bite, the pits and fissures on the tooth surface, and their resistance to decay. Nutrition is one of several factors that help to determine the extent to which these potentials are realized. Chemical insults during pregnancy, including nutrient deficiencies during fetal development, can impair the development of the mouth structures. Severe nutrient deficiencies are not the only cause of abnormalities, but they can result in malformations that will make eating, chewing, and swallowing difficult. Subtle nutrient deficiencies during tooth development can reduce tooth size, interfere with tooth formation, delay the time of tooth eruption, and increase susceptibility of the teeth to caries.

Figure FP3–1 shows the anatomy of a tooth. The cells responsible for creating it are odontoblasts (dentin-forming cells) and ameloblasts (enamel-forming cells). The dentin interior and the outer enamel shell of the tooth are built on protein matrices that are subsequently mineralized—primarily with calcium, magnesium, and phosphorus. For dentin, the protein foundation is a collagen matrix, which requires a variety of substances, including vitamin C, for proper formation. The protein matrix for enamel is keratin, which depends in part on vitamin A for its synthesis. If protein or either vitamin is deficient during tooth development, then an imperfect matrix is laid down, and even with successful mineralization the final structure will be imperfect. Likewise, if the protein matrix is normal but mineralization is not, then the tooth will be poorly formed. Table FP3–1 summarizes some of the effects of nutrient deficiencies on dental development.

The table shows the effects of deficiencies of all of the nutrients just mentioned—protein, the minerals that serve as building materials, and the vitamins that assist in the building of the tooth. In most instances, the effects are easily explained. As would be expected, protein deficiency makes teeth

Figure FP3—1   The Anatomy of a Tooth

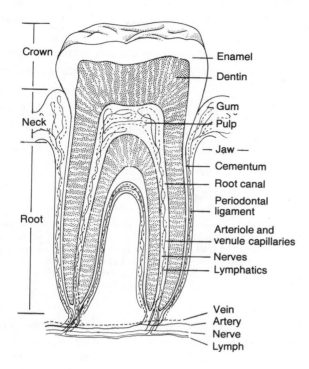

smaller, slower to erupt, and more irregularly shaped than normal.[4] The way in which it makes them susceptible to caries appears to be by reducing salivary flow.[5] Even when fetal and neonatal protein deficiency is later corrected with an adequate diet, reduced salivary flow persists, reflecting an irreversible effect of early protein deficiency on gland function.

Iron deficiency appears to act in the same way. Prenatal iron deficiency, even if marginal, decreases salivary flow and salivary protein content in children.[6] These salivary factors correlate with a high incidence of caries. Suboptimal zinc status prior to tooth eruption is also associated with an increase in dental caries.[7] The last nutrient mentioned in Table FP3—1 is fluoride, known to be important in converting the basic tooth crystal, hydroxyapatite, to the more decay-resistant crystal, fluorapatite. Altogether, nutrition during tooth development clearly has a major influence on future dental health.

Adequate maternal nutrition during pregnancy, with respect to all of these nutrients, is important to permit the optimal development of the child's teeth. Some controversy attends one question, however: whether pregnant women would benefit their children's teeth by taking prenatal fluoride supplements. The Food and Drug Administration prohibits manufacturers from claiming that fluoride supplements will prevent dental caries in infants of women who take supplements during pregnancy. Some researchers believe that because permanent teeth mineralize postnatally, these teeth receive little benefit from

hydroxyapatite (high-drox-ee-APP-ah- tite): the major calcium-containing crystal of bones and teeth. See also **fluorapatite**.

fluorapatite (floor-APP-ah-tite): the stabilized form of bone and tooth crystal (hydroxyapatite), in which fluoride replaces the hydroxy groups of the hydroxyapatite.

Table FP3–1   Nutrient Deficiencies Affecting Tooth Development

Nutrient Deficiency	Effect on Tooth Development
Protein	Small, irregularly shaped teeth, delayed eruption, high caries susceptibility
Vitamin C	Disturbance of collagen matrix of dentin
Vitamin A	Disturbance of keratin matrix of enamel
Vitamin D	Poor calcification, pitting, striations
Calcium	Poor calcification
Phosphorus	Poor calcification
Magnesium	Enamel hypoplasia
Iron	High caries susceptibility
Zinc	High caries susceptibility
Fluoride	High caries susceptibility

Source: Adapted from H. M. Leicester, Nutrition and the tooth, *Journal of the American Dental Association* 52 (1956): 284–289; A. E. Nizel, Preventing dental caries: The nutritional factors, *Pediatric Clinics of North America* 24 (1977): 141–155; J. H. Shaw and E. A. Sweeney, Oral health, in *Nutritional Support of Medical Practice*, ed. H. A. Schneider, C. E. Anderson, and D. B. Coursin, Philadelphia: Harper and Row, 1983.

prenatal supplements. Others point out that fluoride supplementation is most protective when at least part of the preeruptive phase of tooth development is included. If fluoride exposure during preeruptive tooth development is necessary, then prenatal supplementation may indeed be important to protecting primary teeth.

Fluoride does pass through the placenta to the fetus, but whether the placenta can defend against excess fluoride is questionable. Fluoride supplements are therefore not recommended for pregnant women who drink fluoridated water. However, supplementation is ordinarily regarded as safe, and some physicians and dentists do prescribe prenatal fluoride supplements to women who live in communities without fluoridated water. One long-term, well-controlled study reported recently that children of mothers taking prenatal fluoride supplements (2.2 milligrams sodium fluoride, which delivers 1 milligram fluoride) had, at the ages of five and six, teeth that were virtually immune to caries.[8] Their teeth contained greater concentrations of fluoride than those of children whose mothers had used just fluoridated water, and still greater concentrations than the teeth of children whose mothers had used nonfluoridated water during pregnancy.

The 20 primary teeth (sometimes referred to as baby teeth) begin to erupt at around four months of age and continue erupting through the third year of life. Tooth development continues to depend on systemic nutrition—supplied via the vascular system—until the final tooth erupts at around age 13. The formation and mineralization of teeth continues to depend on all of the nutrients named in Table FP3–1.

At the same time, as childhood progresses, the effect of nutrition on the teeth becomes increasingly more environmental than systemic; that is, the presence of food in the mouth increasingly affects the health of the teeth.

Dental Caries

Dental caries is an infectious oral disease that attacks the structure of the teeth. It is a pervasive health problem affecting 95 percent of the population.

The relationship between teeth, food, and caries development is complex and is complicated further by host factors, such as the hormonal and immunological milieux, that affect susceptibility to caries. Additional considerations are the behaviors and lifestyles that influence food selection, eating habits, and oral hygiene.

Caries develops as the result of the metabolism of fuels by microorganisms that reside in plaque on the surface of the teeth. These microorganisms consume carbohydrates, producing organic acids such as lactic acid and pyruvic acid as wastes. These acids cause the pH in the plaque and saliva to fall, and this leads to demineralization of the basic crystal of the enamel, hydroxyapatite. Calcium and phosphorus dissociate from the hydroxyapatite crystals and diffuse into the plaque. Fortunately, salivary fluids dilute and salivary proteins buffer the contents of the mouth; returning the pH to neutral. This results in plaque that is at neutral pH and supersaturated with calcium and phosphorus. A reverse flow of the calcium and phosphorus back into the enamel—that is, a remineralization of the enamel—can now occur. Until recently, caries development was considered to be a continuing demineralization process. Now it is viewed more as a dynamic process—one of alternating phases of demineralization and remineralization. When the net result is demineralization, caries develops.

Research conducted using animals reveals that at least two main ingredients are required to make dental caries: microorganisms and carbohydrates. Without microorganisms, there is no caries; that is, decay does not develop in a germ-free mouth, even with a cariogenic diet. Likewise, without a carbohydrate source, caries does not develop. Teeth remain caries-free when carbohydrate is fed via a tube into the gastrointestinal tract, even when the mouth is infected with microorganisms.

This discussion of caries development begins with the microorganisms that inhabit the mouth, the saliva that influences the oral environment, and the protective role of fluoride. The focus later shifts to the diet, the cariogenicity of foods, and the person's eating habits.

microorganism: small living bodies, such as bacteria, not perceptible to the naked eye.

plaque (PLACK): a sticky, colorless cluster of microorganisms, protein, and polysaccharides that adheres to teeth and gums. Plaque contributes to dental caries and periodontal disease. When calcium combines with the plaque and hardens, it becomes **tartar**.

organic acids: any organic compound containing one or more acid (carboxyl) groups (for example, lactic and pyruvic acids).

buffer: a substance capable of neutralizing both acids and bases.

cariogenic: conducive to caries formation.

Microorganisms

The principal dental plaque-forming, caries-producing microorganism is *Streptococcus mutans*, although other microorganisms have been shown to cause caries. *S. mutans* is found in caries, adheres readily to tooth surfaces, and uses carbohydrate from food to produce acid. Research to develop a vaccine or oral antibiotics against dental caries is focusing on this organism.

In addition to acids, *S. mutans* produces the sticky polysaccharides glucan and fructan from sucrose and other carbohydrates. These polysaccharides allow the microorganisms to adhere to the smooth enamel surfaces, creating the clusters of plaque. As the bacteria continue to metabolize carbohydrates, the acids become concentrated at the site and a carious lesion begins.

S. mutans bacteria are not found in the mouths of infants prior to tooth eruption.[9] Nor are they evident in people who have lost their teeth and do not wear dentures. The bacteria appear shortly after tooth eruption begins, and studies suggest that parents or other caretakers infect the infant's mouth with them.

A relationship is evident between the microbial infection of mothers and that of their children. Mothers with high concentrations of *S. mutans* have children with high concentrations, and mothers with low *S. mutans* concentrations have children with low concentrations. In one study, a preventive program for mothers was implemented that involved diet counseling, professional dental care and instruction, and fluoride treatment.[10] These preventive measures were not offered to their children, but the children were compared with the children of a control group. In both groups, the percentage of infected children increased with age, but it was lower in the experimental group. Only 16 percent of the children in the preventive group developed caries, compared with 43 percent in the control group. Prevention techniques reduced the *S. mutans* population in the mothers as well as in their children, resulting in fewer carious teeth.

Saliva

Most people fail to fully appreciate the complexities and contributions of saliva to their oral health. Fluids secreted by the salivary glands vary according to stimulation, age, sex, time of day, diet, diseases, and drug intake. Approximately 1 liter of saliva is secreted in a day in response to the chewing of food. Salivary flow during other times of the day is small, and during sleep, it is minimal. One of the major actions of salivary fluids is protection against dental caries. Saliva dilutes acid and normalizes pH as mentioned earlier, rinses the mouth, provides minerals, and exerts antibacterial activity.[11] The power to elicit secretion of saliva is one of the factors that determines to the cariogenicity of foods discussed later.

When salivary flow is reduced, the oral environment is less able to defend against caries. Reduced salivary flow may occur as a symptom of a disease, a side effect of medication, or in response to radiation therapy. Fasting also reduces salivary flow. Salivary flow progressively decreases during a 300-kcalorie, 3-liter liquid fast.[12] Researchers note an increase in the rate of plaque formation during fasting. This effect is not simply due to the lack of chewing stimulation, but might be explained by general dehydration.

Fluoride

The effect of prenatal fluoride has already been noted; debated until recently, its importance now appears to be supported by research. The importance of postnatal fluoride, on the other hand, has long been known. Numerous studies have shown that when fluoride is added to the water supply, the children in the community have fewer dental caries than children who drink nonfluoridated water. Children provided with optimally fluoridated water from birth have 50 to 70 percent fewer caries than otherwise expected.

Water fluoridation is the most effective, least expensive way to provide dental care to everyone. It protects the poor, the uninformed, and people who simply do not practice regular preventive measures or seek professional care. However, one-third of the U.S. population is not receiving fluoride because water fluoridation has not been adopted by local communities or the private water companies that serve them.

The National Research Council of the National Academy of Sciences recommends fluoridation of drinking water to approximately 1 part fluoride per million parts of water (1 ppm, which is the same as 1 milligram per liter). Water with 1 ppm fluoride offers the greatest caries protection at virtually no risk of fluorosis. Liquid fluoride supplements are available by prescription, and supplementation is recommended when the natural fluoride concentration in water is below 0.7 ppm. Table FP3–2 lists the American Dental Association's recommended supplement dosages by age.

fluorosis (flur-OH-sis): mottling of tooth enamel caused by excess fluoride.

All food and water supplies naturally contain variable amounts of fluoride in trace quantities.[13] About half of the U.S. population has access to water with an optimal fluoride concentration. Foods are not a major source of fluoride. The fluoride content of foods that are processed with fluoridated water, however, is higher than that of the same foods processed with fluoride-free water. The effect of water fluoridation on the food chain is becoming evident.

As would be expected, the fluoride content of beverages is also higher when they are processed with fluoridated water. The Food and Drug Administration has set limits on the natural and added fluoride content for domestic and imported bottled water. Most teas contain appreciable natural fluoride (contributing about 0.1 milligram fluoride per cup), even when brewed in fluoride-free water. An exception is herbal tea, popularly accepted as a caffeine-free alternative, which has negligible fluoride.

Excess fluoride causes dental fluorosis, a developmental imperfection of the tooth surface. At doses of 2 ppm, the teeth appear extremely white; at doses greater than 4 ppm, brown stains appear. (Stains on the teeth are also produced by other factors. When taken prenatally or during the first eight years of life, tetracycline stains teeth. Like the fluoride stains, tetracycline stains are permanent but do not weaken the tooth structure.) While the brown stains of fluorosis are cosmetically unattractive, dental fluorosis does not threaten health. Studies confirm that drinking water fluoridated to recommended levels poses no adverse health effects.[14]

The *preeruptive* maturation stage of tooth development is the critical time for *systemic* fluoride to offer its benefits in making the tooth resistant to caries throughout life.[15] This stage begins before birth and ends when the last molar

Table FP3–2   American Dental Association's Recommended Fluoride Supplement Dosages for Low-Fluoride Areas

Age	Dosage
0 to 2 yr	0.25 mg/day
2 to 3 yr	0.50 mg/day
3 to 10+ yr	1.00 mg/day

Source: Adapted from Effect of fluoride on dental health, *Nutrition and the M.D.*, December 1980, pp. 3–4.

erupts. It is during this time that the calcium and phosphate in the enamel are combining into hydroxyapatite, and systemic fluoride can convert it into fluorapatite—a combination of calcium fluoride and calcium phosphate. The benefit of this conversion is, as mentioned, that fluorapatite is more resistant than hydroxyapatite to the acid demineralization process that initiates dental caries.

The *posteruptive* maturation phase of tooth development is when *topical* fluoride makes the tooth resistant to caries.[16] Immediately after the tooth erupts and for the following two to three years, the outer enamel surface is immature. This is an ideal time to expose the teeth to the protection of fluoride, because they can take up minerals. (They are also more prone to decay if exposed to harmful substances.) Topical fluoride produces calcium fluoride and fluorapatite compounds. Such fluoride application also disrupts the normal growth and activity of dental plaque bacteria.[17]

Fluoridated drinking water offers both systemic benefits to developing teeth and topical benefits to those teeth already present. Fluoride in the drinking water washes over the teeth during their development, enabling them to continuously incorporate fluoride into their crystals.

Topical fluoride can partially compensate for long periods of enamel formation without fluoride, but this enamel is not as resistant to decay—it contains less fluorapatite. Even after teeth are formed, it is ideal to have fluoride continuously present in the oral environment. Teeth continue to exchange materials with the surrounding fluid all the time. This is why fluoridation of water is preferable to topical fluoride. For children who do not drink fluoridated water, fluoride tablets or drops are an effective method of providing both topical and systemic benefits.

The rate of dental caries in the general population is declining, with major credit going to water fluoridation. Even in communities without fluoridated water, the prevalence of caries is declining. This may be due to the increase of fluoride in the food chain, as already mentioned, because the use of fluoridated water in food processing is becoming increasingly common.[18]

Gum Disease

Although caries is declining, gum disease, or periodontal disease, still poses a large threat to most people, affecting over half of adults over age 45.[19] Gum disease is preventable with diligent oral hygiene, but if left untreated, it leads to bleeding gums, loosening of the teeth, and eventual loss of teeth.

Systemic nutrition may influence periodontal health by way of the immune system, bone metabolism, collagen formation, and epithelial tissue function. Consider, for example, that the oral epithelium has a rapid cell turnover rate, replacing cells every three to seven days. Any stress that compromises this ability to regenerate weakens the defense against microorganisms and, therefore, against gum disease.

The progress of gum disease can be slow and unnoticeable. It may first become evident when gums bleed while a person is brushing teeth. The same plaque that causes dental caries is the major initiating factor in gum disease. The plaque on tooth surfaces collects calcium salts, hardens, and turns into deposits of calculus, or tartar. The gums surrounding the tooth's root become inflamed and infected. If the infection progresses, resorption of the bone below the tooth begins, causing the tooth to lose its anchor.

Many factors contribute to gum disease. The primary cause, of course, is poor oral hygiene, but any irritation of the gums weakens their resistance to infection. Stresses such as bad tooth alignment, tooth loss, and tooth grinding can contribute to periodontal disease development.

Bone resorption may result from an inadequate dietary calcium intake. Results of studies describing the effect of calcium intake, calcium-phosphorus ratio of the diet, and calcium and vitamin D supplements on skeletal osteoporosis are applicable to oral bone and its resistance to resorption. The rate of alveolar bone loss is slowed by a calcium intake of 1000 to 1500 milligrams per day.[20] One study reported that alveolar bone loss in patients receiving a calcium and vitamin D supplement was 36 percent less than in patients receiving a placebo.[21] The effect on the teeth is not as direct as on the bone, but, as noted earlier, alveolar bone resorption causes the teeth to lose their anchor.

Another nutrition connection, not often encountered but worth mentioning, is vitamin C, which has long been associated with the integrity of the gums. Gum deterioration is a classic clinical symptom of acute vitamin C deficiency. The effects of subclinical vitamin C deficiency are less well documented, but a recent study reports that subclinical vitamin C deficiency does influence the early stages of gingival inflammation even under conditions of sustained oral hygiene.[22] Gingival bleeding and inflammation varied directly with changes in vitamin C intake and serum concentrations. Vitamin C depletion did not affect other dental measurements observed, such as plaque accumulation.

calculus: general term for any abnormal concentration of mineral salts, also referred to as **tartar**.

tartar: calcium salts, mucin, and bacteria deposits found on the teeth and gums; also called **calculus**.

gingiva (jin-JYE-va or JIN-jih-va): the tissue surrounding the necks of the teeth and supporting bone; also called the **gums**. Gingival inflammation is known as **gingivitis** (jin-jih-VYE-tis).

Foods and Eating Habits to Foster Oral Health

Healthful eating habits from the nutrition standpoint are not necessarily healthful eating habits from the dental standpoint. A selection of foods may provide all the nutrients in adequate amounts to support overall health, but still may promote caries development. Of course, all meals should be followed by proper oral hygiene, but, realistically, this does not always happen. The question what foods are most and least cariogenic is therefore of interest.

The American Dental Association is trying to develop a rating system for the cariogenicity of foods. Most likely, it will be based on the key factor that results from all the characteristics of a food working together—namely, the amount of acid a food produces in plaque. Guidelines based on cariogenicity may eventually find their way to food labels. In Switzerland, foods that pass the acid-plaque test are labeled with a smiley-faced tooth to signify that the product is "safe for teeth." This positive labeling system encourages consumers to purchase such items for between-meal snacks.

Prime among the relevant characteristics of foods is their carbohydrate content. Carbohydrates are the fuel source for bacteria—carbohydrates of many kinds, not just refined table sugar (sucrose). Honey, molasses, brown sugar, glucose, fructose, and starches all have a strong cariogenic potential.

However, sugar alcohols, which are used as sugar substitutes, are either noncariogenic or have extremely low cariogenicity potential. Some may actually have anticariogenic effects. In experimental studies in rats, partial or total substitution of xylitol for dietary sucrose results in caries reduction.[23] The effect is greater than just the displacement of sucrose—xylitol seems to have a therapeutic effect against caries. Rinsing with a xylitol solution after a sucrose-containing meal reduces the cariogenicity of the diet. Xylitol stimulates salivary flow, increases pH, maintains a high pH, and resists microbial metabolism.

Other sugar substitutes, such as saccharin, aspartame, and cyclamate, are thought to be protective against caries simply because they are not metabolized to acids. However, one study concluded that saccharin actually inhibited caries in rats.[24] Rats fed a saccharin-supplemented diet developed fewer caries than rats fed the same diet without supplementation or with aspartame supplementation. Offsetting this effect of saccharin are other health risks, though, so its use should be moderate.

In addition to the presence of carbohydrate in foods, the retention of those foods in the mouth is critical.[25] Foods that stay in the mouth for a long time yield acid for a long time. Sticky foods are retained on tooth surfaces longer and present a greater risk than foods that are readily cleared from the mouth. For that reason, the sugar in a soft drink is less significant than that in caramels, pastries, or jelly. By the same token, the sugar in a sticky food such as dried fruit is more detrimental than its quantity alone would suggest.

Stickiness is not the only factor affecting food retention. Curiously, sugar speeds up the clearance rate of starchy foods from the mouth. Starchy foods with a high sugar content are removed more rapidly and lower the pH of the plaque for a shorter time than do starchy foods with less sugar.[26]

The sugar content of a food and the amount of acid produced from that sugar do not always parallel the amount of enamel dissolved. Some foods, such as citrus fruits and carbonated beverages, contain acids of their own, and these acids can act directly on the tooth enamel. These dietary acids are strong enough to depress the pH below the point at which bacterial enzymes are active, so no new acid is formed, but the acid already present is strong enough to significantly dissolve enamel.[27]

Interestingly, a high sugar concentration can also depress bacterial growth and activity. Foods with high concentrations of sugar (candies) rapidly leave the mouth and destroy less enamel than do foods with less sugar in combination with starch (breads and cookies).[28] This effect is not simply explained by the stickiness of the foods. A variety of other factors, including fat and salt content, also influence food clearance.[29] Thus, to predict which foods will be cariogenic is not as easy as might be expected. Researchers often isolate one dietary factor to determine the extent of its effect on caries development, but when they do so, the usefulness of the findings is limited because people eat meals that contain multiple dietary factors. Quite often, the findings of such research are variable and inconsistent. Researchers lack standardized reference foods and methods for assessing cariogenic potential. To establish a cariogenicity rating for a food is to rely on many questionable assumptions. Nevertheless, pieces are being collected and analyzed in the hope of assembling a puzzle in which, someday, they will all fit.

The cariogenicity of a food depends on its chemical composition and physical form. The chemical composition of a food includes not only the type of carbohydrate, but also the content of dietary acids, calcium, phosphorus, and fluoride. In addition, the food's ability to stimulate salivary flow is considered. The physical form of a food affects its retention in the mouth.

Some high-fiber carbohydrate foods are an example of anticariogenic foods. In particular, raw vegetables such as celery and carrots are sometimes called "detergent" foods. Their crisp and crunchy texture serves as a mechanical cleanser, removing food particles from teeth. They do not stick to the teeth and they require vigorous, thorough chewing, which stimulates salivary flow. Increased saliva flow helps to clear the food from the mouth and buffer the plaque acid. The person wishing to minimize caries formation could munch on these types of foods at the end of any meal, if brushing was not feasible. Rinsing the mouth with water also helps, of course.

Apples offer an interesting contrast. They are recommended by some as a good food to eat at the end of a meal to help prevent caries, and they have been called "nature's toothbrush" because they stimulate salivary juices and "brush" the surfaces of the teeth. However, while it is true that they stimulate salivary flow, they also liberate sugar after they have been crushed by the teeth; the sugar contributes to acid formation, which soon offsets the buffering effect of the saliva. One study measured the pH changes that occurred when either apples or peanuts were consumed after a lump of sugar.[30] In some individuals, apples caused the pH to fall even lower than the sugar had already done. In contrast, peanuts raised the pH that had been lowered by the sugar. Apples, then, may offer saliva-stimulating benefits, but they still may lower pH, and they do not brush teeth clean at potential caries sites. This example illustrates how foods may have both caries-promoting and caries-preventing effects. The best foods to eat at the end of a meal are those that have a saliva-stimulating effect and do *not* depress pH.

Another contrast is provided by cheese. Cheese is a powerful saliva stimulant, and its proteins also buffer pH in the mouth. Even when eaten immediately after sugary foods, cheese raises plaque pH.[31] A piece of cheese eaten at the end of a meal may therefore reduce the cariogenicity of the meal. A further contribution cheese makes to dental health is its high calcium and phosphorus content.

So far, these factors have been mentioned: the quantity of carbohydrate, the nature of the carbohydrate, its context (such as the stickiness of the food, or acid, fiber, or protein present in it), and its saliva-stimulating effect. Another concern is the *frequency* of its consumption. Carbohydrate eaten between meals poses a greater risk of dental caries than does carbohydrate eaten with meals. Bacteria produce acid for 20 to 30 minutes after an exposure to sugar. So, if a person were to eat three pieces of candy at one time, the teeth would be exposed to approximately 30 minutes of acid demineralization. If that person were to eat three pieces of candy at half-hour intervals, the time of exposure to acid would increase to 90 minutes. Likewise, slowly sipping a sugar-sweetened soft drink between meals may be more harmful than drinking the entire soda at mealtime.

An extreme effect of prolonged tooth exposure to carbohydrate is seen in infants who are put to bed sucking on a bottle of formula, milk, or fruit juice, or who use such a bottle as a pacifier for extended periods of time. They experience extensive and rapid loss of tooth material. Prolonged sucking on such a bottle bathes the upper teeth for long periods in a carbohydrate-rich

nursing bottle syndrome: extensive tooth decay due to prolonged tooth contact with formula, milk, fruit juice, or other carbohydrate-rich liquid offered to an infant in a bottle.

fluid. (The tongue covers and protects most of the lower teeth, although they too may be affected.) Salivary flow, which normally cleanses the mouth and neutralizes the acid, diminishes as the child falls asleep. The result is decayed teeth (nursing bottle syndrome). This syndrome has also been reported in breastfed infants offered the breast for extended times. To prevent it, children should not be given a bottle as a pacifier at bedtime. If a bottle is given, it should be filled with water. In fact, a wise mother would offer her infant water after each feeding to rinse the mouth.

It makes sense to select foods with dental health as well as nutrition in mind. Of course, it is always best to brush and floss the teeth, or at least to rinse the mouth, after eating meals and snacks, but there is no harm in applying some knowledge of the relative cariogenicity of foods as well. For example, the person who likes raisins might be better advised to eat a carrot-raisin salad or raisin muffins with meals after which toothbrushing will follow rather than to eat raisins between meals and let them stick to the teeth. Recommendations from the American Dental Association with respect to foods approved as snacks are provided in Table FP3–3.

Teeth can last a lifetime with proper care. They do not have to loosen and fall out, even with old age. It is evident that diet and nutrition can promote dental health throughout life. The same balanced diet that promotes general health can also contribute to sound dental health, provided that, as the American Dental Association recommends, consumers control the frequency

Table FP3–3   Dietary Recommendations for Controlling Dental Caries

Food Group	Low cariogenicity: Use when teeth cannot be brushed immediately.	High cariogenicity: Do not use unless followed by prompt and thorough dental hygiene.
Dairy	Milk, cheese, plain yogurt	Chocolate milk, ice cream, ice milk, milk shakes, fruited yogurts, eggnog
Meat/alternates	Meat, fish, poultry, eggs, legumes	Peanut butter with added sugar, luncheon meats with added sugar, meats with sugared glazes
Fruit	Fresh, packed in water or juice	Dried, packed in syrup, jams, jellies, preserves, fruit juices and drinks
Vegetable	Most vegetables	Candied sweet potatoes, glazed carrots
Bread/cereal	Popcorn, soda crackers, toast, hard rolls, pretzels, potato chips, corn chips, pizza	Cookies, sweet rolls, pies, cakes, ready-to-eat sweetened cereals as a between-meal snack
Other	Sugarless gum, coffee or tea without sugar	Sugared soft drinks, candy, fudge, caramels, honey, sugars, syrups

with which they eat cariogenic foods, especially when they cannot brush their teeth immediately afterwards. The following guidelines are offered to maximize protection against dental caries and gum disease. Parents can help their children establish good dental habits and health by:

▸ Not allowing their infants to sleep with bottles of carbohydrate-rich liquids.

▸ Watching for hidden sugars in foods they provide their children; using low-sugar or sugar-free products whenever possible.

▸ Restricting sweet treats to mealtimes.

▸ Encouraging their children to practice oral hygiene after eating between-meal snacks.

▸ Limiting the duration of time their children's teeth are exposed to adhesive foods.

▸ Encouraging their children to brush and floss daily, and visit a dentist for regular checkups.

▸ Encouraging their children to rinse with water after eating if brushing and flossing are not possible.

▸ Allowing children to drink fluoridated water; providing fluoride supplements when such water is not available.

▸ Providing their children with a balanced diet composed of a variety of foods that will maintain an adequate nutrition status.

▸ Encouraging their children to eat foods rich in calcium and phosphorus.

▸ Providing their children with a variety of firm, fibrous foods that will stimulate gingival tissues, alveolar bone, and salivary glands.

These measures will serve personal dental health well. For the benefit of the younger generation, it is also important to make efforts to improve the social context so that it will better support their dental health. Unfortunately, much of the effort of the food industry is not directed toward this goal. Printed advertisements and television commercials compete to attract public attention to new items that delight the taste buds, but threaten the teeth. The average television-watching child sees over 21,000 commercials each year; approximately half of those commercials are for foods and beverages, most of which contain sugar.[32] Cereals, candy, and gum lead the list of kinds of foods advertised on the nation's airwaves. Cookies, crackers, desserts, and soft drinks follow close behind. At the bottom of the list are vegetables, citrus fruits and juices, and cheese.

Food companies spend billions of dollars on television advertising. In essence, they try to encourage consumption of the very foods that health experts warn us not to indulge in. The effect of advertising is seen in children's influence on food selections. The tantalizing messages about high-sugar (and therefore low-nutrient) foods take unfair advantage of an impressionable, nutritionally naive audience.

Take a moment to consider this naive audience. Children receive about 70 hours a year learning about foods by way of television commercials—information that is almost invariably misleading. Compare that to the number of hours parents, teachers, and dentists spend each year providing children with sound nutrition and dental care information. Television commercials do not offer nutrition education, nor do they warn of problems certain foods pose to health. The Netherlands require that commercials of sugary foods show an insignia of toothpaste being applied to a toothbrush during the last few seconds of the ad.

Consumers can influence television commercials. When the Surgeon General warned of health problems associated with smoking, antismoking commercials were aired until cigarette advertising was eventually banned. The advertising of sweet foods corrupts good nutrition and dental habits. Parents and health professionals need to continue making efforts to pressure the industry to respond to their concern for healthy teeth.

A poster in a dental office reminds clients, "There is nothing the dentist can do that will overcome what the patient will not do." Professional dental care, in other words, augments but does not replace personal dental hygiene. Learning and practicing good dental hygiene habits early in life will serve a child through adulthood. Parents will want to teach their children how to brush with fluoridated toothpaste and gently floss regularly to remove plaque. When water fluoridation is not available, parents can provide fluoride supplements, lozenges, and rinses. Beyond these strategies, parents can be assertive in helping their children to resist social influences that pull the wrong way, conscientious about providing an adequate diet, and faithful in encouraging eating habits consistent with dental health.

Focal Point 3 Notes

1. Dentistry at the crossroads: The future is uncertain, the challenges are many, *American Journal of Public Health* 72 (1982): 653–654.
2. C. A. Geissler and J. F. Bates, The nutritional effects of tooth loss, *American Journal of Clinical Nutrition* 39 (1984): 478–489.
3. F. B. Glenn, W. D. Glenn, and R. C. Duncan, Fluoride tablet supplementation during pregnancy for caries immunity: A study of the offspring produced, *American Journal of Obstetrics and Gynecology* 143 (1982): 560–564.
4. M. C. Alfano, Effect of diet and malnutrition during development on subsequent resistance to oral disease, *National Symposium on Dental Nutrition*, ed. S. Wei (Iowa City: University of Iowa Press, 1979), p. 23, as cited in M. C. Alfano, Nutrition, sweeteners, and dental caries, *Food Technology* January 1980, pp. 70–74.
5. L. Menaker and J. M. Navia, Effect of undernutrition during the perinatal period on caries development in the rat. V. Changes in whole saliva volume and protein content, *Journal of Dental Research* 53 (1974): 592, as cited in M. C. Alfano, Nurition, sweeteners, and dental caries, *Food Technology* (1980): 70–74.

6. M. C. Alfano, J. Sintes, and D. P. DePaola, Effect of marginal dietary iron deficiency during development on caries susceptibility in rats, *Journal of Dental Research* 58 (special issue A, 1979): 422, as cited in M. C. Alfano, Nutrition, sweeteners, and dental caries, *Food Technology* (1980): 70–74.
7. Increased dental caries in young rats suckled by zinc-deficient rats, *Nutrition Reviews* 37 (1979): 232–233.
8. Glenn, Glenn, and Duncan, 1982.
9. *Streptococcus mutans* and human caries, *Nutrition Reviews* 36 (1987): 107–109.
10. Relation of caries prevention in mothers to the infection of their children's mouths, *Nutrition Reviews* 41 (1983): 341–342.
11. I. D. Mandel, Relation of saliva and plaque to caries, *Journal of Dental Research* 53: (1974): 246–266.
12. I. Johansson, T. Ericson, and L. Steen, Studies of the effect of diet on saliva secretion and caries development: The effect of fasting on saliva composition of female subjects, *Journal of Nutrition* 114 (1984): 2010–2020.
13. G. S. Rao, Dietary intake and bioavailability of fluoride, *Annual Review of Nutrition* 4 (1984): 115–136.

14. V. L. Richmond, Thirty years of fluoridation: A review, *American Journal of Clinical Nutrition* 41 (1985): 129–138.
15. A. E. Nizel, Preventing dental caries: The nutritional factors, *Pediatric Clinics of North America* 24 (1977): 141–155.
16. Nizel, 1977.
17. Nizel, 1977.
18. D. H. Leverett, Fluorides in the changing prevalence of dental caries, *Science* 217 (1982): 26–30.
19. Dentistry at the crossroads, 1982.
20. Diet, nutrition, and oral health: A rational approach for the dental practice, *Journal of the American Dental Association* 109 (1984): 20–32.
21. K. E. Wical and P. Brussee, Effects of a calcium and vitamin D supplement on alveolar ridge resorption in immediate denture patients, *Journal of Prosthetic Dentistry* 41 (1979): 4–11.
22. P. J. Leggott and coauthors, The effect of controlled ascorbic acid depletion and supplementation on periodontal health, *Journal of Periodontology* 57 (1986): 480–485.
23. K. K. Makinen and A. Scheinin, Xylitol and dental caries, *Annual Review of Nutrition* 2 (1982): 133–150.
24. J. M. Tanzer and A. M. Slee, Saccharin inhibits tooth decay in laboratory models,

Journal of the American Dental Association 106 (1983): 331–333.

25. B. G. Bibby and coauthors, Oral food clearance and the pH of plaque and saliva, *Journal of the American Dental Association* 112 (1986): 333–337.

26. Bibby and coauthors, 1986.

27. B. G. Bibby and S. A. Mundorff, Enamel demineralization by snack foods, *Journal of Dental Research* 54 (1975): 461–470.

28. Bibby and Mundorff, 1975.

29. Bibby and Mundorff, 1975.

30. D. A. M. Geddes and coauthors, Apples, salted peanuts, and plaque pH, *British Dental Journal* 142 (1977): 317–319.

31. A. J. Rugg-Gunn and coauthors, The effect of different meal patterns upon plaque pH in human subjects, *British Dental Journal* 139 (1975): 351–356.

32. R. B. Choate, Selling cavities—U.S. style, address presented at the American Dental Association Council on Dental Health Meeting, Miami Beach, Florida, 11 October 1977.

Infants: A Nurtured Beginning

4

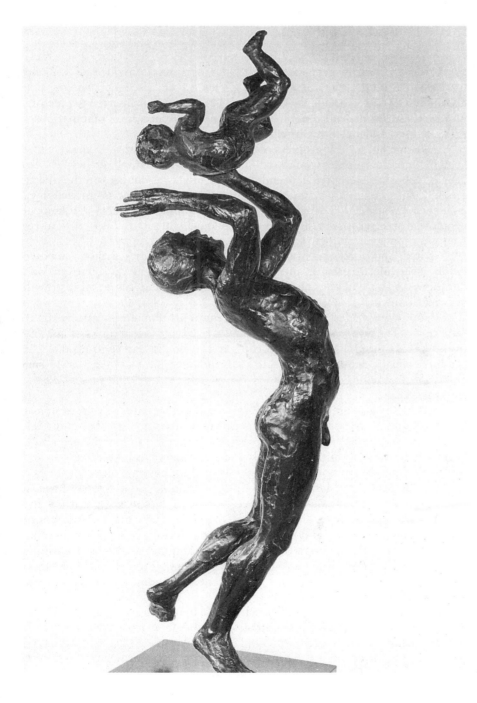

Growth and Development
Nutrient Needs
    Water
    Energy-Yielding Nutrients
    Vitamins
    Minerals
    Vitamin–Mineral Supplements for
        the Infant
    Nutrient Needs of the Preterm,
        Low-Birthweight Infant
Feeding the Infant
    Nutrients in Breast Milk and Formula
    Protection Conferred by Breast Milk
    Introducing Cow's Milk
    Introducing Solids

▶▶ Practical Point: Mealtimes with Infants

▶ **Focal Point:**   Nutrition Care of Sick Infants and Children

153

Father and Son by Paul T. Granlund.

The first year of life is a time of phenomenal growth and development. To attain full potential, the infant requires an abundant supply of nutrients. The infant's high nutrient needs and physical immaturity define the foods most appropriate for the first year of life. Nutrition during that year is the focus of this chapter.

Growth and Development

Physical growth is a diverse and complex phenomenon. It involves not only the progressive increase in size of a living being, but also the changes that accompany this increase. Growth depends on a variety of interrelated factors, of which nutrition is but one. The presence or absence and combination of these factors influence how growth progresses.

Development is "the progress of an egg to the adult state." In many ways, growth and development go hand in hand: as something grows, it also develops. But development is broader than growth, pertaining, on the microscopic level, to qualitative anatomical and physiological changes as well as to an increase in size. On the macroscopic level, development refers to attainment of motor and sensory skills and psychological attributes, as well as to anatomical and physiological changes.[1]

Growth and development are not uniform. Each body system has its own unique schedule of growth and development, varying in rate, pattern, and duration. As you will see, the first year of life is a time of remarkable growth and development.

An infant grows faster during the first year of life than ever again, as Figure 4–1 shows. The infant's birthweight doubles by about four months of age and triples by one year. (If an adult, starting at 150 pounds, were to do this, the person's weight would increase to 450 pounds in a single year.) This tremendous growth is a composite of the differing growth patterns of all the internal organs.

Development proceeds along with growth, and its course in the first year is remarkable. Externally, an observer can note that at birth the infant can hardly see, and cannot roll over; at a year, the infant can talk and crawl and is beginning to walk. At birth, it can only suck; at a year, it can hold a spoon and feed itself. Internal physiological changes parallel the external ones: for the first few months of life, the infant can swallow only liquids, the digestive tract is immature, and the kidneys have a limited capacity to concentrate urine and excrete water and sodium. The internal changes, especially the development of the gastrointestinal tract and kidneys, are of particular relevance to nutrition because they enable the infant to handle more and more complex foodstuffs from plain breast milk or formula at the start of the year to foods from all food groups at the end. A later section, "Developmental readiness," describes these developmental details.

The growth of infants directly reflects their nutritional health, and is a parameter used to assess their nutrition status. Nutrient deficiencies and excesses in early infancy can have long-term, irreversible effects on the growth and development of infants. Throughout the world, undernutrition is by far

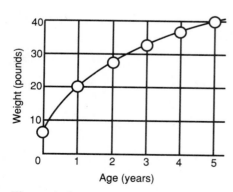

Figure 4–1 Weight Gain of Human Infants in their First Five Years of Life
An infant grows faster during the first year of life than ever again.

the greater of these two problems; thus, many examples of deficiency effects appear in this chapter.

As is true of pregnancy, much of what we know about nutrition during infancy comes from animal studies. One question of critical importance asks whether the effects of malnutrition in infancy or early childhood leave a permanent mark, or can be rectified by subsequent good nutrition. The answer may be either, depending on the time and nature of the deprivation. One study examined the effects of supplying unlimited food to animals that had suffered undernutrition at different ages.[2] Rats malnourished during the first three weeks of life grow more slowly than normal, and continue to grow slowly even when provided an unlimited food supply. They do not catch up in growth to their well-nourished peers, and they become small adults. On the other hand, rats well-nourished until the 9th week of life and then undernourished from the 9th to the 12th week grow rapidly when given unlimited food after that. Their mean weight actually surpasses that of rats that are never malnourished. In both instances, the rats experience three weeks of nutrient deprivation, yet one group's growth potential is never achieved. The critical difference is in the timing of the deprivation.

Severe early malnutrition in human beings can also result in permanent stunting of growth. The long-term consequences of malnutrition are apparent in the short stature and low weight of adult populations who have suffered nutrient deprivation in early childhood.[3]

Depending on each body system's particular schedule of growth, the time of deprivation has different effects on each system. The growth of the brain illustrates this concept. The timing of brain cell replication varies among different species, but in general, it occurs most rapidly just prior to, or immediately following, birth. In human beings, brain cell number, as determined by increase in DNA content, rises rapidly until birth and more slowly until six months of age.[4] Thus, the brain stops its cell replication earlier than the body as a whole does, or than other organs do. Achievement of total adult brain weight occurs at approximately two years of age.

In one rat study, malnutrition during the period of active brain cell division reduced the total brain cell number finally achieved.[5] Based on this information, researchers speculated that if the response to malnutrition in the human brain is similar to that in the rat brain, then the critical postnatal period of cell division would be the first six months of life. The researchers then compared well-nourished infants who died accidentally with infants who had died of severe malnutrition during the first year of life. They examined both brain protein, which reflects the total mass of cells in the brain, and brain DNA, which reflects the number of cells. (The ratio of protein to DNA reflects cell size.) Brain cell sizes were normal in both groups, but the cell number was significantly reduced in the brains of the malnourished infants as reflected by their weight, protein, and DNA contents.[6] Severe early malnutrition, then, can curtail the normal increase in brain cell number in human beings.

The impact of malnutrition during critical periods is evident from these studies. In addition to the timing of the malnutrition episode, the economic and social environment influence the long-term consequences of early malnutrition. The intellectual capacities of young boys who had suffered severe malnutrition (protein deprivation, energy deprivation, or a combination of the two) during their first two years of life were compared with those of a matched group of boys who had never been malnourished. Malnutrition in the context of an unfavorable social and economic environment resulted in intellectual impairment.[7] The effect of malnutrition on intellectual development was negligible, however, against the background of a generally favorable social and economic environment. This study was unique in that it examined the effects of malnutrition during infancy while controlling for living conditions.

Another study examined the effects of severe malnutrition during infancy on intellectual functions as well as subsequent physical growth, but did not control for social and economic variables.[8] The study did, however, produce some interesting results based on a 15-year follow-up of 20 severely malnourished infants. Over the 15 years, evidence of gross, irreversible intellectual impairment was collected. This impairment was not corrected, despite improved nutrition and environmental conditions. The deficits in intellectual function appeared to be permanent. Over the years, with improved nutrition, the difference in mean height between the malnourished group and their well-nourished peers diminished. In contrast, the difference in mean head circumference increased. This does not suggest a correlation between head circumference and intellect, but rather a relation between head circumference and suboptimal brain growth.

These studies indicate that early malnutrition can retard both mental development and physical growth. The extent of growth retardation and mental impairment depends on the timing, severity, and duration of the malnutrition. Fortunately, children have an amazing power to return to their predicted growth curves with adequate nutrition—that is, they can catch up. In physical growth, children show astonishingly rapid rates of catch-up growth. The rate of catch-up growth is influenced by the nature of the initial deficit and the composition of the rehabilitation diet.[9] Catch-up velocity in height can reach four times the normal velocity for chronological age.[10] In mental development, however, catch-up growth appears to be minimal, if it occurs at all.

Malnutrition in human beings generally implies a deficiency of food energy, and thus a deficiency of specific nutrients such as protein. Protein is the single nutrient that most strongly affects the growth rate, but it is difficult to isolate the effects of specific nutrient deficiencies on growth and development. In addition to adequate energy and protein, other nutrients are also vital, including water, the other energy-yielding nutrients, vitamins A, D, E, K, the B vitamins, vitamin C, iron, calcium and zinc. The importance of these nutrients to the infant's growth and development is discussed within the sections on individual nutrients that follow.

Nutrient Needs

Nutrient deficiencies can and do occur in infancy. The effects of these deficiencies confirm the crucial role adequate nutrition has in normal growth and development. The rapid growth and metabolism of the infant demand an ample supply of *all* the nutrients, but the energy-yielding nutrients and those vitamins and minerals critical to the growth process have special importance during infancy. This section emphasizes those nutrients that scientific research

catch-up growth: the acceleration in growth that occurs when a period of growth retardation ends and favorable conditions are restored. It is a self-correcting response that, at best, restores the individual to his or her original growth channel.

has thus far deemed most important to growth and development. Nutrients for which reliable information is lacking, or whose role in growth and development is less well-defined appear in Table 4–1.

Before any discussion of nutrient needs for the infant can begin, it must be acknowledged that the information on which nutrient recommendations for infants are based is incomplete at this point. Much remains to be learned, even as regards such major nutrients as protein and energy. Estimates of vitamin and mineral needs for the infant are based on even more uncertainty. Despite this, we must have a standard on which nutrient adequacy and timing of supplemental foods for the infant can be based. Because of large variations in growth rates, activity level, size, metabolic rate, environment, and other factors, it is impossible to establish an ideal standard for all infants. For this reason, recommendations are often expressed within a specified range. The Recommended Dietary Allowances (RDA), the standard in the United States, and the Recommended Nutrient Intakes (RNI), the standard in Canada, are recommendations for nutrient intakes of population groups, which take into account individual variability (nutrient recommendations appear on the inside front cover and in Appendix B). The standard used in establishing nutrient allowances for infants is the average amount of nutrients consumed by thriving infants breastfed by healthy, well-nourished mothers. Therefore, much of the discussion of infant nutrient needs that follows is a discussion of the nutrient content of breast milk.

During the first year of life the infant's need for most nutrients, based on body weight, is about double that of the adult; for some nutrients it is more than doubled. Figure 4–2 compares a three-month-old infant's needs with those of an adult male. The discussion that follows describes the normal infant's needs, nutrient by nutrient, and the basis on which requirements for individual nutrients are established. At the end is a section on the premature infant's needs.

Water

One of the most essential nutrients for the infant, as for anyone, is water. The younger the infant, the greater the percentage of body weight is water. The water in an infant's body is easily lost because, compared to an adult's body, a larger percentage of it is located in the interstitial (extracellular) and vascular spaces. Conditions that cause fluid loss without replacement, such as diarrhea or vomiting, can result in life-threatening dehydration. During early infancy, breast milk or infant formula normally provides enough water for a healthy infant to replace water losses from the skin, lungs, feces and urine.[11] If an infant is exposed to hot weather, has diarrhea, or vomits repeatedly, however, supplemental water is needed to prevent dehydration. In addition, adults must remember that infants may cry for thirst as well as hunger. Allow infants to drink water until their thirst is quenched.

Supplemental water is required for all infants once the addition of solid foods to the diet has begun. Foods with a high protein content, such as meats and eggs, present the kidneys with a high renal solute load, which requires additional water to ease the burden on the kidneys. The infant's ability to concentrate urine does not reach adult capacity until around a year of age.

renal solute load: a measure of the concentration of all dissolved substances in the urine that result from the feeding of a milk, formula, or diet. As the kidneys mature, they can handle higher solute loads; the low solute load of breast milk is ideal for the infant, especially the premature infant. A formula with too high a renal solute load can cause dehydration by incurring too great an obligatory water excretion. This is a life-threatening condition in the infant.

Table 4–1 Vitamins and Minerals in Infancy

Nutrient	Primary function	Deficiency symptoms	1980 RDA[a]	Significant sources[b]
Vitamin A	Vision; maintenance of cornea, epithelial cells, mucous membranes, skin; bone and tooth growth; reproduction; hormone synthesis and regulation; immunity	Microcytic anemia; night blindness; keratinization; corneal degeneration leading to blindness; rashes; abnormal tooth and jaw alignment	0–6 months: 420 RE 6–12 months: 400 RE	Fortified milk, cheese, cream, butter, fortified margarine, eggs, liver
Thiamin	Part of coenzyme used in energy metabolism; supports normal appetite and nervous system function	Edema; enlarged heart; abnormal heart rhythms; heart failure	0–6 months: 0.3 mg 6–12 months: 0.5 mg	Occurs in all nutritious foods in moderate amounts; pork, ham, bacon, liver, whole grains, legumes, nuts
Riboflavin	Part of a coenzyme used in energy metabolism; supports normal vision and skin health	Cracks at corners of mouth; magenta tongue; hypersensitivity to light; reddening of cornea; skin rash	0–6 months: 0.4 mg 6–12 months: 0.6 mg	Milk, yogurt, cottage cheese, meat, leafy green vegetables, whole-grain or enriched breads and cereals
Niacin	Part of a coenzyme used in energy metabolism; supports health of skin, nervous system, and digestive system	Diarrhea; black; smooth tongue	0–6 months: 6 mg equiv. 6–12 months: 8 mg equiv.	Milk, eggs, meat, poultry, fish, whole-grain and enriched breads and cereals, nuts, and all protein-containing foods
Vitamin B$_6$	Part of a coenzyme used in amino acid and fatty acid metabolism; helps convert tryptophan to niacin; helps make red blood cells	Microcytic anemia; smooth tongue; irritability; muscle twitching; convulsions	0–6 months: 0.3 mg 6–12 months: 0.6 mg	Leafy green vegetables, meats, fish, poultry, shellfish, legumes, fruits, whole grains
Folacin	Part of a coenzyme used in new cell synthesis	Megaloblastic anemia	0–6 months: 30 μg 6–12 months: 45 μg	Leafy green vegetables, legumes, seeds, liver
Vitamin B$_{12}$	Part of a coenzyme used in a new cell synthesis; helps maintain nerve cells	Megaloblastic anemia; smooth tongue; fatigue	0–6 months: 0.5 μg 6–12 months: 1.5 μg	Foods of animal origin (meat, fish, poultry, shellfish, milk, cheese, eggs)

Nutrient	Function	Deficiency	Amount	Sources
Vitamin C	Collagen synthesis (strengthens blood vessel walls, forms scar tissue, matrix for bone growth); antioxidant; thyroxine synthesis; amino acid metabolism; strengthens resistance to infection; helps in absorption of iron	Microcytic anemia; pinpoint hemorrhages; frequent infections; bleeding gums	0–12 months: 35 mg	Citrus fruits, cabbage-type vegetables, dark green vegetables, cantaloupe, strawberries, peppers, lettuce, tomatoes, potatoes, papayas, mangos
Vitamin D	Mineralization of bones (raises calcium and phosphorus blood levels by increasing absorption from digestive tract, withdrawing calcium from bones, stimulating retention by kidneys)	Abnormal growth; joint pain; soft bones; rickets	0–12 months: 10 µg	Self-synthesis with sunlight; fortified milk, fortified margarine, eggs, liver, fish
Vitamin E	Antioxidant (detoxification of strong oxidants); stabilization of cell membranes; regulation of oxidation reactions; protection of PUFA and vitamin A	Red blood cell breakage; anemia	0–6 months: 3 mg; 6–12 months: 4 mg	Plant oils (margarine, shortenings), leafy green vegetables, wheat germ, whole grain foods, butter, egg yolk, milk
Vitamin K	Synthesis of blood-clotting proteins and a blood protein that regulates blood calcium	Hemorrhaging	0–6 months: 12 µg; 6–12 months: 10–20 µg	Bacterial synthesis in the digestive tract; liver, green leafy vegetables, milk
Calcium	Principal mineral of bones and teeth; involved in normal muscle (including heart muscle) contraction and relaxation; proper nerve functioning; blood clotting; blood pressure; immune defenses	Stunted growth	0–6 months: 360 mg; 6–12 months: 540 mg	Milk and milk products, tofu, greens, legumes

Table 4–1   Vitamins and Minerals in Infancy

Nutrient	Primary function	Deficiency symptoms	1980 RDA[a]	Significant sources[b]
Magnesium	Involved in bone mineralization; protein synthesis; enzyme action; normal muscular contraction; transmission of nerve impulses; maintenance of teeth	Growth failure; if extreme, convulsions	0–6 months: 50 mg 6–12 months: 70 mg	Legumes, whole grains, vegetables, seafood
Sodium	Maintains extracellular fluid balance and acid-base balance; nerve impulse transmission	Muscle cramps; loss of appetite	0–6 months: 115–350 mg 6–12 months: 250–750 mg	Moderate quantities in whole, unprocessed foods, large amounts in processed foods[c]
Chloride	Maintains fluid balance; part of the hydrochloric acid found in the stomach, necessary for proper digestion	Growth failure	0–6 months: 275–700 mg 6–12 months: 400–1200 mg	Moderate quantities in whole, unprocessed foods, large amounts in processed foods
Potassium	Facilitates many reactions, including the making of protein; maintains fluid and electrolyte balance, and support of cell integrity; the transmission of nerve impulses; muscle contraction, including the heart	Deficiency accompanies dehydration; causes muscular weakness, paralysis, and possibly death	0–6 months: 350–925 mg 6–12 months: 425–1275 mg	All whole foods; meats, milk, fruits, vegetables, grains, legumes
Iodine	A component of the thyroid hormone thyroxine, which helps to regulate growth, development and metabolic rate	Goiter, cretinism	0–6 months: 40 μg 6–12 months: 50 μg	Seafood, plants grown in most parts of the country and animals fed those plants
Iron	Part of the protein hemoglobin, which carries oxygen in the body; part of the protein myoglobin in muscles, which makes oxygen available for muscle contraction; necessary for the utilization of	Anemia; weakness; pallor; headaches; reduced resistance to infection	0–6 months: 10 mg 6–12 months: 15 mg	Red meats, fish, poultry, shellfish, eggs, legumes, dried fruits

energy as part of the cells' metabolic machinery

Nutrient	Function	Deficiency	Amounts	Sources
Zinc	A working part of many enzymes; present in the hormone insulin; involved in making genetic material and proteins; immune reactions; transport of vitamin A; taste perception; wound healing	Growth failure; sexual retardation; poor wound healing	0–6 months: 3 mg 6–12 months: 5 mg	Protein-containing foods: meats, fish, poultry, grains, vegetables
Copper	Necessary for absorption and use of iron in the formation of hemoglobin; part of several enzymes; helps to form the protective covering of nerves	Anemia	0–6 months: 0.5–0.7 mg 6–12 months: 0.7–1.0 mg	Meats, drinking water
Fluoride	Involved in the formation of bones and teeth; helps to make teeth resistant to decay and bones resistant to loss of their minerals	Susceptibility to tooth decay and bone loss	0–6 months: 0.1–0.5 mg 6–12 months: 0.2–1.0 mg	Drinking water (if naturally fluoride-containing or fluoridated), seafood
Selenium	Part of an enzyme that works with vitamin E to protect body compounds from oxidation	Anemia	0–6 months: 0.01–0.04 mg 6–12 months: 0.02–0.06 mg	Seafood, meat, grains
Chromium	Associated with insulin and required for the release of energy from glucose	Diabetes-like condition marked by inability to use glucose normally	0–6 months: 0.01–0.04 mg 6–12 months: 0.02–0.06 mg	Meats, unrefined foods, fats, vegetable oils
Cobalt	Part of vitamin B_{12} and therefore involved in nerve cell function and in the process of blood formation	Unknown in humans except in vitamin B_{12} deficiency	No RDA	Vitamin B_{12}-containing food (meats, milk)

[a]For some nutrients, ranges of recommended intakes are given because there is less information available on which to base allowances. These nutrients do not appear in the main table of the RDA, but are *Estimated Safe and Adequate Daily Dietary Intakes of Additional Selected Nutrients.*

[b]Breast milk and/or infant formula are sources of all nutrients in infant diets, with the possible exception of vitamin D (low in breast milk) and fluoride, for which supplements are often recommended.

[c]Iodized salt is also a source of sodium, chloride, and iodine, but is not recommended during infancy.

Source: Adapted with permission from E. M. N. Hamilton, E. N. Whitney, and F. S. Sizer, *Nutrition: Concepts and Controversies*, 4th ed. (St. Paul, Minn.: West, 1988).

Figure 4–2   Nutrient Needs of a Three-Month-Old Infant and an Adult Male Compared on the Basis of Body Weight

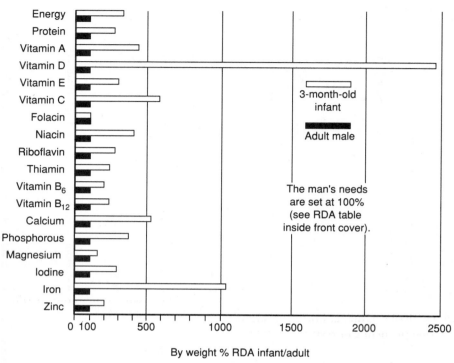

By weight % RDA infant/adult

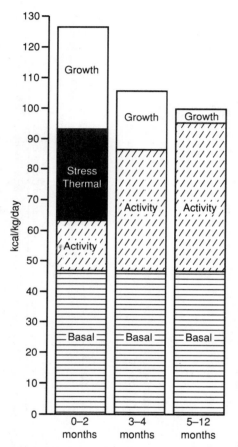

Figure 4–3   Estimated Energy Requirements of the Infant
Energy needs for the infant during the first year vary according to age and weight. As the infant gets older, the growth rate diminishes and the activity level increases.

Source: E. M. Widdowson, Nutrition, in: *Scientific Foundation of Pediatrics*, 2nd ed. (Baltimore, Md.: University Park Press, 1981), pp. 41-53, as cited in M. Gracey and F. Falkner, *Nutritional Needs and Assessment of Normal Growth* (New York: Raven Press, 1985), pp. 23-40.

Without supplemental water, the kidneys are stressed and dehydration becomes a threat. Foods such as fruits and vegetables have a low renal solute load. In addition, water satisfies fluid needs without providing kcalories. Many adults today would no doubt be healthier had they learned early to quench their thirst with water.

Energy-Yielding Nutrients

Energy needs per unit of body weight peak during the first year of life due to the infant's rapid basal metabolic rate and growth. This may not be obvious, for a newborn requires only about 425 kcalories per day, whereas most adults require at least 2000 kcalories per day, but to examine the energy needs per unit of body weight is to see the great differences. Infants require more than 100 kcalories per kilogram body weight per day; most adults require less than 40 (this varies greatly depending on height, body composition, health status, and activity level). Figure 4–3 compares the components of energy need at three different periods within the first year. Until 18 months of age, the energy requirement for basal metabolism is about double that of the adult on a per-pound basis for the healthy infant or child.[12] Note how the infant's daily energy needs for growth are greatest during the early months of life, then decline to a minimum by the infant's first birthday as the energy needs for activity rise.

The National Research Council recommends an average of 115 kcalories per kilogram per day for infants up to 6 months of age, and 105 kcalories per kilogram per day for infants 6 months to 12 months of age.[13] However, actual energy intakes vary widely among both breastfed and formula-fed infants. Measured energy intakes of breastfed infants in North America decrease at a faster rate and at an earlier age than current recommendations.[14] One study reported that infants consume an average of 110 kcalories per kilogram at one month of age, but only 85 kcalories per kilogram by six months of age, considerably less than the current recommendation. In a study of formula-fed infants, energy intakes ranged between 52 and 152 kcalories per kilogram per day.[15] These variations in intake are not surprising, however, considering differences in activity, growth rates, basal metabolic rates, age, and weight. The fact remains that energy needs per unit of body weight during the first year are greater than at any other time of life.

Protein With respect to growth, no single nutrient is more essential than protein. Protein malnutrition during infancy and early childhood can have profound, long-term effects on growth and development. All of the body's cells and most of its fluids contain protein; it is the basic building material of the body's tissues. Nine amino acids are essential for growth, and the absence of any one of them can result in stunted growth. In addition, other amino acids are conditionally essential. That is, an amino acid may be essential for an infant under certain conditions, such as illness, prematurity, or inborn errors of metabolism.

Dietary protein is needed daily to replace the constant body turnover of proteins and amino acids. Knowledge of the protein needs of infants and children has come from dietary surveys, studies of nitrogen balance and creatinine excretion, and measurements of growth at different ages. An adequate protein intake is defined as one that contains all of the essential amino acids in amounts sufficient to meet maintenance and growth needs; thus, the definition considers protein quality as well as quantity.[16] The essential amino acids for the infant are leucine, isoleucine, valine, lysine, threonine, methionine, phenylalanine, tryptophan, and histidine. In addition, premature infants and some term infants require cystine, tyrosine, and taurine.[17] The protein foodstuffs in the normal infant diet in North America, consisting of human milk, infant formula, meat, fish, and eggs, as well as some foods of vegetable origin, supply all of the essential amino acids in reasonably high concentrations relative to their food energy contents.

Dietary allowances for protein for infants are the same as the amounts of protein provided by the quantities of milk required to ensure an adequate rate of growth. Infants consuming 150 to 200 milliliters of breast milk per kilogram body weight per day receive protein in amounts comparable to recommendations.[18] The current recommendations for infants are 2.2 grams per kilogram for the first six months of life, and 2.0 grams per kilogram from six months to a year.[19]

Protein recommendations are designed for healthy, full-term infants. Infection, premature birth, illness, and genetic factors all increase protein requirements. In addition, protein requirements increase with an insufficient food energy intake, which results in use of dietary protein for energy.

Energy

1980 RDA:
   115 kcal/kg (0 to 6 mo).
   105 kcal/kg (6 to 12 mo).

Focal Point 1 discusses the unique nutrient needs of infants with inborn errors of metabolism.

Essential amino acids:

▶ Leucine.

▶ Isoleucine.

▶ Valine.

▶ Lysine.

▶ Threonine.

▶ Methionine.

▶ Phenylalanine.

▶ Tryptophan.

▶ Histidine.

Conditionally essential amino acids:

▶ Cystine.

▶ Tyrosine.

▶ Taurine.

Protein

1980 RDA:
   2.2 g/kg (0 to 6 mo).
   2.0 g/kg (6 to 12 mo).

150 to 200 ml of breast milk contains between 1.8 and 2.4 g of protein.

100 ml is approximately equal to 4 oz or 1/2 c.

protein efficiency ratio (PER): a measure of protein quality assessed by determining how well a given protein supports weight gain in laboratory animals.

$$PER = \frac{Weight\ gain\ (g)}{Protein\ intake\ (g)}$$

Infants consume approximately 750 ml/ day therefore protein intake = 6.75 g protein/ day.

750 ml is approximately equal to 30 oz or about 3 1/2 c.

In breast milk:

Protein = 6% of kcal.
Protein = 0.9 g protein/100 ml.

Excess protein (amino acid) intake causes:

▸ Acidosis.
▸ Dehydration.
▸ Diarrhea.
▸ Elevated blood ammonia.
▸ Elevated blood urea.
▸ Fever.

Hypoglycemia defined by blood glucose level:

Term infant:
  < 30 mg glucose/100 ml (within 72 hr of birth).
  < 40 mg glucose/100 ml (after 72 hr of birth).

Preterm infant:
  < 20 mg glucose/100 ml.

Cholesterol in human milk:

▸ 20 to 30 mg/100 ml.
▸ Approximately 200 mg/day.

Proteins contribute a small percentage of the kcalories in breast milk—about 6 to 7 percent. Breast milk in the quantity normally consumed provides approximately 2 grams protein per kilogram body weight per day for the average 7 1/2 pound infant. The American Academy of Pediatrics recommends that infant formulas provide a minimum of 1.8 grams protein (that is, 7.2 kcalories) per 100 kcalories, with a protein efficiency ratio equal to or greater than that of casein.

The problems associated with protein deficiency in infancy were described in the earlier discussions of malnutrition's influence on growth and development. Excessive dietary protein in an infant's diet can also cause problems. Diarrhea, acidosis, dehydration, fever, and elevated blood urea and ammonia concentrations have occurred in infants with protein intakes greater than 6 grams per kilogram per day.[20] Excessive protein intake, especially in the small infant, produces a buildup of amino acids in the blood. This stresses the kidney and liver, which have to metabolize and excrete these amino acids.

Carbohydrate Carbohydrates provide a readily available source of energy for all human beings and, in doing so, spare protein from being used for energy. The brain relies almost exclusively on carbohydrate for its energy. Carbohydrates contribute almost half of the kcaloric intake in the diets of adults; the U.S. Dietary Goals recommend that they contribute an even larger percent. The portion of carbohydrate kcalories in the diets of infants ranges between 35 and 55 percent. Human milk provides about 39 percent of its energy from carbohydrate; infant formula, about 42 percent. Figure 4–4 illustrates the contribution each energy-yielding nutrient makes toward total kcalories in both human milk and standard infant formula.

In most instances, lactose is by far the major carbohydrate consumed by infants. Lactose makes up about 90 percent of the total carbohydrate in human milk, and contributes most or all of the carbohydrate in standard infant formulas.[21]

A newborn infant is born with a small supply of carbohydrate stored as liver glycogen, but this is rapidly depleted, and hypoglycemia can quickly ensue. Once a feeding begins, under normal circumstances, the digestive tract easily digests and assimilates dietary carbohydrate to replenish glycogen stores and restore glucose homeostasis. The longer the delay in feeding the infant after birth, the greater the risk of hypoglycemia. Hypoglycemia in the newborn infant is critical, since this condition can impair central nervous system function. Hypoglycemia can be easily prevented by feeding the infant either breast milk or formula.

Fat Fat in the body is important in developing the central nervous system and maintaining body temperature. Fat in the milk imparts flavor and satiety and serves as a vehicle for the absorption of the fat-soluble vitamins. Fat provides about 55 percent of the kcalories in human milk and this percentage, presumably, is ideal for infants. Approximately 98 percent of the fat is in the form of triglycerides; the remainder is phospholipids, cholesterol, and free fatty acids.

Human milk is a relatively rich source of cholesterol. Formula manufacturers replace milk fat with vegetable oils, thus lowering the cholesterol content of infant formulas. This raises the question of how much cholesterol infants need. So far, clinical studies show no adverse effects of low-cholesterol formulas, but further research is needed regarding the long-term effects.

Linoleic acid, which is essential for infants, contributes about 7 percent of the kcalories in human milk; infant formula, about 10 percent. Infants develop deficiency symptoms, such as dermatitis and failure to thrive, when linoleic acid provides less than 0.1 percent of the total daily energy intake, but such deficiencies are rare.[22] Linoleic acid deficiencies occur when premature infants with low body fat stores are fed fat-deficient diets.[23]

Vitamins

The extraordinary growth of an infant during the first year of life may not be obvious because each day brings only gradual changes. Yet, internally, the metabolic machinery is fast at work creating new body parts—with the assistance of the vitamins.

Vitamin A Thousands of children in the developing countries of the world go blind each year from vitamin A deficiency. They may also experience stunted growth, decreased appetite, and increased infections and illness. Approximately 20 to 35 percent of all childhood diseases in developing countries are related to vitamin A deficiency.[24] Vitamin A deficiency is an enormous, yet preventable, problem.

In the United States and other developed countries, vitamin A deficiency during infancy is rare, occurring only in infants with impaired fat absorption or in those receiving milk that is not fortified with vitamin A, such as nonfat milk. The earliest clinical sign of vitamin A deficiency is impaired dark adaptation in the retina, which is difficult to detect in infants. As the deficiency progresses, failure to thrive, apathy, anemia, dry skin, and corneal changes appear.

The average retinol content of human milk is about 50 micrograms per 100 milliliters. If a milk consumption of 750 milliliters (30 ounces) per day is accepted as an adequate mean value, then the average intake of vitamin A for the infant is the same as the 1987 recommendation.[25]* This is slightly lower than the 1980 RDA.[26] The reason for the lower recommendation is that the selected reference value for mean breast milk volume for the first six months of life is 750 milliliters rather than the earlier value of 850 milliliters per day.[27]

Vitamin D Vitamin D is similar in structure, metabolism, and mechanism of action to steroid hormones, and is actually considered a hormone rather than a vitamin.[28] Nevertheless, for convenience and historical reasons, it is still called vitamin D.[29] The most important function of vitamin D is the regulation of calcium metabolism, by way of promoting calcium absorption and transport.

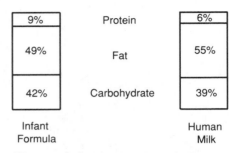

Figure 4–4 Percentages of Energy-Yielding Nutrients in Infant Formula and Human Milk
The proportions of enery-yielding nutrients in breast milk and formula differ slightly.

Source: Ross Laboratories, Columbus, Ohio, January 1979.

retinol: the active form of vitamin A found in milk.

Vitamin A
1980 RDA:
  400 µg/day (0 to 6 mo).
  420 µg/day (6 to 12 mo).

1987 RDI: 375 µg/day (0 to 24 mo).

---

*Appendix B provides an explanation of the RDA controversy and the 1987 Recommended Dietary Intakes (RDI). This book discusses both whenever appropriate to enhance the understanding of establishing recommendations.

In vitamin D deficiency, bone mineralization is impaired, resulting in rickets in children and osteomalacia in adults. The clinical signs of rickets include growth failure, bone deformity, listlessness, and delayed motor development. At one time a common disease, rickets is much less prevalent since the addition of vitamin D to cow's milk. Most milk available in the United States and Canada, including nonfat and low-fat milk, is fortified with vitamin D. In addition, vitamin D forms in response to the action of sunlight on the skin, although the amount formed depends on skin color, duration of exposure, and atmospheric pollution. Fresh air and sunshine provide not only a pleasant outing, but needed vitamin D as well.

Rickets was virtually nonexistent during the 50s, 60s, and early 70s, but medical workers have reported several cases in recent years. In Connecticut, physicians diagnosed four cases of rickets in children between 18 months and 3 years of age within one year.[30] In Philadelphia, physicians reported 24 cases of vitamin D deficiency rickets in the late 1970s; in Chicago, they noted another 10 cases of children with the disease.[31] Based on observation of these children, researchers have identified several risk factors for rickets in infants.[32] These include premature birth, pigmented skin, lack of exposure to sunlight, prolonged unsupplemented breastfeeding, and vegetarian diets.

Pediatricians routinely prescribe vitamin D supplements for breastfed infants in the United States. The vitamin D RDA for infants is 10 micrograms, far exceeding the notoriously low vitamin D content of breast milk (about 0.5 micrograms per liter).[33] Thus, for those breastfed infants not exposed to daily sunlight, vitamin D deficiency can occur in the absence of daily supplements.

Breast milk appears unsuitable as a standard from which to estimate the vitamin D needs of infants. Their needs exceed the amounts of vitamin D that they can obtain from breast milk. The difference can come from sunlight, but in case it does not, infants require supplemental vitamin D (see the section on supplements for infants, later in this chapter).

The question has been raised whether breast milk may contain more vitamin D than early analyses have shown. Researchers have traditionally used the lipid fraction of breast milk to determine its vitamin D content. An unconfirmed report claims that the protein whey fraction of breast milk revealed vitamin D sulfate activity—that is, that an active vitamin D compound existed in the water portion of the milk.[34] More recent reports indicate, however, that vitamin D sulfate in human milk is negligible.[35] Thus, the recommendation that the breastfed infant receive daily vitamin D supplements appears to be in the infant's best interest.

Vitamin D
1980 RDA: 10 µg/day.

Vitamin E The term *vitamin E* refers to two classes of compounds known as tocopherols and tocotrienols. The most biologically active of these is alpha-tocopherol, which is also the most widespread in foods. For these reasons, chemists often use the terms *alpha-tocopherol* and *vitamin E* interchangeably.

Vitamin E is a naturally occurring antioxidant that exerts a major protective role within cell membranes. Blood cells normally produce substances known as oxidant radicals, which attack fats and can disrupt the cell if antioxidants such as vitamin E do not protect it. Being fat soluble, vitamin E is able to penetrate fat-rich red blood cell membranes and detoxify potentially destructive radicals.

antioxidant: a compound that protects others from oxidation by being oxidized itself.

Plasma vitamin E in newborn infants is about one-half that of adults; that of low-birthweight infants is even lower.[36] Thus, all newborns, but especially premature or low-birthweight infants, are relatively deficient in vitamin E. The smaller the infant, the lower the vitamin E levels at birth. Full-term, breastfed infants attain adult values of the vitamin soon after birth, as do infants who consume adequate quantities of commercial infant formula.[37]

The need for vitamin E correlates directly with the amount of polyunsaturated fatty acids (PUFA) in the diet. In addition, the presence of iron in the diet affects vitamin E status. Iron promotes gastrointestinal oxidative destruction of vitamin E.[38] One study showed that infants fed a commercial infant formula with the standard 12 milligrams of iron per quart and a high PUFA-to-vitamin-E ratio suffered hemolytic anemia.[39] To improve the PUFA-to-vitamin-E ratio, formula manufacturers have reduced the level of PUFA and raised the vitamin E content of their products.

Human breast milk contains 1.3 to 3.3 milligrams tocopherol equivalents per liter and is assumed to provide an adequate intake for nursing infants. Infant formula contains about 10 milligrams vitamin E per liter. The RDA for vitamin E for infants is 3 milligrams from birth to six months and 4 milligrams up to one year of age.

Vitamin E
1980 RDA:
3 mg/day (0 to 6 mo).
4 mg/day (6 to 12 mo).

Vitamin K Vitamin K is known as the antihemorrhagic vitamin because it is necessary for the synthesis of prothrombin and three other blood-clotting factors. Vitamin K deficiency results in defective blood coagulation. The best dietary sources of vitamin K are dark-green leafy vegetables. However, it is next to impossible to cause vitamin K deficiency in adults through dietary deprivation alone because about half of the vitamin K present is synthesized by intestinal bacteria.

The newborn infant presents a unique case when it comes to vitamin K nutrition. At birth the sterile intestinal tract of the newborn lacks vitamin K-producing bacteria. At the same time, plasma prothrombin concentrations fall.[40] The combination of a sterile intestine and decreasing clotting factors make newborns, especially premature infants, susceptible to vitamin K deficiency and the resultant occurrence of hemorrhagic disease. The prothrombin concentrations climb back to adult levels as food is consumed and the intestinal tract gradually develops a population of vitamin K-producing bacteria, but this may take weeks. The American Academy of Pediatrics recommends that a single dose of vitamin K be given to infants at birth.[41] In many states, this preventive dose of vitamin K is required by law. The most recent vitamin K recommendation for infants is 10 micrograms, slightly lower than the 1980 RDA of 12 micrograms.[42]

Vitamin K preventive dose
Intramuscular: 0.5 mg to 1.0 mg.
Oral: 1.0 mg to 2.0 mg.

Vitamin K
1980 RDA: 10–20 μg/day.
1987 RDI: 10 μg/day.

The B vitamins The water-soluble B vitamins include thiamin, riboflavin, niacin, vitamin B_6, folacin, vitamin B_{12}, panthothenic acid, and biotin. These vitamins act as cofactors in many different biochemical reactions, and each one plays several metabolic roles. The B vitamins facilitate the release of energy from carbohydrate, fat, and protein. These nutrients are interdependent; a deficiency or excess of one can interfere with the utilization of another, and dietary deficiency of one is usually associated with deficiencies of others.

The body does not store the water-soluble B vitamins to the same extent as it stores the fat-soluble vitamins, so frequent intakes are necessary to avoid deficiency. If infants consume adequate amounts of infant formula or breast milk from healthy women, then their daily requirements for the B vitamins will be met. Normal-weight infants may experience deficiencies if requirements increase as in severe injury or malabsorption. Premature infants may also experience deficiencies because they consume small quantities of breast milk or formula; they may not receive adequate amounts of the B vitamins without supplementation.

Two of the B vitamins, vitamin B_{12} and folacin, deserve special mention for their crucial roles in growth and development. Vitamin B_{12} is required to enable folacin to facilitate the synthesis of DNA and thus support growth. The decreased DNA synthesis that results from vitamin B_{12} deficiency causes all replicating cells in the body to have a megaloblastic (giant cell) appearance. This is usually observed in blood cells and is called megaloblastic anemia.[43]

Vitamin B_{12} is unique among nutrients in that it is present only in foods of animal origin, where it is synthesized by bacteria. A deficiency of this vitamin is rare in infants because they are usually born with stores sufficient for the first year of life, and then receive additional amounts from breast milk or infant formula.[44] The vitamin B_{12} content of breast milk is similar to that present in the mother's serum, and daily output ranges from 0.2 to 0.8 micrograms.[45] Thus, vitamin B_{12} deficiency does not occur in infants who are breastfed by women with adequate serum vitamin B_{12}. However, vitamin B_{12} deficiency has been observed in infants of women who consume strict vegetarian diets.[46] In one case, a breastfed infant suffered severe vitamin B_{12} deficiency when the mother had a marginal deficiency.[47] The mother had avoided all foods of animal origin for the previous eight years, but had not herself shown signs of anemia, probably because she had had a high enough folacin intake to permit new cell synthesis without the help of vitamin B_{12}. The mother's breast milk, with a low concentration of vitamin B_{12}, was the infant's only source of the vitamin. The infant was in a coma by the time treatment with vitamin B_{12} was initiated. The speed and severity with which deficiency developed in this infant emphasizes the importance, and rapid use, of vitamin B_{12} in growth. Based on observations such as these, it is clear that the infant's need for vitamin B_{12} is greater than that of the adult. The 1987 vitamin B_{12} recommendation for infants is 0.3 micrograms, the amount the average infant receives from the breast milk of a healthy woman. Again, this recommendation is lower than the RDA of 0.5 to 1.5 micrograms.

As mentioned, folacin is required for the synthesis of DNA and, in fact, is dependent on the presence of vitamin B_{12} to properly fulfill its role in this process. Folacin deficiency is the most common cause of megaloblastic anemia in infants and children. At birth, an infant's serum folacin is three times maternal concentrations, but infant stores are small, and the rapid growth of the infant depletes these stores. By two weeks of age, serum folacin falls below adult values and stays there for several months.[48]

The folacin needs of infants are adequately met by breast milk or infant formula, but not by goat's milk, which is notoriously low in its folacin content. Human milk and cow's milk contain 50 to 60 micrograms of folacin per liter. The most recent folacin recommendation is 3.6 micrograms per kilogram of body weight, slightly lower than the 1980 RDA which is expressed in terms of micrograms per day.

Vitamin B_{12}

1980 RDA:

0.5 µg/day (0 to 6 mo).

1.5 µg/day (6 to 12 mo).

1987 RDI: 0.3 µg/day.

Folacin

1980 RDA:

30 µg/day (0 to 6 mo).

45 µg/day (6 to 12 mo).

1987 RDI: 3 µg/kg.

Vitamin C Ascorbic acid and dehydroascorbic acid are the two active forms of vitamin C, the more common form being ascorbic acid. Vitamin C is a water-soluble antioxidant, readily donating electrons to oxidants such as iron. The specific metabolic roles of vitamin C are not well defined, but its importance to human beings has been known for 200 years. One of the best-known functions of vitamin C is the hydroxylation of proline in the formation of collagen.[49] It is thought that vitamin C performs similarly in many other metabolic reactions, including wound healing, amino acid metabolism, allergic reactions, and the immune response.[50]

Some animal species are able to synthesize vitamin C, but human beings are not among them. Dietary sources of vitamin C are necessary to prevent the appearance of scurvy, the vitamin C-deficiency disease. The vitamin C requirement of human beings has been a controversial issue for some time, as evidenced by the range of recommended dietary allowances of different countries (20 to 200 milligrams).[51] It is known that as little as 10 milligrams of vitamin C per day can alleviate and cure scurvy in human adults. Scurvy occurs when the body pool of ascorbic acid falls to less than 300 milligrams, and a daily intake of 10 milligrams of ascorbic acid does not maintain a body pool much above 300 milligrams.[52] Thus, the question remains: should the dietary allowance prevent scurvy and provide a small margin of safety, or would greater tissue saturation be desirable? In fact, the most recent vitamin C recommendation is lower for all age groups than the 1980 RDA, in line with the first option.[53]

Scurvy is uncommon in the United States, but it does occur in infants fed exclusively cow's milk for the first 6 to 12 months of life. Symptoms of scurvy in the infant include anorexia, diarrhea, failure to gain weight, irritability, and increased susceptibility to infection.[54] As the disease worsens, hemorrhages under the skin and failure of spontaneous leg movements occur. Dramatic improvement of symptoms is seen with the administration of 25 milligrams of vitamin C four times a day.

Based on an average daily milk output of 750 milliliters, the daily vitamin C output in human milk ranges between 23 and 60 milligrams, depending on the dietary intake of the mother.[55] The 1987 vitamin C recommendation for infants is 25 milligrams per day, based on the amount present in the breast milk of healthy mothers of full-term babies. In 1980, the vitamin C RDA for infants was 35 milligrams per day. This recommendation was based on a higher mean milk volume than the current recommendation.[56] Infant formulas in the United States contain 55 milligrams of vitamin C per liter.[57]

Vitamin C
1980 RDA: 35 mg/day.
1987 RDI: 25 mg/day.

Minerals

Like the vitamins, the minerals are actively involved in the growth and development of infants. Most of the minerals are essential, and each serves a unique function, yet iron, calcium, and zinc are particularly important to infant nutrition.

Iron The rapid growth of infants and children imposes large iron needs on them. Many infants' diets and most toddlers' diets contain a marginal supply of iron. The combination of high need and low intake makes deficiency a likely consequence. In fact, iron deficiency is common in young children throughout

Chapter 5 discusses the nutrition and behavior connection.

the world and ranks as the number one nutrition problem among infants and children in the United States.[58] Only within the last decade or so, has there been a decline in the prevalence of anemia among low-income children in the United States due, in large part, to the positive impact of public health programs.[59]

Iron-deficient infants and children display symptoms of irritability, anorexia, poor weight gain, and behavioral disturbances.[60] Parents, teachers, and physicians often describe these children as disruptive and lethargic. The question of whether nutrient deficiencies influence infant and child behaviors has been extensively explored in recent years.

Evidence of a positive relationship between iron status and behavior has been observed in animals. Lactating mice were fed an iron-deficient diet for 21 days in order to reduce total iron in the brains of their offspring.[61] In response to an adverse, novel environment, the iron-deficient offspring were less responsive. That is, the iron deficient mice reared on their hind legs and stood immobile less frequently than iron-sufficient mice. Further studies indicate that similar long-term effects are observed.

Before a discussion of the results of studies in young human beings, a mention of the problems involved in studies of iron deficiency and infant behavior is in order. The conflicting results of studies that seem on the surface to be similar in design are partially attributable to some of these problems. Researchers have yet to agree on the exact criteria with which to define iron deficiency, oftentimes using different biochemical indices and cutoff points. Researchers relying on only one measure of iron status risk error in the classification of individuals being studied.[62]

In addition to the many problems associated with human research, infant research has specific problems of its own. Researchers encounter difficulty when measuring behaviors and intelligence because infant responses are limited. For example, language as a component of later intelligence is easily measured in an older child, but not in an infant. Despite the shortcomings, tests such as the Bayley Infant Scale of Mental and Motor Development are available to researchers who study infant behavior and motor development. The Bayley scale attempts to establish normal standards for certain behaviors that emerge during infancy, such as reaching for a toy or responding to a voice, and to assign levels of mental development based on these standards.

Iron deficiency and its subsequent resolution during infancy appear to influence mental development. In one study, iron-deficient, anemic infants were treated with either an intramuscular dose of iron or a placebo.[63] Those treated with iron demonstrated significant improvement on the mental portion of the Bayley test. Another study showed significant differences in test performances between iron-deficient, anemic infants and iron-sufficient infants. With iron treatment, the iron-deficient, anemic infants' test scores improved. A study of iron-deficient, nonanemic infants and iron-sufficient infants found no statistically significant differences in mental test performances between the two groups.[64] The iron-deficient infants, however, did show significant test performance improvement after iron treatment.

Inherent in these studies is an important distinction. Iron deficiency and anemia are not one and the same, though they often go hand in hand. Infants may be iron deficient without being anemic. The term *iron deficiency* refers to depleted body iron stores without regard to the degree of depletion or to the presence of anemia.[65] The term *anemia* refers to the hematologic state resulting from a severe deficiency. In the case of iron-deficiency anemia, body iron stores are severely depleted. Iron-deficient infants, with or without anemia, tend to score lower in mental development tests.[66] In summary:

▸ Iron-repletion therapy given to iron-deficient infants results in an improvement in performance on the Bayley Scale of Mental and Motor Development.

▸ The low test performance in iron-deficient infants cannot be attributed to specific mental abilities and skills at this time.

▸ No evidence exists that points to an association between iron deficiency and delayed motor development.

One more observation of iron-deficient infants deserves mention. It seems that at least one researcher has stated that the most noticeable behavioral characteristic of anemic infants is that they are unhappier (irritable and apathetic) than nonanemic infants.[67] The researcher concludes that an iron-deficient infant is a happiness-deficient infant.

Another connection between iron deficiency and central nervous system impairment is the brain's significant iron content. Remember, the critical period for brain development in the human infant occurs early and continues until about six months of age. Thus, iron deficiency during early infancy may impair brain development and central nervous system functioning. Such a deficiency may be evidenced in behavioral disturbances. This period is a susceptible time for irreversible damage to occur.

Exactly how iron deficiency might impair development of the central nervous system, and thus behavior, is not known, but researchers have tried to answer this question based on what is known about iron metabolism.[68] One connection involves the many iron-dependent enzymes that participate in the synthesis and catabolism of neurotransmitters such as norepinephrine and serotonin. The breakdown of these neurotransmitters to their excretion products requires the iron-dependent enzyme monoamine oxidase. When monoamine oxidase activity is depressed, these neurotransmitters are not broken down. In fact, iron-deficient children excrete excessive amounts of norepinephrine in their urine, an abnormality unique to the anemia of iron deficiency and reversible with iron therapy.[69] Thus, researchers theorize that the behavioral abnormalities seen in iron-deficient children may be secondary to abnormal amounts of neurotransmitters in the central nervous system caused by the reduced activity of monoamine oxidase.

The iron deficiency being discussed here develops after birth, for the full-term, newborn infant arrives adequately endowed with iron, at least for the first few months of life. During pregnancy, the fetus receives high priority when it comes to available iron, often at the expense of the mother. In fact, iron stores of newborn infants based on serum ferritin concentrations show negligible differences between infants of iron-deficient, anemic mothers and infants of iron-sufficient mothers.[70] The infant continues to receive high priority for available iron during lactation. The iron status of the mother does not influence the iron concentration of her breast milk.[71]

By four to six months, in full-term infants, iron deficiency can begin to set in.[72] Iron deficiency is most common in children between the ages of six months and three years due to their rapid growth rate and the fact that milk

100 g of cereal is approximately equal to 1/2 c or 4 oz.

Iron

1980 RDA:
  10 mg/day (0 to 6 mo).
  15 mg/day (6 to 12 mo).

1987 RDI:
  6.6 mg/day (3 to 6 mo).
  8.8 mg/day (6 to 12 mo).

Infant food sources of iron are discussed in the Feeding the Infant section of this chapter.

is often a major source of their food energy.[73] Depletion of the iron stores the infant is born with is delayed until then by the consumption of breast milk or iron-fortified formula. Human breast milk contains relatively small amounts of iron (0.5 milligrams per liter), but it has a high bioavailability (50 percent).[74] In contrast, iron-fortified infant formula contains about 12 milligrams of iron per liter, but has a bioavailability of about 4 percent. Full-term, formula-fed infants should be given iron-fortified formula by four months of age, if not sooner. Many pediatricians recommend the use of iron-fortified formula from birth. Between four and six months of age, however, the addition of iron-fortified infant cereal, which contains about 0.45 milligrams of iron per 100 grams, is recommended for all full-term infants.[75]

The infant RDA for iron is 10 milligrams per day up to six months of age, and 15 milligrams per day between six months and three years of age.[76] The Canadian RNI for iron is 0.4 milligrams per day for infants from birth to two months of age (based on the assumption that breast milk is the iron source for the first two months of life), 5 milligrams per day from three to five months of age, and 7 milligrams per day until one year of age. [77]

The length of this discussion on iron accentuates the importance of this nutrient to the infant, especially to the older infant. In view of iron deficiency being the most common nutrient deficiency of infants and children in the United States, Canada, and developing countries as well, knowledge about this nutrient and the practical application of this knowledge should be a high priority for all health professionals involved in the care of young children.

Calcium and phosphorus   Just as iron is an indispensable component of blood, calcium and phosphorus are indispensable components of bone. The adequate intake and proper ratios of these two minerals are critical to the growth and development of bone, as well as to many metabolic reactions. The ratio of calcium to phosphorus in the diet is important because excessive phosphorus inhibits calcium absorption. The calcium to phosphorus ratio of human milk is 2 to 1; the ratio of calcium to phosphorus in commercial infant formulas ranges between 1.3 to 1 and 1.5 to 1, amounts compatible with the American Academy of Pediatrics recommendations that are provided in Table 3–4 of Chapter 3.[78]

Calcium is the most abundant mineral in the body. Ninety-nine percent of the body's calcium is found in the bones and teeth, where it imparts structural strength. The small amounts of calcium present outside of bone—in blood, soft tissues, and extracellular fluids—play vital roles in nerve and muscle excitability, blood coagulation, muscle (including heart muscle) contractility, and intercellular cement integrity.[79]

It is not surprising that calcium needs are greatest during periods of rapid skeletal growth such as infancy. During infancy, the calcium content of the body increases faster with respect to body size than at any other time in the life cycle.[80] By nature's design, milk is both the best source of calcium and the main component of the infant's diet. Human breast milk contains about 300 milligrams of easily absorbed calcium per liter, while standard infant formula contains more calcium (600 to 700 milligrams per liter), that is less readily absorbed.[81] The full-term infant's calcium needs are fully met by either

Calcium

1980 RDA:
  360 mg/day (0 to 6 mo).
  540 mg/day (6 to 12 mo).

breastfeeding or formula feeding. The calcium RDA for infants from birth to six months of age is 360 milligrams per day; for infants six months to one year of age, 540 milligrams per day.[82]

Zinc Zinc requirements of infants are not well defined, but a deficiency of this nutrient causes impaired growth. Zinc participates in many enzymatic reactions, including those involved in DNA and RNA synthesis and protein synthesis. It appears that growth velocity is the main determinant of infant zinc requirements.[83] Thus, zinc needs are highest during early infancy and decline with advancing age. Accordingly, the zinc content of human breast milk declines as lactation progresses, ranging from as high as 20 milligrams per liter in colostrum to less than 2 milligrams per liter during later lactation.[84] Despite this marked decline in breast milk zinc, suboptimal zinc intakes of breastfed infants do not occur as long as maternal zinc intakes are adequate.[85] Availability of zinc from cow's milk is lower than from human milk; and even lower from soy-based formulas. Thus, standard infant formulas are supplemented with zinc, and soy-based formulas with even more.[86]

Vitamin-Mineral Supplements for the Infant

The newborn infant needs no nutrients in supplement form except, possibly, for vitamin D, fluoride, and iron. Breast milk or formula and internal stores should meet all nutrient needs until well into the second half of the first year, and then the introduction of juices and foods should keep up with changing requirements. However, vitamin D may require supplementation if sunlight exposure is infrequent, and fluoride may be needed if the infant's only source of fluoride is breast milk.

As for iron, the pediatrician may find it desirable to begin iron supplements for the breastfed infant at about four months. The use of first foods to add iron to the infant's diet has already been mentioned.

The formula-fed infant's needs for supplementation depend on the particular formula chosen. Formulas contain no fluoride, and so the same considerations apply as for the breast-fed infant. Formulas do contain vitamin D and iron, and when the infant shifts from formula to vitamin D-fortified cow's milk, iron may be needed in supplement form.

The nutrient needs discussed to this point apply to full-term, healthy infants. Preterm, low-birthweight infants present special nutrition concerns.

Nutrient Needs of the Preterm, Low-Birthweight Infant

The terms *preterm* and *premature* were introduced on page 3. They are used interchangeably to refer to a shortened gestation period; they imply incomplete fetal development, or immaturity, of the many body systems. The preterm infant faces physical independence before the growth of some of the organs and body tissues is complete. The rate of weight gain in the fetus is greater during the last trimester of gestation than at any other time in the life cycle.[87] Therefore, a preterm infant is most often a low-birthweight infant as well.

very low birthweight: a birthweight of 1500 g (3⅓ pounds) or less. Low birthweight is 2500 g, or 5½ pounds.

parenteral nutrition: the delivery of nutrients through a vein, bypassing the intestines.
para = opposite
enteron = intestine

hemolytic anemia: anemia characterized by breakage of the red blood cells, with resultant low hemoglobin levels and an increased production of immature red blood cells.
heme = blood
lysis = to break

With a premature birth, the infant is forced to endure the time of maximal growth without the continued nutritional support of the placenta.

The last trimester of gestation is also a time of building nutrient stores. Being born with limited nutrient stores intensifies the precarious situation for the infant. Further compromising the nutrition status of preterm infants is their metabolic immaturity. Nutrient absorption from the immature gastrointestinal tract, especially that of fat and calcium, is impaired.[88] The immature brain and liver are susceptible to high plasma concentrations of certain amino acids, a fact that has implications for protein requirements. Immature renal function and resulting high water requirements also contribute to the precarious nutrition status of the infant. In short, preterm, low-birthweight infants are perfect candidates for nutrient deficiencies. For these reasons, premature infants require special dietary and medical attention.

Few guidelines are available concerning the preterm infant's nutrient requirements. Authorities on infants' and children's nutrition disagree as to how fast the preterm infant should grow and what the body composition should be. In one study, formula-fed preterm infants accumulated more fat than breastfed preterm infants.[89] Whether this is of significance in terms of future growth is not known.

What *is* known about low-birthweight infants, and especially very-low-birthweight infants, is that nutrient deficiencies appear during the first days of life. Deficiencies of vitamin E, folacin, other B vitamins, iron, and calcium are among them.[90]

For the premature infant, the attainment of adequate vitamin E status is difficult. Many of these infants are so small that ingesting adequate breast milk or formula orally is impossible at first. In addition, their immature digestive systems often fail to absorb fat efficiently, and some do not respond to the administration of a water-miscible form of vitamin E either. They may require supplementation by way of parenteral solutions until oral feeding is possible.[91] Vitamin E deficiency in premature infants is associated with hemolytic anemia. Vitamin E deficiency in older infants, children, and adults produces a shortening of the red cell life span in the absence of anemia.[92]

One group of researchers has questioned whether the low plasma vitamin E of low-birthweight infants represents a normal range for these infants, or whether a true deficiency state exists.[93] Based on several measures of vitamin E status, they found that the antioxidant protective role of vitamin E is best attained at plasma concentrations close to adult values. They concluded, therefore, that true vitamin E deficiency exists for most low-birthweight infants at birth.

Premature, low-birthweight infants have small, readily depleted reserves of folacin. At birth, plasma folacin in both premature and full-term infants is higher than in adults, but only temporarily. Plasma folacin concentrations decline in both groups of infants, but in the premature infants, decline is more rapid. Infants with the lowest birthweights experience the greatest declines.[94] A maintenance dose of 50 to 100 micrograms per day is recommended to prevent anemia.[95] As mentioned earlier, premature infants may also experience deficiencies of other B vitamins because they consume small quantities of breast milk or formula; they may require supplementation.

Low-birthweight infants have a greater requirement for dietary iron than do full-term normal-weight infants.[96] These infants have less stored iron on a weight basis to begin with, and their more rapid growth rate exhausts their iron stores sooner. For these reasons, breastfed low-birthweight infants are prescribed ferrous sulfate drops at a dose of 2 to 3 milligrams per kilogram body weight not to exceed 15 milligrams per day, beginning at two months of age.[97] Preterm infants who receive iron-fortified formula do not require supplementation.

Infants who are born eight to ten weeks prior to term have acquired only about 30 percent as much calcium as full-term infants, so their calcium requirements are high.[98] Precise determinations of the mineral needs of preterm infants are not available.

The calcium and phosphorus needs of the preterm infant are not fully met by human breast milk, due to the milk's low content of the minerals, the poor absorptive capacity of the immature digestive tract, and the preterm infant's decreased intake. Formulas designed for the preterm infant contain higher concentrations of calcium and phosphorus than standard formulas. Preterm infants receive these formulas, or human milk supplemented with calcium and phosphorus, to ensure adequate calcium and phosphorus intakes.

Preterm infants miss out on the normal mineralization of bone during the last trimester of gestation. Their inadequate bone mineralization may result in the metabolic bone disease referred to as osteopenia, or rickets of prematurity. The incidence of this condition varies directly with the infant's weight; the smaller the infant, the greater the risk of bone disease.

osteopenia: a metabolic bone disease common in preterm infants; also called **rickets of prematurity.**

Disagreement abounds regarding the best method of feeding the low-birthweight infant. Once the infant can accept enteral feedings, the question at issue is which type of feeding best serves the nutrition needs of the infant: breast milk or formula. Each offers unique advantages, and, in fact, they are often used in combination to nourish preterm infants.

enteral: delivering nutrients into the intestines. Regular breastfeeding and formula feedings, as well as tube feedings, are types of enteral nutrition.

Breast milk does provide protection against infection, but its primary advantage lies in its composition. The composition of breast milk, with its readily digestible fat, low renal solute load, and unique protein profile, makes it particularly suitable to the immature intestine, kidneys, and liver. Despite the obvious advantages, breast milk, even the premature infant's own mother's milk, is sometimes less than ideal. Formulas designed for preterm infants offer the advantages of known composition and precise measurement of intake.

Feeding the Infant

The high nutrient needs of infancy must be met by a limited diet. Infants cannot chew, swallow, and digest the wide variety of foods available to adults. Selection of appropriate foods at the appropriate stage of development is paramount to optimal growth and health.

Infant nutrition and feeding recommendations are much like the infant: constantly changing; in a word, dynamic. Breastfeeding, the age-old way to feed newborns, took a back seat to formula feeding about 50 years ago, and now has returned as the recommended method of feeding. The timing of introducing solid foods to the infant's diet has ranged from a few weeks to three years, and is currently recommended between four and six months of age.[99] On the surface, ever-changing infant feeding recommendations and practices are frustrating and confusing for parents and health care providers alike, but their impact goes much deeper. Such changes occur because new knowledge is being gained about the crucial importance of nutrition during infancy. As discussed earlier in this chapter, undernutrition in the first year of life can have devastating, long-lasting effects. In addition, infancy sets the stage for eating habits that affect nutrition status and health for a lifetime.

The answers to the questions of what to feed infants at what ages can have dramatic consequences. For example, in developing countries, breastfeeding was, until recently, the traditional method of feeding infants for at least a substantial part of the first year. This provided infants with a sterile, steady supply of nutrients and protective factors. As people shifted from a rural to a more urban lifestyle, infant feeding practices changed from breastfeeding to formula feeding. In many instances, formulas were wrongly diluted and unsanitary. As a result, infant malnutrition and disease at early ages became more prevalent. Prior to this change, infant nutrition problems had been delayed until the second year of life, the time of weaning. The remainder of this chapter is devoted to examining what type of milk and food infants are fed, at what ages, and with what consequences.

Nutrients in Breast Milk and Formula

All newborns begin life receiving breast milk, formula, or a combination as their only source of food. Ideally, this continues to be the sole food source until four to six months of age, when solid foods are introduced. Even then, breast milk and formula contribute significantly to infants' diets, providing about half of the day's energy intake.

Chapter 3 discusses factors involved in making the decision to breast or formula feed.

From the nutrition standpoint, breast milk is the preferred choice of infant feeding. The American Dietetic Association advocates breastfeeding "because of the nutritional and immunologic benefits of human milk and physiological, social, and hygienic benefits of the breastfeeding process for the mother and infant."[100] The Committee on Nutrition of the American Academy of Pediatrics (AAP) and the Nutrition Committee of the Canadian Pediatric Society have issued this joint statement: "Breast feeding is strongly recommended for full-term infants, except in the few instances where specific contraindications exist."[101] The AAP also recognizes that the best alternative to breast milk to meet the nutrient needs of infancy is formula.

The recommendations in favor of breast milk arise from its unique nutrient composition and nonnutrient protective factors that promote optimal infant health and development. Acceptance of formula as a reasonable alternative stems from its development as a close copy of breast milk. An examination of breast milk composition will reveal how it best serves a newborn infant.

colostrum (co-LAHS-trum): the secretion from the breast before the onset of true lactation; also referred to as the "first milk."

Colostrum During the first two to three days after delivery, before the onset of true lactation, the breasts produce colostrum. Colostrum is a premilk substance that contains mainly serum with antibodies and white blood cells.

Colostrum differs from mature breast milk in nutrient composition and immunological factors. Colostrum is lower in fat and energy and higher in protein, sodium, chloride, potassium, sulfur, iodine, zinc, copper, and immunological factors than mature breast milk. During the first two weeks of lactation, the concentrations of proteins, immunoglobulins, and fat-soluble vitamins increase. These changes reflect changing infant needs.

Carbohydrate   The carbohydrate in breast milk and cow's milk-based formula is the disaccharide lactose. Lactose facilitates calcium absorption.[102]

Protein   The total protein content of breast milk is less than that of cow's milk, but this is actually beneficial. The low protein concentration contributes to a low renal solute load. The more protein consumed, the harder the kidneys must work to excrete the major end product of protein metabolism, urea. The unique protein quality of breast milk also offers benefits. When compared with cow's milk, breast milk contains a greater proportion of the protein alpha-lactalbumin; cow's milk contains a larger proportion of casein. Digestion and absorption of alpha-lactalbumin is efficient, whereas casein produces tough, hard-to-digest curds in the infant's intestine. Alpha-lactalbumin is also richer in sulfur-containing amino acids than is casein. One of these sulfur-containing amino acids, methionine, is an essential amino acid and another, cysteine, may be essential for premature infants. The enzymes responsible for synthesizing cysteine from methionine are deficient in early infancy.[103]

Breast milk contains all the essential amino acids in appropriate amounts, plus nonprotein nitrogen substances as well. One amino acid, taurine, is abundant in breast milk and has gained attention recently in infant nutrition. Taurine functions in several organ systems. In the central nervous system and muscles, taurine depresses neural excitation, perhaps by decreasing the intracellular calcium concentration.[104] Taurine also functions in the retina, where the process of illumination causes its release. Reduced body pools of taurine are associated with retinal degeneration.[105]

Lipids   The total lipid content of breast milk varies considerably, due partly to differences in sampling techniques, but also to individual differences between milks from different women or from time to time within the same woman. The total fat present in breast milk is not a reflection of the total fat content of the maternal diet, however, except in severely malnourished women. Such is not the case with the fatty acid composition, which changes in response to maternal diet. For example, carbohydrate-predominant diets (70 percent or more) result in higher concentrations of the saturated fatty acids lauric and myristic, which are synthesized in the mammary gland from carbohydrate metabolites.[106]

The lipids in breast milk, cow's milk, and infant formulas provide the main source of energy in the infant's diet. The unique lipid composition of breast milk offers other nutritional advantages as well. The fat in breast milk is more readily and more completely absorbed by the infant than is the fat in cow's milk. The enhanced absorption of breast milk lipids is partially due to the presence of acid-resistant lipases in breast milk. Another advantage is the unique configuration of the triglycerides upon hydrolysis by the lipases. Figure 4–5 illustrates how triglycerides are hydrolyzed at the 1 and 3 positions of the glycerol molecule, leaving a monoglyceride with the fatty acid attached at the 2 position. In breast milk, palmitic acid occupies the 2 position, whereas in

Figure 4–5 Triglyceride Hydrolysis and Fatty-Acid Configuration
Upon hydrolysis, palmitic acid occupies the number 2 position in breast milk, whereas stearic acid occupies that position in cow's milk. Monoglycerides with palmitic acid are more efficiently absorbed than free fatty acids or monoglycerides with stearic acid.

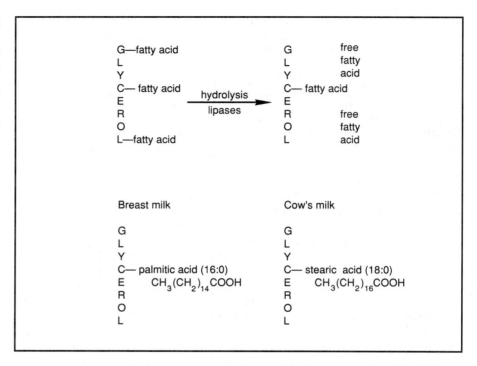

cow's milk, stearic acid is in the 2 position.[107] Monoglycerides with palmitic acid in the 2 position are more efficiently absorbed by the infant than either free fatty acids or monoglycerides with stearic acid in the 2 position.[108]

Triglycerides constitute 98 percent of the lipids present in breast milk, while free fatty acids, cholesterol, and phospholipids make up the remainder. Breast milk contains more than adequate concentrations of the essential fatty acid linoleic acid. Breast milk contains more cholesterol than infant formula, and although the significance of this is still unclear, considerable interest in the subject continues. One group of researchers questioned whether a cholesterol-rich diet during infancy might protect against atherosclerosis in later life.[109] They hypothesized that early high cholesterol consumption may cause reduced cholesterol synthesis and enhanced cholesterol breakdown in later life, responses which might offer protection against atherosclerosis. They tested their hypothesis on male rats by feeding them diets high in cholesterol prior to weaning. These rats had lower serum cholesterol at maturity when compared to rats fed a control diet. Results of further studies, however, are conflicting.

The cholesterol content of infant formulas is only about 10 percent of that in breast milk.[110] Many questions remain unanswered concerning exactly how much cholesterol and other lipids are appropriate in the infant's diet. Cholesterol is essential for normal myelination in the central nervous system, but high serum cholesterol concentrations in later life are a risk factor in the development of atherosclerosis. At the present time, the AAP recommends that breast milk, infant formula, and, after four to six months of age, infant foods are most appropriate during the first year of life.[111] The AAP discourages restriction of fat during infancy even for infants at risk of developing atherosclerosis.

Sodium   Breast milk has a low electrolyte content, which offers at least two nutritional advantages. First, its sodium concentration is low, although it is unclear whether a high sodium intake during infancy predisposes infants to the later development of hypertension. In adults, however, an association between high sodium intake and high blood pressure values does exist. One study of newborn infants compared the effects of dietary sodium on blood pressure.[112] Infants received either a normal-sodium diet or a low-sodium diet, during which time blood pressure was monitored monthly. After six months, the average systolic blood pressure of the low-sodium group was significantly lower than that of the normal-sodium group. Further research in this area is needed before firm conclusions can be drawn, but it appears that the sodium needs of normal, full-term infants are small and are adequately met by breast milk and formulas. Breast milk provides 7 milliequivalents of sodium per liter, while infant formulas contain between 7 and 11 milliequivalents per liter.[113] The current estimated range of safe intakes of sodium is 5 to 15 milliequivalents for the first six months of life, and 11 to 33 milliequivalents for six months to one year.[114] Sodium intakes of infants who are breastfed or fed formula are within the recommended range.

Another advantage of the low electrolyte content of breast milk is the low renal solute load produced. Electrolytes in excess of the infant's need must be excreted via the kidneys. This excretion of waste products requires water. If more water is needed than is available, then the kidneys must concentrate the urine. The concentrating capacity of the kidneys during infancy is more limited than during adulthood. A low renal solute load enables the kidneys to function within their capacity. Water balance during early infancy is fragile because infants can afford less water loss before becoming dehydrated. A low renal solute load is therefore beneficial to the infant's immature kidneys and delicate water balance.

milliequivalent (mEq): the amount of a substance that contains the same number of charges as 1 mg of hydrogen. The number of milliequivalents is a more useful measure than milligrams or grams when considering ions, because what is of interest is the number of charges present. If two solutions contain the same number of milliequivalents, they contain the same number of charges, and exert the same amount of osmotic pressure.

Fluoride   Fluoride is the one mineral not adequately provided in breast milk, formula, or solid foods. Its concentration in breast milk is low, and the breastfed infant normally receives little water, an important source of fluoride, during the first six months of life. The Committee on Nutrition of the American Academy of Pediatrics favors introduction of a fluoride supplement between birth and six months of age for infants who live in areas of nonfluoridated water.[115] For safety and consistency, infant formulas contain no fluoride.

Vitamins   As for vitamins, breast milk from healthy mothers contains all the infant needs for normal growth, with the exception of vitamin D. Until more is known about the vitamin D content of breast milk, supplementation is recommended for the breastfed infant until the time when infant formula or vitamin D-fortified milk is introduced.[116]

The nutritional advantages of breast milk go beyond the nutrient content of the milk. The breastfed infant self-regulates milk consumption, while the formula-fed infant is subject to control by the person offering the bottle. In view of the pervasive concern with childhood obesity, this self-regulation of food intake may be desirable. By recognizing and responding to the infant's cues of satiety, parents strengthen the formula-fed infant's ability to self-regulate food intake.

Protection Conferred by Breast Milk

Protective factors   Parallel to the nutritional benefits of breastfeeding in promoting the infant's health and well-being are the nonnutritional benefits. Breast milk is rich in substances that protect the infant from infection. Bifidus factors, immunoglobulins, lipases, lysozyme, and lactoferrin are among the protective factors in breast milk.[117]

Microbial growth-promoting factors, referred to as bifidus factors, encourage the production of *Lactobacillus bifidus*. They are present in colostrum and breast milk. These bifidus-promoting factors benefit the infant by favoring the growth of the normal bacterial residents of the human gastrointestinal tract, *L. bifidus*. The presence of *L. bifidus* in the digestive tract inhibits the growth of potentially harmful *Escherichia coli* and other bacteria, thereby protecting the infant from intestinal infection.[118]

Researchers have proposed that colostrum may also contain a growth-factor that directly benefits the infant. Newborn rats fed colostrum have higher rates of intestinal cell growth compared with their litter mates who were fed mature milk.[119]

Colostrum is also rich in immunoglobulins. Breast milk also contains immunoglobulins, but in lesser concentrations. Thanks to the unique immune factors in breast milk, the infant's digestive tract is protected against environmental antigens. Most often the mother and infant are exposed to the same antigens. When the antigens reach the mother's digestive tract, they meet with lymphocytes that become sensitized to the antigens and are then transported to the mammary gland, where secretory IgA production begins. Secretory IgA is the major immunoglobulin of colostrum and breast milk. The infant receives these antibodies with the breast milk. Secretory IgA is resistant to proteolysis, so it survives and functions in the infant's digestive tract. It is thought that secretory IgA, in conjunction with lactoferrin and other factors, accounts for the lower incidence of intestinal infection among breastfed infants compared with formula-fed infants.[120]

It now appears that the immunoglobulins in colostrum and breast milk are not alone in offering the breastfed infant antimicrobial protection. In an effort to identify specific factors responsible for the antimicrobial activity of human milk, researchers have identified the lipase activity of breast milk as a strong contender. Some research points to a relationship between the formation of fatty acids and monoglycerides in breast milk and antimicrobial activity. In contrast, cow's milk has a high triglyceride and low monoglyceride content. One classic study attempted to elucidate the antiviral activity of human milk. Milks rich in free fatty acids and monoglycerides exhibited stronger activity against viruses tested, compared with milks rich in triglycerides.[121] Based on these results, the authors suggest that milks used in the manufacture of infant formulas should be fortified with monoglycerides, instead of unsaturated vegetable oils, as is the current practice.

Human milk is richer in the enzyme lysozyme than are other milks. Lysozyme breaks apart bacterial cell walls. It is suggested that lysozyme may therefore have a bacteriostatic function in the digestive tract of breastfed infants, although evidence is limited. Breast milk also contains an amylase enzyme that enables infants to digest their first solid food.

bifidus (BIFF-id-us or by-FEED-us) **factors**: factors in colostrum and breast milk that favor the growth, in the infant's intestinal tract, of the "friendly" bacteria *Lactobacillus bifidus* so that other, less desirable intestinal inhabitants will not flourish.

immunoglobulins: proteins that are capable of acting as antibodies.

antigens: substances foreign to the body that elicit either the formation of antibodies, an inflammation reaction, or both, from immune system cells.

secretory IgA: one of several types of antibodies produced by the human immune system; the predominant antibody of breast milk.

Another protein that contributes to the antimicrobial activity of breast milk is lactoferrin. Lactoferrin appears to successfully compete for iron against iron-demanding bacteria in the intestinal tract, thus inhibiting their growth.[122] Also, lactoferrin may be responsible for the high bioavailability of iron from breast milk compared to that from cow's milk, which contains little lactoferrin.[123] The lower bioavailability of iron from infant formulas is compensated for by the manufacture of iron-fortified formulas, which are effective in preventing iron deficiency.

Like iron, zinc is present at a low concentration in breast milk, but its absorption is exceptionally efficient. The presence of zinc-binding proteins in breast milk enhances zinc's bioavailability.[124]

An epidermal growth factor that stimulates growth of intestinal cells has been discovered in breast milk.[125] The presence of this growth factor allows damaged cells to be replaced more rapidly than normal. The efficient replacement of damaged cells helps keep the infant's digestive tract barrier against infection intact.

Convincing evidence exists in support of breast milk's protecting infants against infection. In developing countries, where the incidence of infection is high, the infection rate among breastfed infants is low. Nevertheless, some skepticism remains with respect to the protective influence of breast milk in industrialized nations.

Several methodological flaws are common among studies that examine the protective properties of breast milk.[126] One of the most basic inconsistencies concerns the definition of the feeding method itself. For example, researchers often fail to precisely define the term *breastfed*. Infants are categorized as "breastfed" or "bottle-fed," without mention of those infants who are partially breastfed, or into what category such infants are placed. Another problem common to infant feeding studies is controlling for confounding variables such as differences in social class, whether the mother smokes, and family size. If these variables are not controlled for during the course of the study, then the results may be inaccurate.

The nutritional and nonnutritional advantages of breast milk are many. The list of the advantages afforded the breastfed infant continues to grow. For example, in addition to protection against infection, it is possible that breast milk protects against the development of allergies as well. When breastfed infants were compared with formula-fed infants, those who had been solely breastfed for six months showed a lower incidence of allergic diseases such as asthma and skin rash.[127] This was especially noticeable among those infants with a family history of allergy.

Breast milk and formula adequately provide most of the nutrients required in the first four to six months of life. With increasing nutrient needs and advancing physical development, solid foods and cow's milk are introduced into the diet.

Introducing Cow's Milk

In the simplest cases, infants are weaned gradually from either breast milk or formula bottles to cow's milk, drunk from a cup, at some time between six months and a year. However, in some cases, infants are weaned from the breast to the bottle, and then to the cup. It is important to mention that if they are weaned from the breast early, before six months, they should not be given whole cow's milk. In some infants, as mentioned earlier, particularly those younger than six months of age, its consumption is associated with intestinal bleeding and iron deficiency; also, whole cow's milk is a poor source of iron. The timing of the introduction of whole cow's milk into the infant's diet remains a controversial issue. Many pediatricians recommend the use of breast milk or iron-fortified formula throughout the first year. The American Academy of Pediatrics currently recommends the introduction of whole cow's milk at any time after six months, or as soon as at least one-third of the infant's energy intake is from a balanced mixture of cereal, fruits, vegtetables, and other foods.[128]

Introducing Solids

Few issues of infant feeding have been debated more than the question of when it is most appropriate to introduce solid foods in the infant diet. As is true with all aspects of infant feeding, recommendations for the timing of the introduction of solid foods have changed repeatedly over the years. At the beginning of this century, introduction of solid foods was delayed until ten months of age or older.[129] In 1958, the AAP suggested that iron-containing foods be introduced during the third month of life.[130] In the 1970s, most infants received beikost by six weeks of age.[131] Currently, the AAP recommends the introduction of solid foods between four and six months of age.

beikost: any nonmilk food given to an infant.

The choice of a later time to introduce solid foods accompanied the resurgence of breastfeeding, probably in the interest of postponing weaning. Studies show a difference in the timing of solid food introduction between breastfed and formula-fed infants: the latter receive solid foods earlier.[132] Survey data indicate that over half of formula-fed infants receive solid foods between two and three months of age, compared with one-fourth of breastfed infants.[133]

Rationale   In practice, the timing of the introduction of solid foods to infant diets should not depend on whether the infant is breastfed or formula fed, or even on the infant's chronological age. It should depend on the individual infant's nutrient needs and developmental readiness. These factors vary from infant to infant due to differences in growth rates, activity, and environmental conditions.

The main purpose of introducing solid foods to infants is to provide nutrients that are no longer supplied adequately by breast milk or formula alone. Solid foods provide an alternative source of nutrients when the needs of the infant exceed what can be provided by a volume of fluid that the infant can easily consume. However, the nutrient needs of the infant cannot be met by solid foods if the infant is developmentally incapable of handling and metabolizing those foods. For the first few months of life, the infant can swallow only liquids, the digestive tract is immature, and the kidneys have a limited capacity to concentrate urine and excrete water and sodium. Inappropriate nutrition can stress the infant's physiological capabilities. Just as it is unrealistic to expect a one-year-old to read and write or ride a bicycle, so it is unrealistic to expect an infant to handle adult foods, or even baby foods, before the physiological capacity exists.

By four to six months of age, infant iron stores are depleted.[134] At the same time, the amounts of energy required for some infants may be greater than can be provided by breast milk or formula alone.[135] Therefore, at about four months of age for some infants, and no later than six months of age for all infants, foods other than breast milk or formula should be making significant energy contributions to the infant diet. It is important, though, that food not displace the infant's most important source of nutrients, milk. Foods should enter the diet only as supplemental foods, given in addition to breast milk or formula, not as replacements for either. Breast milk and formula continue to play important nutritional roles in infant diets during most or all of the first year of life, and breast milk provides some fringe benefits as well. For example, as mentioned earlier, research has shown that breast milk contains an amylase enzyme that may facilitate starch digestion.[136] This point is worth noting because cereals are usually the infant's first solid food.

Research has asked the question whether, for infants less than four months of age, solid food represented a replacement of milk rather than an addition to the diet. A study examining the effect of beikost on the milk intakes of breastfed infants found differing effects depending on the age of introduction.[137] When infants less than four months of age were given beikost, nursing frequency declined; when beikost was introduced later than four months of age, nursing frequency either increased or remained the same. This effect was reflected in lower growth rates of the infants who received beikost early. Other factors, such as differences in nursing styles and infants' digestive capacities, may partially explain the different effects of beikost on infant feeding. The possibility that early beikost introduction may interfere with lactation, rather than appropriately supplement it, however, strengthens the rationale for delaying solids until sometime between four and six months of age.

Infants eat according to energy need, as opposed to amount of food. Energy needs of infants vary greatly; faster growing, larger, or more active infants require additional dietary sources of energy sooner than others. The consumption of nonmilk foods can increase steadily, and breast milk or formula consumption can decrease even more gradually, so that throughout the first year of life, milk foods continue to be a significant part of the infant's diet.

A variety of factors support the rationale to delay the timing of infant feeding until four to six months. These same factors help to define the choice of what foods to offer.

What to introduce first   As energy needs increase with steady growth and increasing activity, the need for other nutrients increases as well. Prominent among nutrients demanding attention at this time is iron. Even though the infant is born with ample supplies of iron, body iron must double as birthweight triples in the first year of life.[138] Iron absorption is minimal during early infancy when iron stores are large. Therefore, no advantage is gained by supplementing the diets of full-term infants with iron during the first four months of life.[139] By four to six months of age, however, iron stores have diminished, and additional dietary sources of iron are needed. For the breastfed infant, iron-fortified cereals are a desirable source of supplemental iron by six months of age. Iron-fortified formula, iron-fortified cereal, or a combination of the two are recommended for the formula-fed infant by four months of age.[140]

Iron-fortified infant cereal is advantageous as the first solid food for several reasons. The needed iron is provided in a convenient, economical form. Cereals readily mix with fluids, so are of a consistency easily swallowed by the infant. They provide energy, calcium, phosphorus, and other vitamins and minerals as well as iron, and most infants accept and tolerate them well.

extrusion reflex: the reflex that causes an infant to push food out, rather than swallowing it.

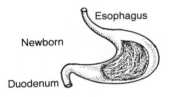

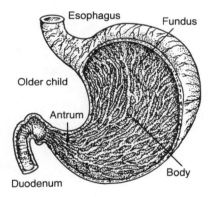

Figure 4–6 Infant and Child Stomachs
The stomach of the normal newborn is more horizontal than that of the older child. The stomach becomes curved and upright as the child assumes a more erect posture. The subdivisions of fundus, body, and antrum are not well defined for the first year of life. The vigorous mixing action of the antrum, which is most involved with the emptying of solids, is apparent in older children but is minimal in the first months of infancy. This difference in stomach anatomy is one reason why solid foods are digested less readily at this time.

Developmental readiness   The exact time to introduce solid foods depends on the developmental readiness of the child. The type and amount of food an infant can swallow, digest, and absorb at any given time varies according to the maturity of the neuromuscular system that controls the gastrointestinal tract.

The full-term, newborn infant is capable of sucking and swallowing at birth, although somewhat inefficiently. Within a few days, however, the infant is better able to coordinate sucking, swallowing, and breathing, so this process becomes more efficient. Until about four months of age, all substances entering the infant's mouth are pushed out through the mouth by the action of the tongue, as when the infant sucks on the breast or bottle. This action is called the extrusion reflex; it prevents foods from being swallowed for the first four to six months of age. Only after the extrusion reflex disappears is the infant able to push food to the back of the mouth for swallowing. Food in the back of the mouth touches the soft palate of the roof of the mouth. This stimulus triggers the swallowing reflex. This is why the nipple has to be well inside the infant's mouth when breastfeeding, and why a spoon has to be well inside when spoon feeding.

Spoon feeding of solid foods promotes proper swallowing movements. In contrast, the use of an infant feeder, which allows an infant to suck pureed food from a bottlelike container, discourages swallowing movements. Sometime after about four months of age, the infant is able to sit alone and has greater control of head movement than previously. Thus, the infant can sit in a high chair and is capable of giving signs of satiety, such as turning the head away when satisfied.

The main role of the stomach is to physically and chemically prepare foods for digestion. As Figure 4–6 illustrates, the infant's stomach is much smaller, shaped differently, and functionally immature, compared with the older child's stomach. During the newborn period, foods move more slowly and are mixed less effectively in the stomach than they are in later infancy. The small capacity and prolonged emptying time of the infant's stomach, together with the large energy requirements of the infant, necessitate that foods consumed be of high energy density. Human milk or infant formula help compensate for the stomach's limited capacities during early infancy.

The concentrations of gastric secretions, such as hydrochloric acid and pepsin, rise throughout infancy. Early on, the low acidity of the infant's stomach prevents some types and large amounts of food from being digested.[141] This explains why the large, tough curds of casein in cow's milk do not readily break down. Similarly, enzymatic secretions of the pancreas and small intestine are low in early infancy, so that the digestion of solid foods is inefficient.

The limited capacity of the infant's renal system during the first few months of life further justifies delaying solid food introduction. Water should be offered to the infant regularly once solid food is added to the diet, to compensate for the higher renal solute load.

Food allergies and sensitivities   The appropriate timing and type of food introduced may also facilitate or prevent the onset of an allergic response. In early infancy, the mucosal barrier of the small intestine is permeable to large molecules.[142] This is advantageous because it allows maternal antibodies to cross the barrier intact, affording the infant protection against infection. If, however, inappropriate protein sources such as those in unmodified cow's milk and some solid foods are fed, undigested proteins may become antigens and induce allergies to these foods.[143] Symptoms of food allergy include nausea, vomiting, abdominal discomfort, respiratory disturbances, and skin rashes.

Chapter 5, which deals with children's nutrition, discusses allergies in detail; this chapter focuses on prevention and early detection. To prevent allergy, and to facilitate its prompt identification should it occur, experts recommend the introduction of single-ingredient foods, one at a time, in small portions, allowing four to five days before introducing the next new food. The gradual introduction of single-ingredient foods permits identification of problem foods. Rice cereal, barley cereal, or other single-ingredient infant cereals are appropriate first foods. Mixed cereals and combination foods can be offered once sensitivity to specific foods has been ruled out.

Because milk makes significant nutrient contributions to infants' and children's diets and because a limited number of nutritionally comparable foods are available, it is especially important to avoid cow's milk allergy. Parents are advised to avoid the use of unmodified cow's milk before six months of age.

Colic during infancy is often attributed to milk intolerance. Milk intolerance can be due to milk toxicity, as can occur when infants less than six months of age are fed large quantities of whole cow's milk. It may be due to milk-protein hypersensitivity (milk allergy) or to lactose intolerance, which results when an individual is unable to completely digest lactose, the carbohydrate in milk.[144] The incidence of milk-protein hypersensitivity in infants is estimated to range from 0.4 percent to 7.5 percent. The actual incidence is difficult to pinpoint because at present no satisfactory, generally accepted way of making the diagnosis exists. Many infants with milk-protein hypersensitivity outgrow it by early childhood.

Other than milk, the foods most often implicated in food allergies in infants include citrus fruits, soy protein, egg whites, and wheat.[145] Some pediatricians recommend delaying introduction of these foods until around nine months of age to coincide with more complete gastrointestinal tract development.

Aside from true food allergies, infants may develop sensitivities or intolerances to foods due to other causes such as reactions to bacterial toxins; reactions to the chemicals in foods such as monosodium glutamate or the natural laxative in prunes; digestive tract disorders such as obstructions or injuries; enzyme deficiencies such as inborn errors of metabolism or lactose intolerance; and even psychological aversions. In some cases it is not possible or necessary to say whether an adverse food reaction is due to allergy or something else, but avoidance of the food, at least for a while, is indicated.

Infants frequently outgrow food allergies and sensitivities within a short time. Avoidance of offending foods, therefore, should not have to be permanent unless a physician confirms the presence of a food allergy.

Commercial infant foods   Infant foods should be selected to provide variety, balance, and moderation. Commercial baby foods offer palatable, nutritious foods, in a safe and convenient form. The wide variety of infant foods available today fall into eight groups: cereals, fruits, fruit juices, vegetables, meats, meat and vegetable combinations, yogurts, and desserts. Most are offered either in dry form to which liquid is added or ready-prepared in jars. In response to consumer concerns during the 1970s, manufacturers have reduced or eliminated salt, sugar, and other additives in commercial infant foods.[146] All infant food ingredients are listed on the label in descending order by weight. In the United States, Food and Drug Administration regulations require that specific nutrients be listed on the label as shown in Figure 4–7.

Iron-fortified infant cereal is usually recommended as the first solid food for the infant.[147] Infant cereal provides needed iron and energy and is convenient, economical, and well tolerated by infants. Rice cereal is usually the first cereal introduced because it is the least allergenic.[148] Infant cereals are available as single-grain or mixed varieties. Single-grain cereals are rice, barley, and oatmeal. Mixed cereals include mixed-grain varieties and cereals mixed with fruit. Ready-prepared cereals in jars usually contain fruit, as do the dehydrated, canned varieties. Dry cereals are prepared by adding water, breast milk, or formula to obtain the desired consistency, which should be almost liquid at first. Cereals and other solids should be fed by spoon and offered once a day in small quantities (1 to 2 tablespoons) until the infant becomes accustomed to the food and spoon.

The infant's diet, for the most part, contains nonheme iron rather than the heme iron found primarily in meat. Heme iron is well absorbed, regardless of the nature of the meal. In contrast, the absorption of nonheme iron is influenced by the presence of other foods consumed at about the same time. For example, vitamin C greatly enhances the absorption of nonheme iron. Once the infant is consuming a variety of foods, the inclusion of vitamin C-rich fruits and vegetables in an iron-containing meal will further promote the iron nutrition of the infant.

Fruits are often the second food introduced in infant diets. Commercially prepared infant fruits are fortified with vitamin C and may provide up to half of the infant RDA of this vitamin per serving. Because of their sweet taste, fruits are well liked by most infants. Baby food fruits are made from fresh fruits or concentrates. Some of the more tart, acidic, prepared fruits contain small amounts of added sugar, while others such as apples and pears do not. Some infant fruits contain a little modified starch to improve consistency. Modified starches include corn, tapioca, potato, or wheat starch treated in such a way as to improve palatability, product stability, and shelf life.[149] The use of modified starches in baby foods has been extensively studied by the Food and Drug Administration and the AAP and is considered safe as practiced.[150]

Figure 4–7   Nutrition Information on a Baby Food Label and Cap

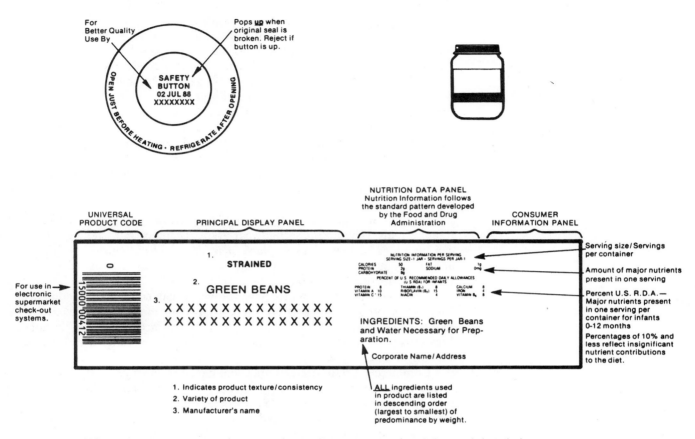

NOTE: Nutrient information may vary among manufacturers due to crop variety, formulations, analytic methods.

Source: Baby Foods: A report by the American Council on Science and Health (Summit, N.J.: American Council on Science and Health, 1987).

Fruit juices prepared for infants are also fortified with vitamin C. Fruit juices contain no added sugar and are prepared from pressed, whole fruits or concentrates. Several brands of regular, adult fruit juices are prepared similarly and may be offered to the infant. Fruit juices are useful both to increase fluid intake and to provide vitamin C. Fruit juice can be introduced in a cup about the same time as solid foods are introduced. Infants enjoy their taste, so juices are a good choice for introducing the cup and avoiding the use of a juice bottle at the same time. Juices should be used moderately in the infant diet, so as not to displace other foods. After about six months of age, the infant can receive one meal a day with vitamin C-fortified juice as the beverage in place of formula or breast milk.[151] The meal should contain iron-fortified cereal to take advantage of the enhancement of iron absorption by the vitamin C in the juice. Breast milk or formula can be offered later in the day, then, as a snack in place of juice.

Commercially prepared baby food vegetables, like all vegetables, are good sources of vitamins and minerals, especially vitamin A and the B vitamins. In the past, the introduction of vegetables in infant diets usually followed fruits, but the opposite order may better favor vegetable acceptance. Once an infant is accustomed to the sweet taste of fruits, the taste of some vegetables may be less appealing than if they had been offered prior to the fruits.

Meats for infants are prepared with broth. They are excellent sources of protein, B vitamins, and iron. Meat and vegetable combinations contain less protein per serving than single-ingredient meats. This is a satisfactory option for parents who want to introduce meat into their infant's diet. In most cases, protein from meat sources is not critical to an infant's diet. Adequate protein is available from breast milk, formula, and cereal. Meats are generally introduced between eight and ten months of age. They may be less readily accepted than other foods at first. As long as the infant is consuming iron-fortified cereal and breast milk or formula daily, the iron and protein contribution of meats is less critical than when these other foods are absent.

Children in vegetarian families should be encouraged to eat iron-fortified infant cereals well into the second year of life. Legumes and whole-grain foods can be added to their diets in place of meat. Children who eat no foods of animal origin will require vitamin B_{12} supplements as well as calcium- and vitamin D-fortified food sources or supplements.

Commercial infant yogurts have a lower sugar content than adult fruit-flavored yogurts and are good sources of calcium and protein. Plain or reduced-sugar varieties of regular yogurt are also acceptable for the infant. Yogurt is a popular food for infants, and is often introduced around eight months of age.

Commercial infant desserts are usually made from a custard or fruit base. They are intended as energy supplements for infants whose needs are greater than those supplied by a regular diet of milk, cereal, fruits, vegetables, and meats, such as underweight and seriously ill infants. They provide more kcalories and fewer nutrients than other infant foods. These foods should be limited in most infant diets.

Homemade infant foods   Homemade infant foods can be as nutritious as commercially prepared ones as long as nutrient losses are minimized during preparation. Ingredients for homemade baby food recipes should be fresh, whole foods without added salt, sugar, or seasonings. Pureed food can be frozen in ice cube trays, which provides convenient-sized blocks of food that can be thawed, warmed, and fed to the infant. Precautions to guard against food poisoning or infection must be taken; hands and equipment must be clean.

Over the years, many claims have been made connecting infant feeding practices with health in later life. In most cases, however, long-term, direct relationships between what or how an infant is fed and future health remain controversial or unsubstantiated. A classic example is the association between a high food energy intake in infancy and obesity in later life.[152] (This subject is discussed in full in Focal Point 5.) Despite doubts about the direct effects of infant nutrition on later health and disease, however, one thing is certain.

Eating habits acquired during infancy and childhood influence the overall food attitudes of the individual throughout life.

The provision of foods in accordance with an infant's nutrient needs and developmental readiness promotes sound nutrition and health. The nurturing of an infant, however, involves more than nutrition. In light of the developmental and nutrient needs of one-year-olds, and in the face of their often contrary and willful behavior, a few feeding guidelines may be helpful (see Practical Point: Mealtimes with Infants). It is the responsibility of those who care for infants to provide not only nutritious milk, foods, and water, but also a safe, loving, secure environment in which they may grow and develop.

▸▸ **PRACTICAL POINT**

Mealtimes with Infants[a]

The following are several problem situations that may be encountered when feeding infants with some suggestions for handling them:

▸ *He stands and plays at the table instead of eating.* Don't let him. This is unacceptable behavior and should be firmly discouraged. Put him down, and let him wait until later to eat again. Be consistent and firm, not punitive. If he is really hungry, he will soon learn to sit still while eating. An infant's appetite is less keen at a year than at eight months, and his energy needs are relatively lower. A one-year-old will get enough to eat if he lets his own hunger be his guide.

▸ *She wants to poke her fingers into her food.* Let her. She has much to learn from feeling the texture of her food. When she knows all about it, she'll naturally graduate to the use of a spoon.

▸ *He wants to manage the spoon himself, but can't handle it.* Let him try. As he masters it, withdraw gradually until he is feeding himself competently. This is the age at which an infant can learn to feed himself and is most strongly motivated to do so. He will spill, of course, but he'll grow out of it soon enough.

▸ *She prefers sweets—candy and sugary confections—to foods containing more nutrients.* Human beings of all races and cultures have a natural inborn preference for sweet-tasting foods. Limit them strictly. If they are kept in the house, keep them out of sight. There is no room in an infant's daily 1000 kcalories for the kcalories from sweets, except occasionally.

These recommendations reflect a spirit of tolerance that serves the best interest of the child emotionally as well as physically. The wise parent of a one-year-old offers nutrition and love together.

---

[a] Adapted with permission from E. M. N. Hamilton, E. N. Whitney, and F. S. Sizer, *Nutrition: Concepts and Controversies*, 4th ed. (St. Paul, Minn.: West, 1988).

Chapter 4 Notes

1. D. Sinclair, *Human Growth after Birth*, 4th ed. (New York: Oxford University Press, 1985), pp. 1–22.
2. E. M. Widdowson, Early nutrition and later development, in *Diet and Bodily Constitution*, Ciba Foundation Study Group (Boston: Little, Brown, 1964), pp. 3–11; R. A. McCance, Some effects of undernutrition, *Journal of Pediatrics* 65 (1964): 1008–1014.
3. K. Satyanarayana and coauthors, Effect of nutritional deprivation in early childhood on later growth—A community study without intervention, *American Journal of Clinical Nutrition* 34 (1981): 1636–1637.
4. M. Winick, Changes in nucleic acid and protein content of the human brain during growth, *Pediatric Research* 2 (1968): 352–355.
5. M. Winick and A. Noble, Cellular response in rat during malnutrition at various ages, *Journal of Nutrition* 89 (1966): 300–306.
6. M. Winick and P. Rosso, The effect of severe early malnutrition on cellular growth of human brain, *Pediatric Research* 3 (1969): 181–184.
7. S. A. Richardson, The relation of severe malnutrition in infancy to the intelligence of school children with differing life histories, *Pediatric Research* 10 (1976): 57–61.
8. M. B. Stoch and P. M. Smythe, 15-year developmental study on effects of severe undernutrition during infancy on subsequent physical growth and intellectual functioning, *Archives of Disease in Childhood* 51 (1976): 327–336.
9. A. Ashworth and D. J. Millward, Catch-up growth in children, *Nutrition Reviews* 44 (1986): 157–163.
10. A. Prader, J. M. Tanner, and G. A. von Harnack, Catch-up growth following illness or starvation, *Journal of Pediatrics* 62 (1963): 646–659.
11. Committee on Nutrition, American Academy of Pediatrics, *Pediatric Nutrition Handbook*, 2nd ed. (Elk Grove Village, Ill.: American Academy of Pediatrics, 1985), p. 31.
12. G. H. Lowrey, Nutrition in normal growth, in *Growth and Development of Children*, 8th ed. (Chicago: Year Book Medical Publishers, 1986), pp. 383–410.
13. Food and Nutrition Board, Committee on Dietary Allowances, *Recommended Dietary Allowances*, 9th ed. (Washington, D.C.: National Academy of Sciences, 1980), p. 27.
14. R. G. Whitehead and coauthors, A critical analysis of measured food energy intakes during infancy and early childhood in comparison with current international recommendations, *Journal of Human Nutrition* 35 (1981): 339–348.
15. R. A. Stewart, *Infant and Child Feeding* (New York: Academic Press, 1981), pp. 123–133.
16. Food and Nutrition Board, 1980, pp. 39–54.
17. J. A. Sturman, D. K. Rassin, and G. E. Gaull, Minireview: Taurine in development, *Life Science* 21 (1977): 1–21.
18. L. A. Barness, Nutrition for healthy neonates, in *Nutritional Needs and Assessment of Normal Growth* (New York: Nestle Nutrition and Raven Press, 1985), pp. 23–40.
19. Food and Nutrition Board, 1980, pp. 39–54.
20. L. A. Barness, Nutritional requirements of the full-term neonate, in *Textbook of Pediatric Nutrition*, ed. R. M. Suskind (New York: Raven Press, 1981), pp. 21–28.
21. K. Brostrøm, Human milk and infant formulas: Nutritional and immunological characteristics, in *Textbook of Pediatric Nutrition*, ed. R. M. Suskind (New York: Raven Press, 1981), pp. 41–64.
22. Brostrøm, 1981.
23. Z. Friedman and coauthors, Rapid onset of essential fatty acid deficiency in the newborn, *Pediatrics* 58 (1976): 640–649.
24. U.S. House of Representatives, Select Committee on Hunger, *Vitamin A: An Urgent Nutritional Need for the World's Children* (Washington, D.C.; Government Printing Office, 1985), pp. 1–20.
25. J. A. Olson, Recommended dietary intakes (RDI) of vitamin A in humans, *American Journal of Clinical Nutrition*, 45 (1987): 704–716.
26. Food and Nutrition Board, 1980, pp. 55–60.
27. Olson, 1987.
28. H. L. Henry and A. W. Norman, Vitamin D: Metabolism and biological actions, *Annual Review of Nutrition* 4 (1984): pp. 493–520.
29. R. H. Herman, Disorders of fat-soluble vitamins A, D, E, and K, in *Textbook of Pediatric Nutrition*, ed. R. M. Suskind (New York: Raven Press, 1981), pp. 65–111.
30. M. Rudolf, K. Arulanantham, and R. M. Greenstein, Unsuspected nutritional rickets, *Pediatrics* 66 (1980): 72–76.
31. S. Bachrach, J. Fisher, and J. S. Parks, An outbreak of vitamin D deficiency rickets in a susceptible population, *Pediatrics* 64 (1979): 871–877; D. V. Edidin and coauthors, Resurgence of nutritional rickets associated with breast-feeding and special dietary practices, *Pediatrics* 65 (1980): 232–235.
32. Rudolf, Arulanantham, and Greenstein, 1980.
33. Committee on Nutrition, 1985, pp. 37–48.
34. D. R. Lakdawala and E. M. Widdowson, Vitamin-D in human milk, *Lancet* 1 (1977): 167–168.
35. L. E. Reeve, R. W. Chesney, and H. F. DeLuca, Vitamin D of human milk: Identification of biologically active forms, *American Journal of Clinical Nutrition* 36 (1982): 122–126.
36. J. G. Bieri, Vitamin E, in *Present Knowledge in Nutrition*, 5th ed. (Washington, D.C.: Nutrition Foundation, 1984), pp. 226–240.
37. F. A. Oski, Vitamin E in infant nutrition, in *Textbook of Pediatric Nutrition*, ed. R. M. Suskind (New York: Raven Press, 1981), pp. 145–151.
38. M. L. Williams and coauthors, Role of dietary iron and fat in vitamin E deficiency anemia of infancy, *New England Journal of Medicine* 292 (1975): 887–890.
39. Oski, 1981.
40. Herman, 1981.
41. Committee on Nutrition, 1985, p. 40.
42. J. A. Olson, Recommended dietary intakes (RDI) of vitamin K in humans, *American Journal of Clinical Nutrition* 45 (1987): 687–692.
43. V. Herbert, Nutritional anemias of childhood—folate, B_{12}: The megaloblastic anemias, in *Textbook of Pediatric Nutrition*, ed. R. M. Suskind (New York: Raven Press, 1981), pp. 133–143.
44. Herbert, 1981.
45. V. Herbert, Recommended dietary intakes (RDI) of vitamin B-12 in humans, *American Journal of Clinical Nutrition* 45 (1987): 671–678.
46. M. C. Higginbottom, L. Sweetman, and W. O. Nyhan, A syndrome of methyl-

malonic aciduria, homocystinuria, mega-loblastic anemia and neurologic abnormalities in a vitamin-B_{12} deficient breastfed infant of a strict vegetarian, *New England Journal of Medicine* 299 (1978): 317–323

47. Higginbottom, Sweetman, and Nyhan, 1978.
48. V. Herbert, Recommended dietary intakes (RDI) of folate in humans, *American Journal of Clinical Nutrition* 45 (1987): 661–670.
49. M. J. Barnes, Function of ascorbic acid in collagen metabolism, *Annals of New York Academy of Science* 258 (1975): 264–277.
50. J. A. Olson and R. E. Hodges, Recommended dietary intakes (RDI) of vitamin C in humans, *American Journal of Clinical Nutrition* 45 (1987): 693–703.
51. M. I. Irwin and B. K. Hutchins, A conspectus of research on vitamin C requirements of man, *Journal of Nutrition* 106 (1976): 823–879.
52. J. S. Flier and L. H. Underhill, New concepts in the biology and biochemistry of ascorbic acid, *New England Journal of Medicine* 314 (1986): 892–902.
53. Olson and Hodges, 1987.
54. H. L. Greene, Disorders of the water-soluble vitamin B-complex and vitamin C, in *Textbook of Pediatric Nutrition* ed. R. M. Suskind (New York: Raven Press, 1981), pp. 113–131.
55. L. Salmenpera, Vitamin C nutrition during prolonged lactation: Optimal in infants while marginal in some mothers, *American Journal of Clinical Nutrition* 40 (1984): 1050–1056.
56. Olson and Hodges, 1987.
57. Brostrøm, 1981.
58. F. A. Oski and J. A. Stockman, Anemia due to inadequate iron sources or poor iron utilization, *Pediatric Clinics of North America*, 27 (1980): 237–252.
59. R. Yip and coauthors, Declining incidence of anemia among low-income children in the United States, *Journal of the American Medical Association* 258 (1987): 1619–1623.
60. Oski and Stockman, 1980.
61. J. Weinberg, Behavioral and physiological effects of early iron deficiency in the rat, in *Iron Deficiency: Brain Biochemistry and Behavior*, ed. E. Pollitt and R. L. Leibel (New York: Raven Press, 1982), pp. 93–123.
62. E. Pollitt and coauthors, Iron deficiency and behavioral development in infants and preschool children, *American Journal of Clinical Nutrition* 43 (1986): 555–565.
63. F. A. Oski and A. S. Honig, The effects of therapy on the developmental scores of iron-deficient infants, *Pediatrics* 92 (1978): 21–25; T. Walter, J. Kovalskys, and A. Stekel, Effect of mild iron deficiency on infant mental development scores, *Journal of Pediatrics* 68 (1983): 828–838.
64. F. A. Oski and coauthors, Effect of iron therapy on behavior performance in nonanemic, iron-deficient infants, *Pediatrics* 71 (1983): 877–880.
65. E. Pollitt and R. L. Leibel, Iron deficiency and behavior, *Journal of Pediatrics* 88 (1976): 372–381.
66. Pollitt and coauthors, 1986.
67. T. Walter, J. Kovalskys, and A. Stekel, Effect of mild iron deficiency on infant mental development scores, *Pediatrics* 102 (1983): 519–522.
68. R. L. Leibel, Behavioral and biochemical correlates of iron deficiency, *Journal of the American Dietetic Association* 71 (1977): 398–404.
69. M. L. Voorhees and coauthors, Iron deficiency anemia and increased urinary norepinephrine excretion, *Journal of Pediatrics* 86 (1975): 542–547.
70. E. D. Rios and coauthors, Relationship of maternal and infant iron stores as assessed by determination of plasma ferritin, *Pediatrics* 55 (1975): 694–699.
71. B. Lonnerdal, C. L. Keen, and L. S. Hurley, Iron, copper, zinc, and manganese in milk, *Annual Review of Nutrition* 1 (1981): 149–174.
72. Committee on Nutrition, 1985, pp. 213–220.
73. Committee on Nutrition, 1985, p. 41
74. G. H. Johnson, F. A. Purvis, and R. D. Wallace, What nutrients do our infants really get?, *Nutrition Today*, July/August 1981, pp. 4–10, 23–26.
75. Committee on Nutrition, 1985, p. 42.
76. Food and Nutrition Board, 1980, pp. 137–144.
77. Bureau of Nutritional Sciences, Committee for the Revision of the Dietary Standard for Canada, *Recommended Nutrient Intakes for Canadians* (Ottawa: Canadian Government Publishing Centre, 1983), pp. 126–127.
78. Brostrøm, 1981.
79. Food and Nutrition Board, 1980, pp. 125–133.
80. Food and Nutrition Board, 1980, pp. 125–133.
81. Food and Nutrition Board, 1980, pp. 125–133.
82. Food and Nutrition Board, 1980, pp. 125–133.
83. N. F. Krebs and K. M. Hambridge, Zinc requirements and zinc intakes of breast-fed infants, *American Journal of Clinical Nutrition* 43 (1986): 288–292.
84. Food and Nutrition Board, 1980, pp. 144–147.
85. Krebs, 1986.
86. Brostrøm, 1981.
87. O. G. Brooke, Nutrition in the preterm infant, *Lancet* 1 (1983): 514–515.
88. O. G. Brooke, Nutritional requirements of low and very low birthweight infants, *Annual Review of Nutrition* 7 (1987): 91–116.
89. B. Reichman and coauthors, Diet, fat accretion, and growth in premature infants, *New England Journal of Medicine* 305 (1981): 1495–1500.
90. Brooke, 1983; J. Senterre and J. Rigo, Nutritional requirements of low-birthweight infants, in *Nutritional Needs and Assessment of Normal Growth*, ed. M. Gracey and F. Falkner (New York: Raven Press, 1985).
91. Bieri, 1984.
92. P. J. Leonard and M. S. Losowsky, Effect of alpha-tocopherol administration on red cell survival in vitamin E-deficient human subjects, *American Journal of Clinical Nutrition* (1971): 388–393.
93. G. R. Gutcher, W. J. Raynor, and P. M. Farrell, An evaluation of vitamin E status in premature infants, *American Journal of Clinical Nutrition* 40 (1984): 1078–1089.
94. M. S. Rodriguez, A conspectus of research on folacin requirements of man, in *Nutritional Requirements of Man: A Conspectus of Research* (Washington, D.C.: Nutrition Foundation, 1980), pp. 397–489.
95. E. E. Ziegler, R. L. Biga, and S. J. Fomon, Nutritional requirements of the premature infant, *Textbook of Pediatric Nutrition*, ed. R. M. Suskind (New York: Raven Press, 1981), pp. 29–39.
96. P. R. Dallman, M. A. Siimes, and A. Stekel, Iron deficiency in infancy and childhood, *American Journal of Clinical Nutrition* 33 (1980): 86–118.
97. Committee on Nutrition, 1985, p. 43.
98. M. I. Irwin and E. W. Kienholz, A conspectus of research on calcium requirements of man, in *Nutritional Requirements of Man: A Conspectus of Research* (Washington, D.C.: The Nutrition Foundation, 1980), pp. 135–211.
99. Spady, 1977; Committee on Nutrition, 1985, p. 42.

100. American Dietetic Association, Position of the American Dietetic Association: Promotion of breastfeeding, *Journal of the American Dietetic Association* 86 (1986): 1580–1585.

101. American Academy of Pediatrics, Committee on Nutrition and the Nutrition Committee of the Canadian Pediatric Society, Breastfeeding: A commentary in celebration of the international year of the child, *Pediatrics* 62 (1978): 591–601.

102. E. M. E. Poskitt, Infant feeding: A review, *Human Nutrition: Applied Nutrition* 37A (1983): 271–286.

103. Poskitt, 1983.

104. K. C. Hayes and J. A. Sturman, Taurine in metabolism, *Annual Review of Nutrition* 1 (1981): 401–425.

105. T. A. Picone, Taurine update: Metabolism and function, *Nutrition Today,* July/August 1987, pp. 16–20.

106. M. W. Borschel and coauthors, Fatty acid composition of mature human milk of Egyptian and American women, *American Journal of Clinical Nutrition* 44 (1986): 330–335.

107. Brostrøm, 1981.

108. Poskitt, 1983.

109. R. Reiser and Z. Sidelman, Control of serum cholesterol homeostasis by cholesterol in the milk of the suckling rat, *Journal of Nutrition* 102 (1972): 1009–1016, as cited in Cholesterol and the Reiser hypothesis, *Journal of Nutrition Education,* March 1983, p. 27.

110. Spady, 1977.

111. American Academy of Pediatrics, Committee on Nutrition, Toward a prudent diet for children, *Pediatrics* 71 (1983): 78–79.

112. A. Hofman, A. Hazebroek, and H. A. Valkenburg, A randomized trial of sodium intake and blood pressure in newborn infants, *Journal of the American Medical Association* 250 (1983): 370–373.

113. Food and Nutrition Board, 1980, pp. 169–172.

114. Food and Nutrition Board, 1980, pp. 169–172.

115. Committee on Nutrition, 1985, p. 42.

116. Committee on Nutrition, 1985, p. 41.

117. Lonnerdal, 1985; J. K. Welsh, I. J. Skurrie, and J. T. May, Use of semliki forest virus to identify lipid-mediated antiviral activity and anti-alphavirus immunoglobulin A in human milk, *Infection and Immunity,* February 1978, pp. 395–401.

118. Lonnerdal, 1985.

119. C. L. Berseth, L.M. Lichtenberger, and F.H. Morriss, Comparison of the gastrointestinal growth-promoting effects of rat colostrum and mature milk in newborn rats in vivo, *American Journal of Clinical Nutrition* 37 (1983): 52–60.

120. M. G. Kovar and coauthors, Review of the epidemiologic evidence for an association between infant feeding and infant health, *Pediatrics* 74 (1984): 615–638.

121. Welsh, Skurrie, and May, 1978.

122. J. J. Bullen, H. J. Rogers, and L. Leigh, Iron-binding proteins in milk and resistance to *Escherichia coli* infection in infants, *British Medical Journal* 1 (1972): 69–75, as cited in B. Lonnerdal, Biochemistry and physiological function of human milk proteins, *American Journal of Clinical Nutrition* 42 (1985): 1299–1317.

123. J. A. McMillan, S. A. Landaw, and F. A. Oski, Iron sufficiency in breast-fed infants and the availability of iron from human milk, *Pediatrics* 58 (1976): 686–691.

124. C. D. Eckhart, Isolation of a protein from human milk that enhances zinc absorption in humans, *Biochemical and Biophysical Research Communications* 130 (1985): 264–269.

125. G. Carpenter, Epidermal growth factor is a major growth-promoting agent in human milk, *Science* 210 (1980): 198–199.

126. H. Bauchner, J. M. Leventhal, and E. D. Shapiro, Studies of breast-feeding and infections: How good is the evidence, *Journal of the American Medical Association* 256 (1986): 887–892.

127. U. M. Saarinen and coauthors, Prolonged breast-feeding as prophylaxis for atopic disease, *Lancet* 2 (1979): 163–166.

128. Committee on Nutrition, American Academy of Pediatrics, The use of whole cow's milk in infancy, *Pediatrics* 72 (1983): 253–255.

129. D. M. Paige, Infant growth and nutrition, *Clinical Nutrition* 2 (1983): 14–18.

130. R. A. Stewart, Supplementary foods: Their nutritional role in infant feeding, *Infant and Child Feeding,* ed. J. T. Bond and coeditors (New York: Academic Press, 1981), pp. 123–133.

131. S. J. Fomon, Reflections on infant feeding in the 1970's and 1980's, *American Journal of Clinical Nutrition* 46 (1987): 171–182.

132. D. W. Marlin, M. F. Picciano, and E. C. Livant, Infant feeding practices, *Journal of*

the *American Dietetic Association* 77 (1980): 668–675; D. L. Yeung and coauthors, Infant feeding practices, *Nutrition Reports International* 23 (1981): 249–260.

133. Fomon, 1987.

134. P. R. Dallman, M. A. Siimes, and A. Stekel, Iron deficiency in infancy and childhood, *American Journal of Clinical Nutrition* 33 (1980): 86–118.

135. Poskitt, 1983.

136. T. Lindberg and G. Skude, Amylase in human milk, *Pediatrics* 70 (1982): 235–238.

137. S. A. Quandt, The effect of beikost on the diet of breastfed infants, *Journal of the American Dietetic Association* 84 (1984): 47–51.

138. Dallman, Siimes, and Stekel, 1980.

139. Dallman, Siimes, and Stekel, 1980.

140. Committee on Nutrition, 1985, p. 41.

141. The gastrointestinal tract: Development and nutrition, in *Dynamics of Infant Physiology and Nutrition,* ed. L. J. Filer (Bloomfield, N.J.: Health Learning Systems, 1982), pp. 1–16.

142. W. A. Walker, Antigen handling by the gut, *Archives of Disease in Children* 53 (1978): 527–531.

143. Committee on Nutrition, 1985, p. 34.

144. N. W. Solomons, An update on lactose intolerance, *Dairy Council Digest,* July–August 1985, pp. 1–3.

145 *Baby Foods,* A report by the American Council on Science and Health (Summit, N.J.: American Council on Science and Health, 1987).

146. *Baby Foods,* 1987.

147. D. L. Yeung, Commercial baby foods, in *Infant Nutrition: A Study of Feeding Practices and Growth from Birth to 18 Months* (Ottawa, Canada: Canadian Public Health Association, 1983), pp. 132–149.

148. Yeung, 1983.

149. American Council on Science and Health, 1987.

150. H. M. Barry, Addressing confusion over role of modified starches, *Food Engineering* 58 (1986): 56–57.

151. C. Briggs, Recent developments in infant feeding and nutrition, in *Nutrition Update: Volume 1,* ed. J. Weininger and G. M. Briggs (New York: John Wiley and Sons, 1983), pp. 227–261.

152. E. M. E. Poskitt and T. J. Cole, Do fat babies stay fat? *British Medical Journal* 1 (1977): 7–9.

▶ *Focal Point 4*

Nutrition Care of Sick Infants and Children

The emphasis of this text is on wellness and the prevention of disease, but even children who are generally in good health get sick on occasion. This discussion examines some of the common symptoms that most children experience at one time or another—infections and fever, diarrhea, and constipation. It then continues with a look at the special needs of any child who requires hospitalization.*

A healthy, well-nourished child can easily slip into poor nutrition status with an illness. Serious illness can affect a child's nutrition status in several ways. An illness can alter:

▶ Appetite.

▶ Chewing and swallowing abilities.

▶ Digestion and absorption.

▶ Metabolism.

▶ Excretion.

Any or all of these effects can occur during illness and compromise nutrition status. Competent medical care includes attention to nutrition.

Infections and Fever

Each day, the body confronts an environment teeming with disease-causing organisms. The body's remarkable capacity to survive such an environment is a tribute to its immune system. The immune system has no central organ of control, but rather depends on various organs and white blood cells. Their interactions and secretions defend the body against infectious organisms, such as bacteria and viruses. Figure FP4–1 summarizes the action of the immune system; the miniglossary defines related terms. The immune system recognizes these organisms and destroys or otherwise neutralizes them. When organisms do manage to penetrate the immune defenses, an infection, or an even more damaging disease, develops. Still, for every successful penetration of foreign organisms, the immune system averts thousands of attempts.

---

*Parts of this discussion have been adapted with permission from E. N. Whitney, C. B. Cataldo, and S. R. Rolfes, *Understanding Normal and Clinical Nutrition*, 2nd ed. (St. Paul, Minn.: West, 1987).

Figure FP4–1 The Immune System

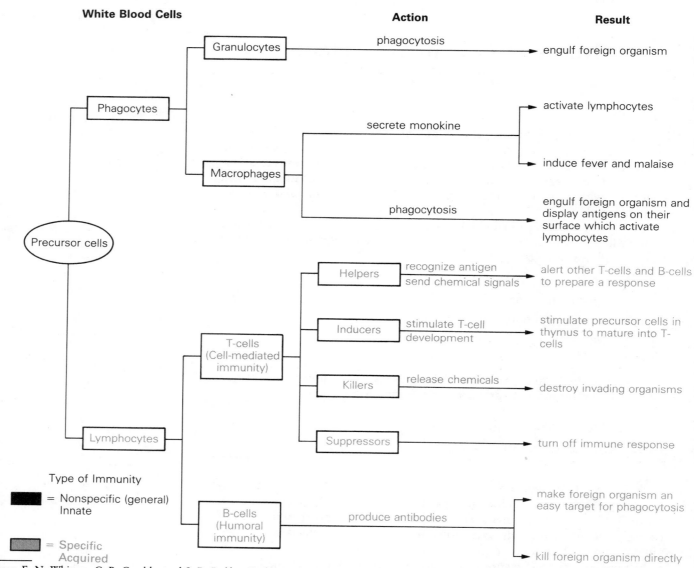

Source: E. N. Whitney, C. B. Cataldo, and S. R. Rolfes, *Understanding Normal and Clinical Nutrition*, 2nd ed. (St. Paul, Minn.: West, 1987). Used with permission.

Malnutrition alters immune system components in ways that compromise their function, thus impairing the defense against infecting organisms. It is little wonder that malnourished children develop more infections than well-nourished children. Infection is a major cause of mortality and morbidity in children with protein-energy malnutrition. A vicious cycle develops in which malnutrition reduces resistance to infection, and infection further aggravates malnutrition. This synergistic relationship between malnutrition and infection threatens a child's survival.

synergism: the effect of two factors operating together in such a way that their combined actions are greater than the sum of the actions of the two considered separately.

Miniglossary of Immunity Terms

acquired immunity: immunity directed at specific organisms (also called *specific immunity*). The lymphocytes mediate this type of immunity, which depends on prior exposure, recognition, and reactions to invading organisms. Two types of specific immunity are *cell-mediated immunity* and *humoral immunity.*

antibody: a protein produced by the B-cells in response to invasion of the body by a foreign protein.

antigen: a substance foreign to the body that elicits the formation of antibodies or an inflammation reaction from immune system cells.

cell-mediated immunity: immunity conferred by the actual reaction of T-cells to an invading organism.

granulocytes: a type of phagocyte.

helper T-cells: the T-lymphocytes capable of recognizing antigens and alerting other T-cells to prepare to mount a response.

humoral immunity: immunity conferred by antibodies secreted by B-cells and carried to the invaded area by way of the body fluids.

immune system: the body's natural defense system against foreign materials.

immunity: the body's ability to recognize and eliminate foreign materials.

inducer T-cells: T-lymphocytes that stimulate precursor cells in the thymus to develop into mature T-cells.

innate immunity: immunity directed at foreign organisms in general (also called *nonspecific immunity*). The skin, mucous membranes, and phagocytes are a part of this type of immunity.

killer T-cells: T-lymphocytes that release chemicals that can destroy an invading organism. Also called *cytoxic T-cells.*

lymphocytes: white blood cells that originate from precursors in the bone marrow and mature into two distinct types of lymphocytes—B-cells and T-cells—upon their release.

macrophage: the type of phagocyte that secretes *monokines.*

monokines: various proteins secreted by phagocytes that help mediate the immune response, such as interferon and interleukin-1.

nonspecific immunity: see *innate immunity.*

phagocytes: cells that have the ability to engulf and destroy foreign materials.

phagocytosis (FAG-oh-sigh-TOE-sis). the process by which some cells (phagocytes) engulf and destroy foreign materials.
phagein = to eat
kytos = cell
osis = intensive

precursor cell: a simple cell that matures. Precursor white blood cells are capable of maturing into three different types of cells.

specific immunity: see *acquired immunity.*

suppressor T-cells: T-lymphocytes that slow down the immune response and eventually turn it off.

fever: an increase of body temperature of more than 1° F above normal (98.6° F).

The course of an infection generally progresses as follows. Disease-causing organisms invade the body, overcoming initial immune defenses. A few days after exposure to these infective organisms, symptoms begin to appear, with fever developing shortly thereafter.

People fear fever and rush to treat it because it accompanies many dangerous diseases, but the fever itself may actually assist the immune system.[1] Clearly, fever stresses the body—it raises the heart rate and increases the tissues' demand for oxygen. High temperatures (over 104° F or, in some cases, lower) can cause convulsions and demand medical attention not only to control the fever, but to determine and treat the underlying condition. Moderate temperatures (between 102° F and 104° F) may be cause for concern and require a consultation with a health care provider. Generally, though, a mild fever should be allowed to do its job of assisting the immune system.[2] Fever causes the T-cells of the immune system to proliferate, thus enhancing the system's activity.[3] When researchers suppress fever experimentally, sick animals are more likely to die from infection than when fever is allowed to run its course. Furthermore, animals kept continuously at fever temperatures resist viruses better than nonfeverish ones.

After the onset of fever, catabolic changes begin. The body loses nitrogen (from protein catabolism) and intracellular electrolytes. These losses are great enough to result in negative balances. If diarrhea and vomiting accompany the infection, the body's losses are even greater.

Fever is a major factor in determining the energy needs of an infected child. The basal metabolic rate increases (roughly 10 to 13 percent for each 1 degree centigrade; 7 percent for each 1 degree Fahrenheit) as the temperature rises above normal (98.6° F; 37° C). Additional food energy may be needed to support physical activity—for example, if a child is restless, coughing, crying, or the like.

The scientific name for the centigrade temperature scale is Celsius. To convert from centigrade to Fahrenheit (and vice versa) use these equations:

$$t_F = 9/5 \; t_C + 32.$$
$$t_C = 5/9 \; (t_F - 32).$$

sodium salicylate: a compound used as an analgesic and antipyretic; aspirin is acetylsalicylic acid.

interleukin-1: a protein released by the immune system that mediates many responses to infection.

Ironically, during this time of heightened energy needs, appetite diminishes. Infection-related anorexia aggravates negative nutrient balances and contributes to weight loss. Researchers have questioned whether this anorexia is a result of the fever itself.[4] When they blocked the fever of infected rats with sodium salicylate, appetite remained depressed. Additional investigation revealed that interleukin-1, a protein released by the immune system in response to infection, both induces fever and suppresses food intake.

The immune system functions best when protein status is optimal. The protein requirements of a child with an infection depend primarily on total energy consumption. At a minimum, protein intake should meet the RDA for age, weight, and gender. With fever, protein allowances increase above the RDA by 10 percent per 1 degree centigrade (5.5 percent per 1 degree Fahrenheit) of fever.

All the nutrients appear to play some role in the functioning of the immune system. Changes in immune function have been associated with deficiencies of folacin, iron, and zinc, and with excesses of vitamin E and essential fatty acids. Furthermore, clinical reports suggest that changes in immune function accompany deficiencies of vitamins A, B_6, B_{12}, and C; deficiencies of pantothenic acid; and elevated blood cholesterol levels. Studies in animals link the concentrations of many vitamins, minerals, trace elements, amino acids, fatty acids, and cholesterol with immunologic changes. Table FP4–1 lists nutrients reported to influence immune function, with the effect of each.

Table FP4–1   Effects of Selected Nutrients on the Immune System

Nutrient Deficiency	Effects
Vitamin A	Depletion of T-lymphocytes[a]; increased frequency and severity of some infections[a]; increased incidence of infections (human beings)[b]
Vitamin B$_6$	Depressed cell-mediated and humoral immunity[a]; reduced antibody responses to vaccines (human beings)
Folacin	Impaired response to skin tests; lymph tissue atrophy[a]; reduced numbers of white blood cells[a]; impaired cell-mediated and humoral immunity[a]
Pantothenic acid	Depressed antibody responses (human beings)
Vitamin B$_{12}$	Some reduction of phagocytosis by granulocytes (human beings)
Vitamin E[c]	Depressed antibody responses[a]; impaired response to skin tests[a]
Iron	Atrophy of lymph tissue; impaired response to skin tests; defective phagocytosis (human beings)
Zinc	Atrophy of lymph tissues; abnormalities in cell-mediated and humoral immunity (human beings)
Individual amino acids	Impaired humoral immunity[a]

[a]Information is from animal studies.
[b]Some reports support this finding, but more information is needed.
[c]Vitamin E excess can cause inhibition of multiple immune functions in human beings.

Source: E. N. Whitney, C. B. Cataldo, and S. R. Rolfes, *Understanding Normal and Clinical Nutrition*, 2nd ed. (St. Paul, Minn.: 1987). Used with permission.

Maintaining fluid balance is of particular concern during an infection. In some infectious diseases, especially those that involve vomiting, diarrhea, or considerable sweating, fluid needs may be as high as 3 to 4 liters per day. If the child does not drink fluids at this rate, dehydration can quickly develop. On the other hand, the child may retain water due to the hormonal changes that accompany fever. In the rare case that a child's fluid intake is excessive, water intoxication can develop. Table FP4–2 lists the symptoms associated with dehydration and water intoxication.

dehydration: loss of too much fluid from the body.

water intoxication: the condition in which body water content is too high.

Little information is available regarding specific vitamin and mineral requirements during infection. The need for B vitamins increases with increasing energy and protein intakes, but remains consistent with the RDA. Foods can generally cover the vitamin and electrolyte losses incurred during catabolism. Children who have lost their appetites or are feeling nauseated may prefer liquids to solid foods. Liquids are an acceptable alternative to solid foods provided that the caretaker selects those that offer energy, vitamins, and minerals. Drinking liquids also prevents dehydration, of course.

Children with infections may develop a type of anemia referred to as the anemia of infection. At the onset of the infection, the blood concentration of iron rapidly declines as iron moves into the liver for storage. This shift of iron from the blood to the liver helps to fight the infection by making the body's

anemia of infection: a condition in which iron moves from the blood to the liver to help fight infection, resulting in a decline in hemoglobin synthesis.

Table FP4–2   Dehydration and Water Intoxication Symptoms

Dehydration Symptoms	Water Intoxication Symptoms
Thirst	Low plasma sodium concentrations
Muscle cramps	Headache
Weakness, fatigue, exhaustion	Muscular weakness and fatigue
Delirium	Lack of concentration, poor memory, delirium
Death	Loss of appetite
	Seizure
	Death

iron unavailable for the infecting bacteria, which require iron to perform their metabolic functions.[5] However, iron in storage is also unavailable for hemoglobin synthesis, so anemia results. This type of anemia is the body's normal physiological response to infection and does not respond to iron, folacin, or vitamin B_{12} supplements, nor to any other dietary or medical treatment. Instead, the situation corrects itself; iron returns to the blood from the liver as the infection resolves.

Physicians' primary concerns for children with infections are to identify and eliminate the infecting organisms. Quite often, they prescribe antibiotics, but these can interfere with nutrient absorption, thus compromising nutrition status (see Table A–3 of the Assessment Appendix).

When the infection ends, a well-balanced diet best restores the body to its normal status. The time it takes to reach a positive balance and the duration of positive balance depend on the extent of nutrient deficiencies, the quality of the diet, and the quantity of food intake. A well-balanced diet that restores the nutrient reserves also helps to defend against future infections. In some cases, physicians may prescribe a multivitamin-mineral supplement to augment nutrient intake.

Quite often, a child with a fever does not require medical attention, but may benefit from tender loving care. The child's caretaker can comfort the child by:[6]

▶ Helping the child's body to maintain its own body temperature by keeping the room temperature moderate and bed coverings to a minimum.

▶ Sponging the child with lukewarm water to increase heat loss by evaporation.

▶ Providing the child with plenty of fluids.

▶ Providing the child with acetaminophen if a physician recommends drug intervention.

Fever is the body's signal that something is wrong and it is trying to defend itself. In many cases, the body is successful without medical attention, but infants with any degree of fever and older children with fevers of 103 degrees Fahrenheit or greater require medical attention. In addition, fevers that go away and recur, that persist for more than 72 hours, or that accompany a rash or marked irritability and confusion require consultation with a physician.

acetaminophen: an antipyretic, analgesic drug used to reduce fever or relieve pain.

Pediatricians recommend acetaminophen instead of aspirin because of aspirin's association with Reye syndrome, a rare disease that primarily affects children and adolescents, generally following flu or chicken pox. Symptoms begin with tiredness and vomiting, progress to permanent brain damage, and result in death in 20 to 30 percent of the cases.[7]

Diarrhea

Diarrhea is characterized by frequent, loose, watery stools. Such bowel movements indicate that the chyme has moved too quickly for the intestines to absorb enough fluids from it, or that it has drawn water from the cells lining the intestinal tract. In both cases, the result is the same—extensive fluid and electrolyte losses. If diarrhea continues without treatment, an infant or young child can quickly become dehydrated and malnourished. The smaller and younger the child, the more dramatic are the effects.

Nearly every child suffers from diarrhea at one time or another. Many times an acute case of diarrhea develops and remits in 24 to 48 hours. Well-nourished children with acute diarrhea can usually endure the uncomfortable symptoms without medical treatment. Caretakers can support children during such episodes of diarrhea by eliminating food irritants from the diet and offering clear liquids. Fruit juices aggravate diarrhea and are therefore inappropriate beverages to offer. Children may enjoy such clear liquids as gelatin dessert, carbonated beverages, and Popsicles, but these treats fall short of correcting for dehydration. Their low electrolyte content and high osmolality make them unsuitable for rehydration therapy.[8]

Nutrient reserves of well-nourished children protect them from the detrimental effects of diarrhea for a short while. The availability of medical treatment and high-quality food in industrialized countries offers children the opportunity to recover, both from fluid and electrolyte losses and from growth losses.

The story is quite different in developing countries. Acute diarrhea in a malnourished child threatens life and requires immediate medical attention. In developing countries, more children suffer from malnutrition, and acute diarrhea seriously threatens their tenuous nutrition status. With repeated episodes of diarrhea falling close together, these children's recovery time becomes limited. Without full restoration of nutrients, children are progressively less able to defend against future infections.

Diarrhea is the most common cause of dehydration and malnutrition among children in developing countries.[9] Millions of children die from the complications of diarrhea each year. With reduced dietary intake, impaired intestinal absorption, and the increased nutrient requirements that accompany diarrhea, malnutrition is inevitable.

Children with diarrhea eat less, and therefore their energy intakes are low, averaging between 15 and 50 percent less than their usual intakes.[10] Factors interfering with food intake include anorexia, nausea, and vomiting. In addition, parents or health care workers may withhold food in an effort to resolve the diarrhea. (The wisdom of such a practice is discussed in upcoming paragraphs.)

Maldigestion and malabsorption accompany diarrhea. Normally, hormones and nerves orchestrate the digestive and absorptive processes by signaling several organs to respond at the appropriate times with contractions that move the intestinal contents along, secretions that dismantle nutrients into absorbable molecules, and receptors that transport these molecules into the body. When the contents of the intestine pass too rapidly, digestion is

Diarrhea that results from an accelerated movement of fluids and electrolytes from the intestinal capillaries into the lumen of the intestine is called **secretory diarrhea**. When unabsorbed water and electrolytes cause diarrhea by increasing the osmolarity of the intestinal contents, then **osmotic diarrhea** exists.

The term **acute** describes diseases or conditions that develop rapidly, have severe symptoms, and are of short duration. A disease or condition that develops slowly, shows little change, and lasts a long time is said to be **chronic**. Severe, chronic diarrhea is often called **intractable diarrhea**.
acutus = sharp
chronos = time

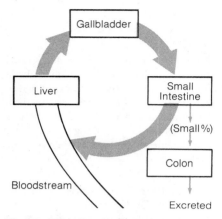

Figure FP4–2 Enterohepatic Circulation
The recycling of nutrients through the intestine and liver is known as **enterohepatic circulation**.

enteron = intestine
hepat = liver

steatorrhea (stee-ah-toe-REE-ah): fatty diarrhea characteristic of fat malabsorption; stools are foamy, greasy, and malodorous.

oral rehydration therapy (ORT): the administration of a simple solution of sugar, salt, and water taken by mouth, to treat dehydration caused by diarrhea.

incomplete. When intestinal cells that allow the transport of nutrients into the body are damaged, absorption is limited. Absorption of protein, carbohydrate, and fat in children with diarrhea can be 10 to 30 percent less than in healthy children.[11] On the positive side, 70 to 90 percent of these nutrients *is* getting absorbed, a fact that emphasizes the value of feeding children with diarrhea. Without food intake, pancreatic function and intestinal cell production and maturation remain low, thus limiting the supply of enzymes for digestion and the surface area for absorption.

Clinicians focus on the most appropriate way to minimize and replace nutrient losses incurred by diarrhea. Controversy surrounds the question of whether to withhold or provide nutrients during episodes of diarrhea. The advantages of both delayed feeding and continued feeding are worthy of consideration.

The traditional practice of withholding food is based on the premise that the bowel needs to rest and that ingested food is malabsorbed. Malabsorption results from the rapid intestinal transit time and damage to the intestinal mucosa. Injuries to the intestine diminish mucosal surface area, alter villus structure, and lower enzyme concentrations. Lactose intolerance is a common, usually temporary, consequence of diarrhea. The intestinal cells that produce lactase are located on the delicate fringe of microvilli that form the brush border of the intestinal villi. Any condition (such as diarrhea) that damages the brush border can lead to lactose intolerance. For this reason, dairy products are reintroduced into the diet gradually following diarrhea.

The obvious consequence of malabsorption is the loss of potential nutrients, but unabsorbed nutrients in the intestine present other complications as well. For one, they have an osmotic effect, drawing water and electrolytes into the gut; this can intensify the diarrhea beyond that caused by the original infection.[12] Unabsorbed nutrients in the intestine may also bind with bile acids, thus preventing their normal conservation via enterohepatic circulation. (Figure FP4–2 illustrates the normal conservation of nutrients via enterohepatic circulation.) Such losses deplete the bile acid pool, and can contribute to steatorrhea.

Diminished absorption capacity is not the only consequence of damaged intestinal cells. Absorption of whole proteins is another concern. Some researchers speculate that ingestion of whole proteins during acute diarrhea may induce food sensitivities; however, evidence of this possibility is lacking.[13]

Even considering the problems of malabsorption, the argument in favor of feeding the child appears to weigh more heavily. For well-nourished children, short-term fasting may be appropriate therapy, but for malnourished children, fasting throughout the course of diarrhea can be devastating. Consider that the annual prevalence rate of diarrhea in children under the age of three in Bangladesh is 55 days a year.[14] To fast for close to two months a year is to lose a significant percentage of a year's nutrient intakes. It is unreasonable to expect that the diet during times without diarrhea could replace losses incurred by such prolonged fasting. Health care providers argue that "suboptimal absorption of some food is preferable to no malabsorption of no food."[15]

The potential for accelerated deterioration of nutrition status demands rapid replacement of fluids and nutrients.[16] Health care workers around the world are treating diarrhea with oral rehydration therapy (ORT). Table FP4–3 lists the World Health Organization (WHO) standards for ORT formulas. The

Table FP4–3 World Health Organization ORT Formula

The World Health Organization (WHO) recommends the following ORT formula:	
Sodium	90 mmol/l
Chloride	80 mmol/l
Potassium	20 mmol/l
Glucose	111 mmol/l
Citrate tribasic or bicarbonate	30 mmol/l

components of ORT formulas provide needed energy and electrolytes. Except in cases of severe dehydration, ORT can replace the traditional treatment of intravenous (IV) fluid therapy. Intravenous therapy is still most valuable in treating severely dehydrated children; ORT is useful in treating mild to moderate cases and following initial IV therapy.[17]

ORT provides an electrolyte solution with an optimal glucose concentration, which favors rapid intestinal absorption of water and sodium.[18] This solution reverses dehydration, but may not correct the diarrhea. If diarrhea continues, the child receives water and the solution alternately. Infants with diarrhea usually tolerate breast milk well, and breastfeeding can alternate with supplements of the solution.

Perhaps the most significant value of ORT is that it is oral—it does not require hospitalization, as with intravenous or parenteral feedings. In addition, if the specific WHO recommended solution is unavailable, caretakers can make other suitable ORT solutions. A mother who lives miles from the nearest pharmacy or clinic and who does not have the resources to purchase medicines anyway can prepare a solution to refeed her dehydrated infant. A properly prepared rice powder solution facilitates the absorption of electrolytes and water, as well as limiting the duration of diarrhea. The primary role of health care providers then becomes one of educating those who care for children. The people of a community must learn how to prepare a rehydration solution from ingredients available locally. They must learn to measure ingredients carefully and to use sanitary water. Parents will also want to learn how to recognize diarrhea and dehydration symptoms.

The success of ORT in developing countries is central to the WHO's effort to counter the dehydration and death commonly associated with diarrhea. Yet, in developed countries, physicians are reluctant to adopt ORT, recommending IV fluids instead.[19] In some cases, the practice of giving IV fluids serves as the only justification to hospitalize a child. However, treating well-nourished children in developed countries with ORT is as effective as, and less expensive and invasive than, IV therapy.

Once rehydrated, children can resume eating foods. At first, they tolerate frequent, small meals best. If food consumption intensifies the diarrhea and threatens dehydration, then they should again go without food temporarily. Clinical observation and the child's willingness are often the best determinants of whether to offer food.

The nutrient needs of an undernourished child with diarrhea are exceptionally high. Convalescence time must include food consumption of greater quantity and higher quality than normal to replenish nutrient losses and to

intravenous (IV) fluid therapy: the administration of nutrient solutions through a vein.

A simple recipe: 1 c boiling water
2 tsp sugar
a pinch of salt

allow for catch-up growth. The nutrient intake must compensate for impaired intestinal absorption, support a raised metabolic rate, repair damaged tissue, and make up for growth losses. A conservative goal during convalescence is to provide at least 25 percent more energy than the average requirement for healthy children.[20] A protein intake twice as high as the recommendation for healthy children covers the catabolic and malabsorption losses incurred and the inefficient use of protein when energy intake or absorption is inadequate. These recommendations serve as guidelines and should be adjusted according to the child's growth response.

Constipation

constipation: the condition of having painful or difficult bowel movements (elapsed time between movements is not relevant).

The consequences of constipation are far less life-threatening than those of diarrhea. Each child's digestive tract responds to food uniquely, with its own rhythm. When a child receives the signal to defecate and ignores it (as active children having fun will do), the signal may not return for several hours. During this time, the intestine continues withdrawing water from the fecal matter, so that when the child does take time to defecate, the bowel movement is dry and hard. Bowel movements that are hard and passed with difficulty, discomfort, or pain define constipation. The amount of time that has elapsed since the previous bowel movement is irrelevant. In the case of painful bowel movements, a parent will want to consult with a physician in order to rule out the presence of organic disease.

Some fibers attract water into the digestive tract, thus softening the stools and preventing or relieving constipation. For this reason, increased fluid intake should accompany increased fiber intake. Wheat bran is one of the most effective stool-softening fibers, although convincing a child to eat bran regularly can be a challenge. One group of pediatricians recommends one to two quarts of popped popcorn per day to relieve constipation.[21] They found this "treatment" to soften stools and increase stool volume, thus providing an enjoyable and inexpensive solution to the problem of constipation. Fluids also help to relieve constipation by augmenting stool weight and softness. Children may prefer fruit juices to water, and these are acceptable alternatives.

The Hospitalized Child

At times, children may require hospitalization. Health care providers encounter unique problems when feeding children in the hospital. To effectively solve these problems, they need an understanding of the concepts underlying diet therapy and child development. This discussion does not examine the specific dietary treatments of diseases, but does recognize a child's developmental needs.

To work effectively with an infant or child, a health care provider must work effectively with the family and community. Family members must feel comfortable and be able to communicate openly with hospital staff. Their participation in the child's care helps family members to feel needed and the child to recover.

Mealtimes

Much of the discussion in Chapter 5 on feeding children applies to hospitalized children as well. Hospitalized children require careful attention to ensure that their nutrient needs are met. Health care providers and parents must also be sensitive to the child's emotional needs. Pointers from people experienced in working with hospitalized children include:

▶ Notice the child's posture. Body language can indicate fear, pain, or discomfort.

▶ Touch the child often and lovingly. Touch communicates more than words.

▶ Allow the child to choose what foods to eat as much as possible. If permissible, foods brought from outside the hospital can help stimulate appetite.

▶ Encourage the child to eat the food; putting it in front of a child is not enough. Notice the quantities and types of food not eaten.

▶ Stay with the child during the meal, or make sure a caring person is present. The child will eat and digest food better if someone is nearby to soothe anxieties and loneliness.

▶ Encourage the child to eat the most needed foods first. This ensures that the child will receive valuable nutrients before becoming too full to complete the meal.

▶ Allow children to eat with other children, if possible. They will enjoy mealtimes more, accept more food, and eat for a longer period.

▶ Avoid painful procedures near mealtimes. The stress of pain or fear shuts down digestion and turns off interest in food.

▶ Serve small servings of well-liked foods.

▶ Serve foods attractively, selecting a colorful variety of foods. Cut foods into different shapes. Arrange foods in patterns such as faces or vehicles.

Even though its effects may not be immediately obvious, nutrition care contributes importantly to a child's recovery. Providing nourishment is sometimes not as simple as serving a meal. Special circumstances may require providing nourishment through alternative methods.

Tube Feedings

Tube feedings nourish children who have functioning digestive tracts but are unable to orally ingest enough nutrients to meet their needs. This may be due to a physical problem that impairs chewing or swallowing, lack of appetite, coma, or intense nutrient requirements. Physicians determine the most appropriate formula and feeding route for each case, after completing a thorough nutrition assessment (see Appendix A).

At first glance, tube feedings may appear to be a horrible experience. A closer inspection of the procedure reveals that tube feedings offer lifesaving nutrition in many critical situations. When health care providers select the correct size and type of tube and prepare the child for the procedure, there is little discomfort. They can explain the tube insertion and feeding procedure to a child by using dolls or stuffed animals. They can alleviate parental discomfort in handling the child or fears of causing pain or dislodging the feeding tube by showing parents how to hold and move the child.

For infants and young children, especially small feeding tubes minimize discomfort and interference with the airways. Removal of the feeding tubes after each feeding frees the infant's airways between feedings and reduces the risk that formula will back up into the esophagus and enter the lungs. The feeding route for infants is usually from the mouth to the stomach, rather than from the nose (as is common for older children and adults). This route allows infants to breathe more easily because infants breathe through their noses, not their mouths.

An infant's stomach is small, and gastric emptying is slow. For these reasons, the quantity of formula in a tube feeding must be small. If too much formula empties into the stomach at one time, complications can quickly arise. Health care workers who continually monitor the formula's concentration, infusion rate, and volume help to ensure tolerance and avoid problems.

Children are not simply growing, they are also developing. They learn new skills as they grow. Health care workers must always be aware of the developmental age of a child. Self-feeding skills missed at the appropriate age may be difficult to learn at a later age. Infants fed by tube feedings should have partial feedings by bottle, if possible. Using a pacifier during a tube feeding helps to maintain an association of sucking and swallowing with eating and fullness. Likewise, older infants must learn to use and accept food by spoon, even when primary nourishment is from tube feedings. A therapist can help stimulate appropriate development when problems occur in cases of long-term tube feedings.

At times, physicians use infusion pumps to administer tube feedings to young children. Such a procedure requires additional precautions. The bright lights, interesting sounds, and many controls of the pump stimulate a child's curiosity. To ensure safety to the child and to the pump, health care workers must position it a safe distance from the child's bed.

Adolescents are more likely to physically tolerate and adapt to tube feedings than are younger children. However, their social and psychological development may interfere with their acceptance of tube feedings. The prospect of tubes feeding them can horrify teenagers, particularly those overly concerned with appearances. These suggestions might help:

► Encourage teens to be as active as possible.

► Allow teens to dress in their own clothes and to bring their favorite personal items from home, when possible.

► Explain the tube feeding procedure and its importance.

► Include teens in decisions. Allow them to arrange daily schedules and help with feedings, when possible.

► Encourage time with friends and favorite activities.

Health care workers best serve teenagers by being available to listen to their fears and their problems.

Tube feedings offer an alternative when children are unable to eat regular meals. When the digestive tract cannot handle meals or tube feedings, intravenous nutrition must be employed.

Intravenous Nutrition

Intravenous nutrition is required when the digestive system is not functioning. Many of the concerns that arise with tube feedings also arise when infants and children receive IV feedings. For example, it is important to involve parents in the child's care, develop the child's skills at the appropriate age, maintain a safe distance between the child and the infusion pump, and ease the child's and family's fears with proper instructions.

To feed an infant intravenously poses additional problems. The particular nutrient needs of each infant, especially of premature infants, are difficult to determine. To feed a mixture of water, glucose, electrolytes, amino acids, fats, vitamins, and trace elements that will adequately promote growth without overloading an immature body is a challenge. Such mixtures may omit substances that naturally occur in foods and that infants require, but that are still unknown.

The infant's renal system is immature and cannot adjust to changes in the blood's composition as rapidly as can an adult's renal system. Furthermore, an infant's body contains a larger percentage of fluid, so fluctuations cause major problems. Delivering too much or too little of any solution constituent directly into an infant's vein leads to immediate imbalances. Too much fluid can quickly stress the infant's immature renal system; too little can quickly cause dehydration. Too much glucose can rapidly lead to hyperglycemia, with severe consequences; ceasing a feeding or dislodging the tube too rapidly can precipitate hypoglycemia. The list of such possible complications could go on for virtually every substance found in the IV solution. Health care workers must explore all possible sources of any complications that may arise.

The care of children in times of sickness requires careful attention to their nutrition needs. To feed children is to provide them with much more than nutrients and fluids alone. Foods carry both a physical and an emotional comfort. Chicken noodle soup does offer fluids, some energy, a little protein, and a variety of vitamins and minerals, but its healing power also comes from the caretaker's concern about the child. Children given tender loving care recover more quickly than those deprived of it. As Dr. F. W. Peabody of Harvard University said, "The secret of the care of the patient is in the caring for the patient."

Focal Point 4 Notes

1. M. S. Kramer, L. Naimark, and D. G. Leduc, Parental fever phobia and its correlates, *Pediatrics* 75 (1985): 1110–1113.

2. H. D. Jampel and coauthors, Fever and immunoregulation III: Hyperthermia augments the primary in vitro humoral immune response, *Journal of Experimental Medicine* 157 (1983): 1229–1238.

3. E. Atkins, Fever: The old and the new, *Journal of Infectious Diseases* 149 (1984): 339–348.

4. D. O. McCarthy, M. J. Kluger, and A. J. Vander, Suppression of food intake during infection: Is interleukin-1 involved?, *American Journal of Clinical Nutrition* 42 (1985): 1179–1182.

5. American Academy of Pediatrics, Nutrition and infection, in *Pediatric Nutrition Handbook*, eds. G. B. Forbes and C. W. Woodruff (Elk Grove Village, Ill.: American Academy of Pediatrics, 1985), pp. 267–273.

6. A. Hecht, Fever: What to do—and what not to do—when the heat is on, *FDA Consumer* November 1985, pp. 16–18.

7. Reye syndrome: New research, regulation, *FDA Consumer* March 1986, pp. 2–30.

8. J. D. Snyder, From Pedialyte to Popsicles: A look at oral rehydration therapy used in the United States and Canada, *American Journal of Clinical Nutrition* 35 (1982): 157–161; Z. Weizman, Cola drinks and rehydration in acute diarrhea (letter), *New*

England Journal of Medicine 315 (1986): 768.

9. L. M. Roberson, A. J. McLaughlin, and J. K. Lund, Promoting oral rehydration therapy for acute diarrhea, *Journal of the American Dietetic Association* 87 (1987): 496–497.

10. *Nutritional Management of Acute Diarrhea in Infants and Children,* Subcommittee on Nutrition and Diarrheal Diseases Control, Committee on International Nutrition Programs, Food and Nutrition Board, Commission on Life Sciences, National Research Council, National Academy Press, Washington, D.C.: 1985.

11. *Nutritional Management of Acute Diarrhea in Infants and Children,* 1985.

12. K. H. Brown and W. C. MacLean, Jr., Nutritional management of acute diarrhea: An appraisal of the alternatives, *Pediatrics* 73 (1984): 119–125.

13. Brown and MacLean, 1984.

14. R. E. Black and coauthors, Longitudinal studies of infectious diseases and physical growth of children in rural Bangladesh: Incidences of diarrhea and association with known pathogens, *American Journal of Epidemiology* 115 (1982): 315–324 as cited in Brown and MacLean, 1984.

15. Brown and MacLean, 1984.

16. *Nutritional Management of Acute Diarrhea in Infants and Children,* 1985.

17. T. I. Bhutta, Oral rehydration for diarrhea (letter), *New England Journal of Medicine* 307 (1982): 952.

18. Roberson, McLaughlin, and Lund, 1987.

19. M. Santosham and coauthors, Oral rehydration therapy of infantile diarrhea: A controlled study of well-nourished children hospitalized in the United States and Panama, *New England Journal of Medicine* 306 (1982): 1070–1076.

20. *Nutritional Management of Acute Diarrhea in Infants and Children,* 1985.

21. D. Chen and B. Sullivan, Constipation (letter), *Pediatrics* 77 (1986): 933.

Children: Eating, Growing, and Learning

5

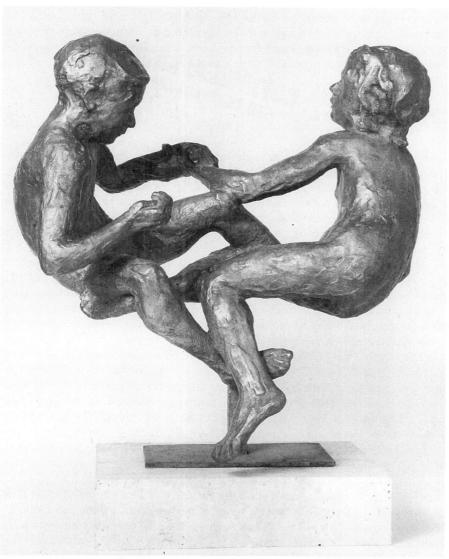

Children by Paul T. Granlund.

The quantities of nutrients a child needs continue to change throughout the growing years. Individual variables such as genetic constitution, rate of growth, gender, and previous nutrition and health status continue to influence the body's requirements. When nutrient supplies fall short of needs, growth, health, and behavior are all affected.

To deliver nutrients in the form of meals and snacks that are nutritious and delicious to children is a challenging task. Children, easily influenced by their peers, the media, and their taste buds establish their likes and dislikes without regard to nutrient quality. Yet, of a food's many qualities, it is the nutrients that have the greatest impact on a child's health. Childhood is the time of continuing to develop food habits that were rooted in infancy—habits that will be carried into the future—for better or for worse. This chapter explores the world of nutrition for preschool and school-age children.

Growth and Development

Rule of thumb: To approximate a child's eventual adult height, double the height at age 2.

Childhood obesity is the subject of Focal Point 5.

After the first year of life, growth begins to slow down. A child grows approximately 5 inches in height between the ages of one and two.[1] Thereafter, the rate slows to about 2 inches per year. Like growth in height, growth in weight settles into a steady annual increase. A child adds approximately 5 to 6 pounds per year until the onset of adolescence. Of course, weight gains may exceed the requirements of growth and reflect overeating. Obesity is a major nutrition problem that follows many children into adulthood.

Increases in height and weight are only two of the many dramatic changes growing children experience. At age one, children can stand alone and are beginning to toddle; by two, they can walk and are learning to run; by three, they can jump and are climbing with confidence.[2] The accumulation of a larger mass and greater density of bone and muscle tissue makes these new accomplishments possible.

The development of fetal bones into those of an adult involves a series of well-coordinated dynamic processes. Bone tissue is continually being remodeled, with new tissue forming on the outer bone surfaces and other tissue being resorbed from the inner surfaces. This turnover of skeletal tissue varies with age. During the growing years, formation exceeds resorption. The relationship between bone formation and resorption can be determined by examining the calcium balance. When bone formation dominates, calcium is retained, thus creating a positive balance.

The growth of skeletal muscles involves increases in muscle fiber size and number. Muscle mass is determined by measuring the amount of creatinine excreted in the urine, since muscle tissue is the site of creatinine production.[3] The lengthening of bones and development of muscles are reflected outwardly in the child's growth. Other tissues such as connective tissues, teeth, body fat, skin, and nervous system are also growing. Growth continues unevenly and rather slowly until adolescence.

As children enter the second year of life, growth slows compared with infancy, but development progresses rapidly. The brain and central nervous system mature at a tremendous pace, as evidenced by increasing muscle control, coordination, and the ability to perform new skills. By the age of two,

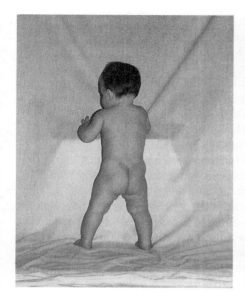 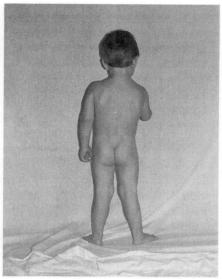

One-year-old and two-year-old shown for comparison of body shape. The two-year-old has lost much of the baby fat; the muscles (especially in the back, buttocks, and legs) have firmed and strengthened, and the leg bones have lengthened.

most of the primary teeth have erupted and control of the jaw muscles is voluntary.[4] During the second year of life, children can handle significantly more types of foods than they could at age one.

At the same time, after a year of age, children who as infants were more than willing to taste anything and everything, whether it was food or not, are learning ever so quickly to be assertive and selective about what they will ingest and how they will do it. This behavior reflects children's psychological development.

Children's Nutrient Needs

Growth during childhood necessitates gradually increasing intakes of all nutrients. The RDA table and the RNI for Canadians list nutrient averages for each span of three years. Recommended nutrient allowances for children are, for the most part, extrapolated from studies conducted on infants and adults. These allowances consider body size and growth needs. Beyond their roles of maintaining a healthy body, most of the nutrients actively contribute to growth. Consider, for example, the growth of a bone. Vitamin A is required for the resorption process; vitamin C helps form the collagen matrix on which the bone is formed; and vitamin D, calcium, phosphorus, magnesium, and fluoride are required to mineralize the bone. For many nutrients, the roles they perform during growth involve a variety of body systems. For example, in addition to its contributions to bone growth, vitamin A helps manufacture red blood cells.

Energy and Protein Needs

A one-year-old child needs perhaps 1000 kcalories a day; a three-year-old needs only 300 to 500 kcalories more. At age ten, a child needs about 2000 kcalories a day. Total energy needs increase slightly with age, but when the child's size is considered, the energy needs are actually declining gradually. The wide variation in the physical activity of children creates big differences in their energy needs. Inactive children can become obese even when consuming diets that are below average in kcalories. Like energy needs, total protein needs increase slightly with age, but when the child's body weight is considered, the protein requirement actually declines gradually. The estimation of protein needs considers the requirements for maintaining nitrogen balance, the quality of protein consumed, and the added needs of growth.[5]

Different malnutrition problems characterize different stages of the life cycle. To review for a moment, the last chapter focused on those nutrition disorders that were particularly severe or had particular impact in infancy. Foremost among the severe diseases for infants are protein-energy malnutrition (PEM) and iron deficiency; Vitamin A and D deficiencies are beginning to set in. PEM and iron deficiencies continue to take a toll throughout childhood, and vitamin A and D deficiencies grow more severe. Foremost among the diseases with impact on infants are those that infants are not physiologically prepared to withstand—protein excess (because their kidneys are immature), linoleic acid and vitamin E deficiency (because their fat stores are limited), vitamin K deficiency (because their GI tract bacteria are not yet established), vitamin B_{12} deficiency (if they enter life without adequate stores built up prior to birth). The distinction between malnutrition problems of infancy and childhood is somewhat artificial; they grade into each other just as the periods of life do, but the emphasis here reflects the diseases that remain or first become severe in childhood.

Protein-energy malnutrition, which takes a heavy toll both domestically and worldwide, continues to afflict children after the first year of life, even in the United States. Poverty is its precursor and other nutrient deficiencies accompany it.

Results of the 1985 Continuing Survey of Food Intakes by Individuals (CSFII) conducted by the U.S. Department of Agriculture (USDA) showed that low-income children's mean intakes of energy, calcium, iron, and zinc failed to meet the RDA.[6] When families who received food stamps were considered separately from those who did not, the results of this survey change slightly. The diets of children in families who received food stamps had intakes below the RDA only for zinc and iron. The difference in nutrient intakes between children who received food stamps and those who did not emphasizes the importance of food assistance programs to the nutritional health of low-income families in the United States. This has become all too apparent in the years since 1982 when cutbacks in federal nutrition programs such as the Food Stamp Program and the school lunch program were initiated.[7]

Hunger in the United States, which was practically eliminated during the 1970s, is on the rise. Using the medical community's generally accepted concept of a hungry person as one who is chronically short of the nutrients needed for growth and good health, it is staggering to realize that 12 million children in America are hungry. Specific nutrient deficiencies cause a variety of deficiency diseases affecting every body system. The malnourished child is weak, lethargic, and vulnerable to disease. Malnourished children are susceptible to colds and ear infections, which cause school absences, thus handicapping social, intellectual, and emotional development. As discussed in the upcoming section on lead toxicity on page 216, malnourished children are also vulnerable to poisoning by lead and other environmental toxins.[8]

The nutrition status of average-income children is not so severe as that of low-income children. A Canadian survey typifies the situation: it examined the nutrient intakes of close to 200 preschool children 3 1/2 to 4 years of age.[9] Energy intake of the children was sufficient to support normal growth. Average nutrient intakes were above current Canadian recommendations. With the exception of iron, nutrient intakes were above U.S. recommendations as well. Preschoolers' vitamin C intakes in this survey far exceeded recommendations. Two-thirds of these children were taking vitamin supplements, which partially explains the excess. Even without the supplements, however, the children's vitamin intakes were sufficient according to Canadian recommendations.

All of the children in the survey were eating three meals a day and at least one snack. Dinner was the most important meal, providing the most energy and protein. Milk and milk products provided the main source of energy, protein, fat, and calcium. Breakfast supplied the most iron, with cereals and cereal products representing the primary iron food sources. Snacks were less energy dense than meals, but still made a substantial contribution to daily energy intake. Without them, energy intake would have been insufficient to support normal growth.

Iron Needs

In all surveys, children's iron intakes are below recommended levels. Iron is a problem nutrient for young children, and for this reason, deserves special attention. Iron-deficiency anemia is the most prevalent nutrient deficiency among children in the United States.[10] Almost one out of every ten children between the ages of one and two is iron deficient.[11] The prevalence of iron deficiency is slightly less (approximately 1 out of every 15) in children between the ages of three and ten. The high iron needs of growth combined with typically low iron intakes leave many children with marginal iron status.

The food intakes of children between the ages of one and two provide about half of their RDA for iron; children between the ages of three and five receive about three-fourths of their RDA.[12] Iron intakes for older children satisfactorily meet their RDA.

The apparent improvement after age three is partly explained by the change in RDA, which becomes abruptly lower for the older age group. Iron recommendations for children are expressed on the basis of age at the present time. Some researchers suggest that iron recommendations for children should be based on adequate body weight for age.[13]

Iron
1980 RDA: 10–15 mg/day (1–9 yr).
1987 RDI: 10 mg/day (1–9 yr).

Appendix A describes how to calculate iron absorption from a meal.

Critical to the discussion of dietary iron intake and iron status is the amount of iron available for absorption. The RDA assume that 10 percent of dietary iron is available, yet less than that may be available in children's diets because the percentage of iron they receive from the more absorbable heme iron is small.[14]

The body's iron status reflects its ability to conserve and recycle iron once it has been absorbed. Thus, iron status reflects more than dietary intake alone, but diet is more critical to iron balance in children than it is in adults. In adult males, about 95 percent of the required iron is recycled and only 5 percent need come from the diet. In children, the percentages are 70 and 30, respectively.[15]

Supplements for Children

Many parents provide their children with vitamin and mineral supplements, relying on them as insurance against possible dietary insufficiencies. Supplements are reasonably inexpensive and available without a prescription. Most children's vitamin supplements are of two kinds: the first contains vitamins A, C, and D and the second contains vitamins A, B_6, B_{12}, C, D, E, thiamin, folacin, riboflavin, and niacin. Both kinds are available with or without iron. A few children's supplements include other minerals as well.

Routine supplement use for most children, when growth is slowing down, is unnecessary. Diets of normal, well-fed children generally supply sufficient amounts of vitamins, so that supplements do not improve their nutrient status.[16] In the case of iron, fortification of foods seems effective in remedying possible deficiencies—certainly in children over five, in any case. However, particular groups of children may benefit from supplementation.[17] These groups include:

▸ Children who suffer from malnutrition.

▸ Children with anorexia or poor eating habits.

▸ Children adhering to restricted diets, such as regimens to control obesity or to abstain from foods of animal origin.

The treatment of choice for most cases of iron deficiency is oral ferrous sulfate administered between meals for maximum absorption. Blood measures should indicate improvement within two months, and iron stores should be replete within five months. Unfortunately, disadvantaged children, who most need more food or supplements to provide the essential nutrients they lack, are the ones most likely not to have access to them. For children who do take them, the kind chosen should be any multivitamin-mineral product that provides a complete array of vitamins and minerals at approximately the RDA levels.

Appendix E provides a comparison of children's supplements.

Little effort is required to convince a child to take a vitamin supplement. Fruit-flavored, chewable vitamins shaped like cartoon characters entice young children to accept them eagerly. These cute, flavorful tablets also have the potential to cause poisoning in children. Of most concern are the supplements that contain iron. Iron-containing supplements should be packaged in child-proof containers and labeled with a warning to parents to keep out of reach of children. A mild overdose of iron-containing vitamins causes gastrointestinal distress, nausea, and black diarrhea. More severe overdoses result in bloody diarrhea, shock, liver damage, coma, and, in some cases, death.[18] The ingestion of 30 milligrams of iron per kilogram of body weight is toxic and vomiting should be induced immediately.

Fluoride is discussed in more detail in Focal Point 3.

Supplements with fluoride are available on prescription for children living in areas without water fluoridation. Regular exposure of the teeth to low doses of fluoride is beneficial to caries prevention. Fluoridation of the community water supply is the most effective and cost-beneficial way to reduce caries. However, in the absence of fluoridated water, fluoride supplements are recommended to all children. The recommended fluoride dosage varies from

0.25 to 1.0 milligrams per day depending on the child's age and the fluoride concentration of the water.[19]

Signs of Malnutrition

The effects of malnutrition during childhood are not limited to growth impairment. They are diverse and numerous, and include behavioral as well as physical effects.

If a child looks unhealthy and acts abnormally, consider that the cause *may* be malnourishment. This may sound obvious, but, surprisingly, parents and medical practitioners often overlook the possibility that malnutrition may account for abnormalities of appearance and behavior. Any departure from normal, healthy appearance and behavior is a possible sign of poor nutrition. Figure 5–1 shows the physical signs to watch for in assessing nutrition status.

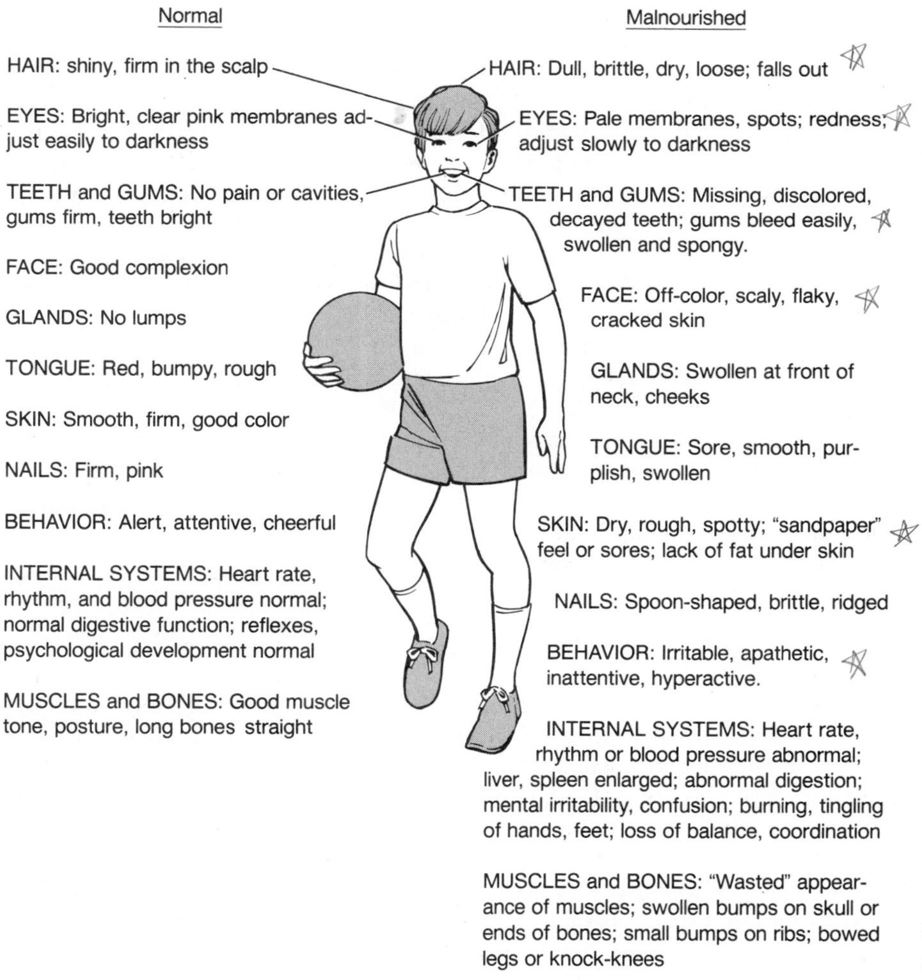

Normal

HAIR: shiny, firm in the scalp

EYES: Bright, clear pink membranes adjust easily to darkness

TEETH and GUMS: No pain or cavities, gums firm, teeth bright

FACE: Good complexion

GLANDS: No lumps

TONGUE: Red, bumpy, rough

SKIN: Smooth, firm, good color

NAILS: Firm, pink

BEHAVIOR: Alert, attentive, cheerful

INTERNAL SYSTEMS: Heart rate, rhythm, and blood pressure normal; normal digestive function; reflexes, psychological development normal

MUSCLES and BONES: Good muscle tone, posture, long bones straight

Malnourished

HAIR: Dull, brittle, dry, loose; falls out

EYES: Pale membranes, spots; redness; adjust slowly to darkness

TEETH and GUMS: Missing, discolored, decayed teeth; gums bleed easily, swollen and spongy.

FACE: Off-color, scaly, flaky, cracked skin

GLANDS: Swollen at front of neck, cheeks

TONGUE: Sore, smooth, purplish, swollen

SKIN: Dry, rough, spotty; "sandpaper" feel or sores; lack of fat under skin

NAILS: Spoon-shaped, brittle, ridged

BEHAVIOR: Irritable, apathetic, inattentive, hyperactive.

INTERNAL SYSTEMS: Heart rate, rhythm or blood pressure abnormal; liver, spleen enlarged; abnormal digestion; mental irritability, confusion; burning, tingling of hands, feet; loss of balance, coordination

MUSCLES and BONES: "Wasted" appearance of muscles; swollen bumps on skull or ends of bones; small bumps on ribs; bowed legs or knock-knees

Figure 5–1   The Well-Nourished versus the Malnourished Child

Physical Signs of Malnutrition

A healthy, well-nourished child has shiny hair that is firm in the scalp. Hair that is dull, brittle, and loose and that falls out is indicative of malnutrition, especially protein deficiency. The eyes of the well-nourished child are bright and clear with no dark circles. The iron-deficient child has pale eye membranes and dark circles. In vitamin A deficiency, the eyes adjust slowly to dark and the skin is dry. The teeth of the well-nourished child are bright and healthy, and the gums are firm. Bleeding gums can be a symptom of vitamin C deficiency, due to its role in production and maintenance of collagen, the base for all connective tissue in the body. Strong, straight bones are indicative of adequate vitamin D nutrition.

A wasted appearance of muscles occurs with energy deprivation, as the body breaks down its own protein for energy. As a result, protein deficiency is an indirect effect of energy lack. In fact, protein deficiency and energy deficiency go hand in hand so often, especially in developing countries, that the pair are called protein-energy malnutrition (PEM). Protein deficiency alone is kwashiorkor, while energy deficiency is marasmus. PEM is the world's most widespread malnutrition problem. The protein-deficient child ceases to grow, becomes apathetic and weak, and loses skin color. Fluid balance is disturbed, causing it to accumulate in the belly and legs. The child becomes an easy target for infection so that intestinal infections are common, further depleting nutrients. Measles, which might make a healthy child sick for a week or so, kills the kwashiorkor child within days. The marasmic child has wasted muscles, slow metabolism, and a weakened heart. Marasmus occurs most often in children between 6 and 18 months of age, especially in city slums. Although such extreme malnutrition is less common in developed countries than in developing ones, nutrient deficiencies can and do occur in children everywhere. People who care for children, in any capacity, should be aware that poor nutrition is reflected in physical appearance as well as behavioral symptoms.

The assessment of children's iron status is discussed in Appendix A.

The effects of iron-deficiency anemia are evident in physical, mental, behavioral, and biochemical signs. These signs are listed in Table 5–1.

Zinc is essential to many biochemical functions, including the metabolism and synthesis of proteins. Zinc deficiency in children is associated with growth retardation, poor appetite, and impaired taste acuity.[20]

Behavioral Signs of Malnutrition

Many different effects of nutrition on behavior have been suggested in recent years. Among them are nutrient deficiencies, allergies to food, reactions to food additives, reactions to sugar, stimulation by caffeine, and more. While reading the information presented here, remember that while poor nutrition does affect behavior, causing a multitude of symptoms, abnormal behavior is equally likely to be the result of a variety of factors.

tension-fatigue syndrome: apparent hyperactivity produced in a child by the combination of lack of sleep and overstimulation with anxiety.

All children at times become excitable, rambunctious, and unruly. The most common cause of such "hyper" behavior is not nutrition but the tension-fatigue syndrome, which arises from a combination of factors: lack of exercise, a craving for attention, lack of sleep, overstimulation, and too much

Table 5–1 Signs of Iron Deficiency

Effects on muscular work:

▸ Reduced work productivity.

▸ Reduced tolerance to work.

▸ Reduced voluntary work.

Reduced physical fitness; weakness, fatigue.
Reduced resistance to cold, inability to regulate body temperature.
Reduced resistance to infection (lowered immunity).
Itching of skin.
Pale nailbeds, eye membranes, palm creases; concave nails.
Pica (clay eating, ice eating).
Lactose intolerance, and possibly intolerance to other sugars.
Impaired wound healing.
Increased risk of lead and cadmium poisoning.
Impaired cognitive function (children):

▸ Reduced learning ability.

▸ Imparied visual discrimination.

▸ Increased distractibility (inability to pay attention).

Impaired reactivity and coordination (infants).

Source: Adapted from L. Hallberg, Iron absorption and iron deficiency, *Human Nutrition: Clinical Nutrition* 36C (1982): 259–278; N. S. Scrimshaw, Functional consequences of iron deficiency in human populations, *Journal of Nutrition Science and Vitaminology* 30 (1984): 47–63.

television. This syndrome can be relieved by giving more consistent care to the child's welfare. It helps especially to insist on regular hours of sleep, regular mealtimes, and regular outdoor exercise.

A nutrition-related condition that does *not* cause behavioral abnormalities—except for the general misery associated with any sickness—is food allergy. Another condition is not even nutrition related, although often thought to be so: the learning disability known as attention-deficit disorder with hyperactivity. Both of these disorders have been wrongly blamed on diet, and both are treated in this chapter. Food allergies are real, need diagnosis, and demand dietary treatment; they have a later section of their own. Learning disabilities are also real and need diagnosis; they do not require dietary treatment (although the general health of any child may be improved by attention to diet); and the idea that they do is debunked in an upcoming subpart of this section.

A dietary factor that does not cause behavioral abnormalities in children is sugar—except as it contributes to nutrient deficiencies by displacing nutrients in the diet. The following section describes the effects of nutrient-poor diets on children's behavior, and especially the effect of iron-deficient diets, which are known to affect many children.

Signs of iron deficiency Iron deficiency presents the best-known and most widespread effects on behavior. Most people are familiar with the role of iron in carrying oxygen in the blood, but iron also moves oxygen around within cells, which use it to help produce energy. A lack of iron not only causes an energy crisis, but also directly affects behavior, mood, attention span, and learning ability. Iron is involved in the functioning of many molecules in the brain and nervous system. Deficiencies of iron produced experimentally in animals have caused abnormal synthesis and degradation of neurotransmitters, most notably those that regulate the ability to pay attention, which is crucial to learning.[21]

Iron deficiency is usually diagnosed by use of iron indicators in the *blood* when it has progressed all the way to overt anemia. A child's *brain*, however, is sensitive to slightly lowered iron levels long before the blood effects appear. Iron's effects are hard to distinguish from the effects of other factors in children's lives, but it is likely that iron deficiency manifests itself in a lowering of the "motivation to persist in intellectually challenging tasks," a shortening of the attention span, and a reduction of overall intellectual performance. Anemic children perform less well on tests and have more conduct disturbances than their classmates.[22]

Iron is only one of several dozen nutrients that can be displaced in a diet high in empty-kcalorie foods. Any of the others may be lacking as well, and the deficiencies of those nutrients may also cause behavioral as well as physical symptoms, as Table 5–2 shows.

A child with the behavioral symptoms of nutrient deficiencies might be irritable, aggressive, disagreeable, or sad and withdrawn. One might label such a child "hyperactive," "depressed," or "unlikeable" when, in fact, the cause for these behaviors may be marginal malnutrition. In any such case, inspection of the child's diet by someone knowledgeable about children's nutrient needs is clearly in order. Should suspicion of dietary inadequacies be raised, *no matter what other causes may be implicated*, the people responsible for feeding the child should take steps to correct those inadequacies promptly.

Signs of lead toxicity   Another nutrition factor influencing children's behavior is lead toxicity, which is widespread—1 out of every 20 children suffers the consequences of high blood-lead levels.[23] The signs of mild lead poisoning are nonspecific, including such symptoms as diarrhea, irritability, and lethargy. With higher levels of lead, the symptoms become more pronounced yet still difficult to pinpoint to a cause. Children lose their general cognitive, verbal, and perceptual abilities, developing learning disabilities and behavior problems.

Infant formula and evaporated milk are still available in cans. Industry programs to reduce the lead content of these products have been in effect since 1974, and lead contents of these products have declined. Despite the decline, canned milk continues to be a major source of lead intake for infants and children. Other common sources include dirt contaminated by leaded gasoline and peeling lead paint, either deliberately or inadvertently ingested during play.

Lead absorption is greatest during times of rapid growth.[24] Therefore, infants and young children are more susceptible to lead poisoning and absorb five to ten times as much lead as adults do. Indeed, lead toxicity is highest in children less than six years old. Adverse effects appear primarily in the nervous system, kidney, and bone marrow.[25]

High blood-lead concentrations are associated with iron, calcium, or zinc deficiencies—nutrient deficiencies that are common in young children. Iron deficiency cannot be held totally accountable for the high blood-lead concen-

Table 5–2 Behavioral Symptoms of Nutrient Deficiencies

▸ Protein-energy deficiency—apathy, fretfulness, lack of energy, lack of interest in food.

▸ Thiamin deficiency—confusion, uncoordinated movements, depressed appetite, irritability, insomnia, fatigue, general misery.[a]

▸ Riboflavin deficiency—depression, hysteria, psychopathic behavior, lethargy, and hypochondria are evident before deficiency can be detected by clinical symptoms.[b]

▸ Niacin deficiency—irritability; agitated depression; headaches, sleeplessness, memory loss, emotional instability (early signs of pellagra onset), and mental confusion progressing to psychosis or delirium.

▸ Vitamin B_6 deficiency—irritability, insomnia, weakness, mental depression, abnormal brainwave pattern; convulsions, the mental symptoms of anemia, fatigue, headache.[a]

▸ Folacin deficiency—the mental symptoms of anemia, tiredness, apathy, weakness, forgetfulness, mild depression, abnormal nerve function, irritability, headache, disorientation, confusion, inability to perform simple calculations.[c]

▸ Vitamin B_{12} deficiency—degeneration of peripheral nervous system, anemia.

▸ Vitamin C deficiency—hysteria, depression, listlessness, lassitude, weakness, aversion to work, hypochondria, social introversion, possible iron anemia, fatigue.

▸ Vitamin A deficiency—anemia.

▸ Iron deficiency—fatigue, weakness, headaches, pallor, listlessness, irritability—and the mental symptoms of anemia.

▸ Magnesium deficiency—apathy, personality changes, hyperirritability.

▸ Copper deficiency—iron-deficiency anemia.

▸ Zinc deficiency—poor appetite, failure to grow, iron-deficiency anemia, irritability, emotional disorders, mental lethargy.[d]

[a]Symptoms of thiamin and vitamin B_6 deficiency are from marginal vitamin deficiency, *Nutrition and the MD*, July 1983, p. 3.
[b]Symptoms of riboflavin deficiency are from R. Sterner and W. Price: Restricted riboflavin: With subject behavioral effects in humans, *American Journal of Clinical Nutrition* 26 (1973): 150–160.
[c]Symptoms of folacin deficiency are from J. H. Pincus and coauthors, Subacute combined system degeneration with folate deficiency, *Journal of the American Medical Association* 221 (1972): 496–497. (Possibly, because folacin is required for many steps in amino acid metabolism, its lack causes altered amino acid levels in the blood, and therefore altered neurotransmitter levels in the brain. Neurological disease in folic acid deficiency, *Nutrition Reviews* 39 (1981): 337–338.)
[d]Symptoms of zinc deficiency are from A. S. Prasad, Clinical, biochemical and nutritional spectrum of zinc deficiency in human subjects: An update, *Nutrition Reviews* 7 (1983): 197–206.

Source: Unless otherwise cited, all of the listed symptoms can be found in R. S. Goodhart and M. E. Shils, *Modern Nutrition in Health and Disease*, 6th ed., ed. (Philadelphia: Lea and Febiger, 1980).

trations, but it does impair the body's defenses against absorption of lead. A child with iron-deficiency anemia is three times as likely as a child with adequate iron stores to have elevated blood lead concentrations.[26] Not only does iron deficiency contribute to lead toxicity, lead toxicity contributes to iron deficiency. One of lead's actions is to interfere with iron's incorporation into heme, resulting in symptoms of anemia. Thus, the combination of iron deficiency and lead toxicity is greater than the effect of either alone.

Similarly, a low-calcium diet is associated with a high lead burden. A significant, inverse relationship between dietary calcium and blood lead levels has been observed.[27] It is possible that inadequacy of calcium intake renders the body susceptible to lead absorption and retention.

Zinc status also appears to influence lead toxicity.[28] Serum zinc concentrations are frequently low in children with elevated lead levels.[29]

General hunger effects   Not only content, but also timing, of meals makes a difference in children's behavior. Children who eat no breakfast perform poorly in tasks of concentration, their attention spans are shorter, and they even show lower IQs on testing than their well-fed peers.[30] Common sense dictates that it is unreasonable to expect anyone to learn and perform work when no fuel has been provided. By the late morning, discomfort from hunger may become distracting even if a child has eaten breakfast.

The problem that arises for children who attempt morning schoolwork on an empty stomach appears to be at least partly due to hypoglycemia. The average child up to the age of ten or so needs to eat every four to six hours to maintain a blood glucose concentration high enough to support the activity of the brain and nervous system.[31] A child's brain is as big as an adult's— and the brain is the body's chief glucose consumer. A child's liver is considerably smaller—and the liver is the organ responsible for storing glucose (as glycogen) and releasing it into the blood as needed. A child's liver cannot store more than about four hours' worth of glycogen; hence the need to eat fairly often. Teachers aware of the late-morning slump in their classrooms wisely request that a midmorning snack be provided; it improves classroom performance all the way to lunchtime.[32]

hyperactivity syndrome in children: a cluster of symptoms in which "the essential features are signs of developmentally inappropriate inattention, impulsivity, and hyperactivity." Other important features are: onset before age 7, duration of 6 months or more, and proven absence of mental illness or mental retardation. Other names associated with hyperactivity: attention deficit disorder, hyperkinesis, minimal brain damage, minimal brain dysfunction, minor cerebral dysfunction.

syndrome: a cluster of symptoms.

learning disability: a disorder in one or more psychological processes involved in understanding or using language, which manifests itself in an imperfect ability to listen, think, speak, read, write, spell, or do mathematical calculations.

Hyperactivity: a nondietary disorder   True hyperactivity, or attention deficit disorder with hyperactivity (ADDH), is not caused by diet. It is a type of learning disability that occurs in 5 to 10 percent of young school-age children—that is, 1 or 2 in every classroom of 20 children. It can lead to academic failure and major behavior problems.[33] Parents and teachers need to deal effectively with it wherever it appears in order to avert the grief that can otherwise result.

The idea that hyperactivity might be caused by diet became popular in 1973, when Dr. Benjamin Feingold proposed that hyperactive children suffer adverse reactions to natural salicylates (compounds with a chemical structure similar to aspirin) and the artificial flavors and colors in foods. The Feingold diet eliminates foods with high levels of natural salicylates (apples, berries, tomatoes, and peaches, for example) and foods with artificial flavors and colors. However, when controlled, double-blind experiments with additive-containing and additive-free foods are conducted, the benefits of the Feingold diet do not materialize as they do in some individual family situations. In family situations, diet is not the only thing that changes. Children receive special attention, along with the special diet, and this may well have beneficial effects on their behavior. Both the children and their parents and teachers are likely to be influenced by the hope that the experiment will work—and by suggestibility, a factor that is difficult to rule out.[34]

The dietary approach to hyperactivity seems to work mostly by suggestion, if it works at all.[35] A child who has been deemed hyperactive "learns" that the food causes the hyperactive behavior. From now on the child and family are going to eat differently—no more junk foods, no more processed convenience foods, no more casual snacks. Foods will be prepared from scratch at home and eaten together. The whole family's lifestyle will change, and the child's behavior is expected to improve. It does improve—but in response to what? Not only is the family eating differently, they are living differently, and the child is receiving more attention, more parental energy, and more structure than before. It appears not to be the additive-free nature of the diet that works, but the changed lifestyle that the diet demands.[36]

One method physicians use to diagnose hyperactivity is to conduct a trial with stimulant drugs. If the child responds by calming down, then drugs are used to help control the behavior problems. *In children who are responsive,* prescription medication is considered an integral part of treatment. Such treatment is accepted by the medical profession as a safe and effective means to treat hyperactivity in children. The most common side effects, insomnia and anorexia, usually disappear within a week or two.[37]

Caffeine   Caffeine is often overlooked as a source of "hyper" behavior in children, but it is a matter of some concern to pediatricians. A 12-ounce cola beverage may contain as much as 50 milligrams of caffeine; two or more such beverages are equivalent in the body of a 60-pound child to the caffeine in eight cups of coffee for a 175-pound man. Chocolate bars also contribute caffeine. Children who are troubled by sleeplessness, restlessness, and irregular heartbeats may need to control their caffeine consumption. A survey of over 1000 children found that 77 percent of those between one and seventeen years of age were caffeine consumers. [38]

One study examined behavioral differences between children previously determined to be either "high" caffeine consumers (more than 500 milligrams of caffeine per day) or "low" consumers.[39] Both groups of children were given 5 milligrams of caffeine twice a day or a placebo for two weeks. While receiving the caffeine, low consumers were perceived by their parents as more emotional, inattentive, and restless, while high consumers were rated as unchanged when receiving the caffeine. When the high consumers were not receiving the caffeine, they had higher scores on an anxiety questionnaire than the low consumers. As long as undeniably attractive temptations such as cola beverages and candy bars surround children, barriers against their abuse have to be provided by concerned adults until the children learn to control consumption themselves.

Feeding Children

Feeding children requires not only providing a variety of nutritious foods, but also nurturing their self-esteem and well-being. Parents face a number of challenges in preparing meals that appeal to their children's tastes as well as providing needed nutrients. The interactions between parents and children regarding food intake set the stage for lifelong attitudes and habits.

Eating Patterns

To provide all the needed nutrients, a variety of foods from each of the food groups is recommended. Table 5–3 offers a daily food pattern for children. The serving sizes increase with the child's age. To estimate portions for meat, fruits, and vegetables, a serving is loosely defined as 1 tablespoon per year. Thus, at four years of age, a serving of any of these foods would be 4 tablespoons (1/4 cup). Because the serving sizes adjust as the child grows older, this rule of thumb is appropriate from age two to the teen years.

Careful food selection is essential to ensure adequate nutrition. Some food intakes that seem fairly nutritious are not, as the comparison demonstrates. Consider the following two (A and B) sample days' menus for two fairly typical 5-year-old children. Both children's parents were conscientious in supplying three meals and snacks delivering nutrients from all four food groups.

Sample Menu A
▶ *Breakfast*: 1/2 cup of cereal with 1/2 cup of 2 percent milk; 1/2 banana; 3/4 cup orange juice.
▶ *Snack*: 2-ounce raisin/pumpkin seed mixture.
▶ *Lunch*: Peanut butter and jelly sandwich with 1 tablespoon of peanut butter and 1 tablespoon jelly on 2 slices of whole-wheat bread; 1 cup of 2 percent milk; 3 small carrot sticks; 1 small apple.
▶ *Snack*: 6-ounce fruit yogurt.
▶ *Supper*: Two fish sticks with 1 tablespoon catsup; 1/4 cup macaroni and cheese; 3/4 cup apple juice; 1/4 cup broccoli with 1 tablespoon butter.
▶ *Snack*: 2 peanut butter cookies.

Sample Menu B
▶ *Breakfast*: One glazed doughnut and 1 cup of 2 percent milk.
▶ *Lunch*: Peanut butter and jelly sandwich with 1 tablespoon of peanut butter and 1 tablespoon of jelly on 2 slices of white bread; 1 cup of lemonade; 1 small apple; 10 potato chips.
▶ *Snack*: One 6-ounce fruit yogurt.
▶ *Dinner*: Two fish sticks with 1 tablespoon catsup; 10 large french fries with 1 tablespoon catsup; 1/2 cup of applesauce; 6 ounces of grape soda.
▶ *Snack*: 1 ounce jelly beans

Figure 5–2 shows that sample menu A provided adequate amounts of all the recommended nutrients, while sample menu B fell short of supplying some important nutrients.

A comparison between the recommended food pattern in Table 5–3 and the two sample menus shows some foods missing in menu B, which account for the lacks identified in Figure 5–2. The child's intake of foods in the milk and cheese group fell short of the recommended three servings. The cereal food

Table 5–3 Children's Daily Food Pattern for Good Nutrition

Food Group	Servings per Day	Average Size of Serving		
		1 to 3 Years	*4 to 5 Years*	*6 to 12 Years*
Milk and cheese (1 oz cheese = 1 c milk)	4	½–¾ c	¾ c	¾–1 c
Protein foods	3 or more			
Eggs		1	1	1
Lean meat, fish, poultry, legumes (liver once a week)		2 tbsp	4 tbsp	2–4 oz
Peanut butter		0–1 tbsp	2 tbsp	2–3 tbsp
Fruits and vegetables	4; more recommended			
Vitamin C source (citrus fruits, berries, tomatoes, cabbage, cantaloupe)	1 or more	⅓–½ c	½ c	1 medium orange
Vitamin A source (green or orange fruits/vegetables)	1 or more	2–3 tbsp	4 tbsp	¼–⅓ c
Other vegetables (including potatoes)	2	2–3 tbsp	4 tbsp (¼ c)	⅓–½ c
Other fruits		¼–⅓ c	½ c	1 medium
Cereals (whole grain or enriched)	4; more recommended			
Bread, buns, pizza		½–1 slice	1½ slices	1 to 2 slices
Ready-to-eat cereals		½–¾ oz	1 oz	1 oz
Cooked grains (cereals, macaroni, grits, rice)		¼–⅓ c	½ c	½–¾ c
Fats and sugars	*Optional* These foods can be used to meet energy needs when the required servings of nutritious foods do not. Serving sizes listed here are maximum.			
Butter, margarine, mayonnaise, oils	1	1 tbsp	1 tbsp	2 tbsp
Desserts and sweets (100-kcalorie portions)[a]	1	1–1½ portions	1½ portions	3 portions

[a]⅓ c pudding or ice cream; 2 to 3 cookies; 1 oz cake; 1⅓ oz pie; or 2 tbsp jelly, jam, honey, sugar.

Source: Adapted from B. B. Alford and M. L. Bogle, *Nutrition during the Life Cycle* (Englewood Cliffs, N.J.: Prentice-Hall, 1982), pp. 60–61. Originally from Behrman and Nelson *Textbook of Pediatrics,* 13th ed., 1987; Table 3–7.

Figure 5–2 Sample Menus A and B Compared

These graphs show that sample menu A provides adequate amounts of the recommended nutrients, while sample menu B falls short of supplying several nutrients.

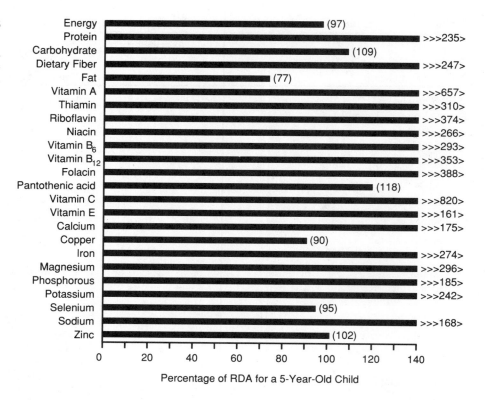

Percentage of RDA for a 5-Year-Old Child

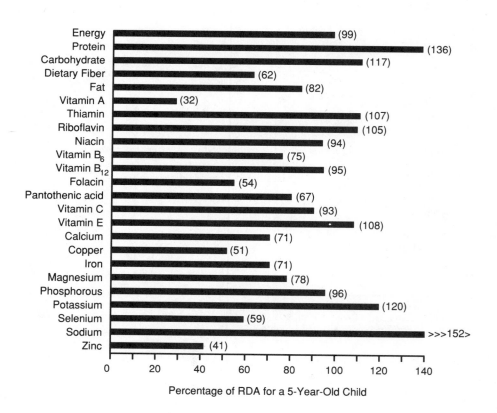

Percentage of RDA for a 5-Year-Old Child

group was inadequately represented as well; as a consequence, iron and zinc were lacking for the day. An additional small serving of whole-grain cereal or bread, and an additional serving of legumes or meat would have boosted the intakes of these nutrients considerably. Fruits and vegetables were minimal on this day, consisting of an apple, applesauce, and french fries. Had this child eaten at least two more servings of fruits and vegetables as recommended in Table 5–3, the folacin and vitamin A intakes provided by this day's meals would have improved. The foods in menu A provided more nutrients for a similar energy intake and offered a greater variety of foods; in the long run, they did a lot more than the foods in menu B in promoting healthful eating habits. A little extra effort and planning can make a big difference in a child's day-to-day nutrient intake.

The child represented by menu B did have three meals and a snack on this day. Imagine how much worse the picture is when a child skips breakfast, or when more sugary foods take the place of some of the nourishing ones. Chances are, the nutrients missed from a skipped breakfast will not be "made up" at lunch and dinner, but will be completely left out that day.

Experimentation with children's food patterns shows that candy, cola, and other concentrated sweets must be limited in a child's diet if the needed nutrients are to be supplied. (Table 5–3 notes that these optional high-kcalorie foods may be included only in addition to the required servings of nutritious foods, and then only in small portions.) A nonobese, active child can enjoy the higher-kcalorie nutritious foods in each category: ice cream or pudding in the milk group, cake and cookies (whole-grain or enriched only, however) in the bread group. These foods, made from milk and grain, carry valuable nutrients and encourage a child to learn, appropriately, that eating is fun. However, children cannot be trusted to choose nutritious foods on the basis of taste alone; the preference for sweets is innate. If such foods are permitted in large quantities, there are only two possible outcomes: nutrient deficiencies and/or obesity.

To meet the RDA for iron, food choices must be carefully made. Iron-rich foods, such as those listed in Table 5–4, should be included in snacks and

Table 5–4   Selected Iron-Rich Foods

Meats	Nonmeats[a]
Liver sausage	Baked beans, limas, peas
Small pieces of lean meat	Raisin bran cereal
Eggs	Cream of wheat cereal (can be served hot or sweetened with fruit parfait-style with a favorite pudding)
Any meat cooked in ironware	
	Prunes or prune juice
	Raisins
	Strawberries
	Watermelon
	Apple juice (check the label)
	Any nonmeat cooked in ironware

[a]All items in this list should be served along with a vitamin C source (like citrus). Vitamin C triples the absorption of iron present in the same meal.

meals. Foods or beverages that inhibit iron absorption should be restricted, and those that enhance absorption should be encouraged. Tea, for example, is a potent inhibitor of iron absorption.[40] Foods and beverages rich in vitamin C enhance iron absorption from a meal by two- to fivefold. Meat, fish, and poultry also enhance the absorption of nonheme iron. Dairy products are important sources of energy, protein, calcium, and riboflavin in children's diets, but excessive consumption can displace other foods that make equally important nutrient contributions. Milk and milk products are poor iron sources.

Children above the age of one or so are no longer passive recipients of food from spoons held by parents, but are active in feeding themselves (see Practical Point: Developing Healthy Eating Behaviors for ways to support the learning of desired behaviors).

▸▸ PRACTICAL POINT

Developing Healthy Eating Behaviors

Children's appetites often diminish around the age of one year, in line with the reduction in their growth rates. Overenthusiastic parents, unaware that their one-year-old is slowing down, may force food on a child who does not want (or even need) to eat. Thereafter, appetite fluctuates; at times children seem to be insatiable, and at other times they seem to live on air and water. Parents need not worry about varying appetites; children need and demand more food during periods of rapid growth than during slow periods. In children of normal weight, appetite regulates the energy intake so that it is appropriate for each stage of growth. Unfortunately, many people mistakenly believe it is necessary to control children's portion sizes in order to regulate energy intake. An innovative study showed otherwise.[a] Researchers wanted to determine how much lunch children would eat if given snacks of different energy value before lunch. The children ate puddings that contained either 40 kcalories or 150 kcalories, but were otherwise identical. The children were then given lunch. They compensated for the kcaloric difference: those who had eaten the high-kcalorie pudding ate less lunch than those who had eaten the low-kcalorie pudding. (Overweight children, however, may eat in response to external cues, disregarding appetite regulation signals.)

Not surprisingly, feeding problems often arise during the second or third year of life, when children are asserting their independence. Many of these problems arise from the conflict between children's inclinations and their parents' wishes. Children's developmental stages and capabilities promote their making their own choices, while parents attempting to do what they think is best for their children try to control every aspect of eating. Such conflicts can harm children, disrupting their abilities to regulate their own food intakes and to determine their own likes and dislikes. The end result is usually far from the desired one. For example, many people share the misconception that children must be persuaded or coerced to try new foods. Research with children indicates the opposite. When children are pushed to try new foods, even by way of rewards, they are less likely to try those foods again than children who are left to decide for themselves.[b]

One authority on children's eating behaviors makes a point relevant to the research just discussed.[c] The parent is responsible for what the child is offered to eat, the child is responsible for *how much* and even *whether* to eat.

Parents should help children become independent and learn self-control by allowing them to do things for themselves. At the same time, children must be protected from repeated failures and destructiveness. In other words, parental control is necessary, but continual punishment of toddlers as they strive for independence will promote feelings of self-doubt in their abilities to make decisions and humiliation in their incompetence. Threatening or forcing young children to behave in a certain way requires no forethought or skill. It takes patience and understanding, however, to guide them toward developing self-control and pride in themselves for accomplishing it.

Toddlers must be allowed to explore and satisfy their curiosity about the world around them. This is as true with respect to food as it is with other aspects of their lives. Parents who expect their toddlers to eat and behave at the table as adults do, or even as older children do, are setting themselves up for difficult times and disappointment. Young children learn about food with all their senses; this includes feeling it as well as tasting and smelling it. Table manners can be taught with time. Young children make messes while eating. They are learning new skills and should be allowed to feed themselves and drink from a cup when the interest arises, even if much of the food or beverage ends up on the floor. The parents should gently guide them in learning these skills and protect them while doing so by ensuring that they consume adequate amounts of nutritious food.

It is desirable for children to learn to like nutritious foods in all the food groups. With one exception, this liking usually develops naturally. The exception is vegetables, which young children frequently dislike and refuse.[d] Even a tiny serving of spinach, cooked carrots, or squash may elicit an expression that registers the utmost in negative feelings (as well as great pride in the ability to make an ugly face). Since most youngsters need to eat more vegetables, the next few paragraphs are addressed to this problem.[e]

Try to remember how you felt when first offered a cup of vegetable soup, a serving of runny spinach, or a pile of peas and carrots. If the soup burned your tongue, it may have been years before you were willing to try it again. As for the spinach, it was suspiciously murky looking. (Who could tell what might be lurking in that dark, stringy stuff?) The peas and carrots troubled your sense of order. Before you could eat them, you felt compelled to sort the peas onto one side of the plate and the carrots onto the other. Then you had to separate, into a reject pile, all those that got mashed in the process or contaminated with gravy from the mashed potatoes. Only then might you be willing to eat the intact, clean peas and carrots one by one—perhaps with your fingers, since the peas, especially, kept rolling off the fork.

Why children respond in this way to foods that look uninviting or messy to them is a matter for conjecture. Parents need only be aware that this is how many children feel and then honor those feelings. Researchers attempting to explain children's food preferences are met with contradictions. Children describe liking colorful foods, yet vegetables are often rejected and brown peanut butter and white potatoes, apple wedges, and breads are among their favorites. Raw vegetables are better accepted than cooked ones, so it is wise to offer vegetables that are raw or slightly undercooked and crunchy, bright in color, served separately, and easy to eat.[f] They should be warm, not hot, because a child's mouth is much more sensitive than an adult's. The flavor should be mild. A child has more taste buds and they are more sensitive than those of an adult. Strong flavors offend them. Smooth foods such as mashed potatoes or pea soup should have no lumps in them (a child wonders, with some disgust, what the lumps might be). Irrational as the fear of strangeness may seem, the parent must realize that it is practically universal among children. Children prefer foods that are familiar to them.[g] One study showed that the more times two-year-old children are exposed to a new food, even if they do not taste the food each time, the higher the preference for the food becomes.[h]

When feeding children, parents must always be alert to the dangers of choking. A choking child is a silent child. An adult knowledgeable about what to do if choking does occur should be present whenever a child is eating. Encouraging the child to sit when eating is also a good practice. The possibility of choking is more likely when a child is running or falling. Round foods such as grapes, nuts, hard candies, and hot-dog pieces are the foods most likely to choke a child. They are difficult to control in a mouth with few teeth and can easily become lodged in the small opening of a child's trachea. Other potentially dangerous foods include tough meat, hard pieces of fruit or vegetables, popcorn, chips, and peanut butter. Parents of toddlers need to remember that topical anesthetics used to numb gums when the child is teething interfere with the ability to chew and swallow.

Wise parents allow children to help make the family's choices, including sometimes giving them the right to say their favorite word (No!)—at the same time, of course, sensibly preventing them from dominating the family. Allowing children to help plan and prepare the family's meals provides enjoyable learning experiences that encourage children to eat the foods they have prepared. Vegetables are pretty, especially when fresh, and provide opportunities to learn about color, about growing things and their seeds, about shapes and textures—all of which are fascinating to young children. Measuring, stirring, decorating, cutting, and arranging vegetables are skills even a young child can practice with enjoyment and pride.

Before sitting down to eat, small children should be helped to wash their hands and faces thoroughly. Ideally, outdoor playtime will have preceded the meal. If fun and games *follow* the meal, children are likely to hurry out to play, leaving food on their plates that they were hungry for and otherwise would have eaten.

Little children like to eat at little tables and to be served little portions of food. Teaching children how to serve themselves the quantity they will eat minimizes waste. Parents need to remember that food is wasted not only when it is dumped in the garbage, but also when it is stored as excess fat on the child's body. Never force children to clean their plates. This practice can lead to behaviors that encourage obesity. Instead, allow children to stop eating when they are full; encourage them to listen to their bodies. The remaining food can be recycled as leftovers for another meal or as food for the family pet. One word of caution is in order: children who are too full to eat their dinner must also be too full to eat dessert.

Children like to eat with other children and have been observed to stay at the table longer and eat much more when in the company of their peers.

Children are also more likely to eat nonpreferred foods when their peers are eating those foods.[i] Eating is fun. It is healthy to look forward to and enjoy meals.

When introducing new foods at the table, parents are advised to offer them one at a time—and only a small amount at first. The more often a food is presented to a young child, the more likely the child will like that food. Whenever possible, the new food should be presented at the beginning of the meal, when the child is hungry. Offer the new food and allow the child to make the decision. Whether the child accepts or rejects the new food is irrelevant. Never make an issue of food acceptance, not even to reward acceptance. Parents often mistakenly use rewards or bribes to train their children to eat specific foods. "When you finish eating your spinach, you will be allowed to watch television." Children learn that they must work to earn the reward. In this case, the "work" is spinach, and if it is work, it must not be desirable. The end result is a decreasing preference for the food, in this case, spinach.[j] Sometimes parents use foods as rewards to train their children to perform specific tasks. "When you finish putting your toys away, you will be allowed to eat ice cream." In this case, the child learns to give ice cream an enhanced preference.[k]

Parents may find that their children often snack so much that they are not very hungry at mealtimes. Some parents find they can live with the philosophy not of teaching children *not* to snack, but of teaching them *how* to snack. Provide snacks that are as nutritious as the foods served at mealtime. Milk and water are appropriate beverages at snack time. Sweet drinks contribute to problems of dental caries and obesity. Snacks can even be mealtime foods that are served individually over time, instead of all at once on one plate. When providing snacks to children, a smart parent thinks of the four food groups and offers pieces of cheese, tangerine slices, carrot sticks, and peanut butter on whole-wheat crackers. Snacks need to be easy to prepare and readily available to children. This is particularly important to children who return home after school without parental supervision.

A bright, unhurried atmosphere free of conflict is conducive to good appetite. Parents who serve meals in a relaxed and casual manner, without anxiety, provide the climate in which a child's negative emotions will be minimized. Conflicts can be promoted by unaware parents, even if they have the best of intentions. Parents who beg, cajole, and demand that their child eat deny the child an opportunity to develop self-control. Instead, the child enters a battle that takes on more importance than hunger. The power struggle almost invariably results in a confirmed pattern of resistance and a permanently closed mind on the child's part. Mealtimes can be nightmarish for the child who is struggling with personal and parental problems. If, as a child sits down to the table, a barrage of accusations are shouted—"Your hands are filthy . . . your report card . . . and clean your plate! Your mother cooked that food!"— mealtimes may be unbearable. The stomach may recoil because the body, as well as the mind, reacts to stress of this kind.[l]

In an effort to practice these many tips, parents may overlook perhaps the single most important influence on their child's food habits—their own example. Parents who do not eat carrots should not be surprised when their children refuse to eat carrots. Likewise, parents who comment on the odor of brussels sprouts do not convince children that these vegetables are delicious.

Much of the learning a child accomplishes is through imitation. By setting an example, parents can show children how to enjoy nutritious foods.

At each age, food can be served and enjoyed in the context of encouraging emotional as well as physical growth. If the beginnings are right, children will grow without the confusion over food that can lead to nutrition problems. In the interest of promoting both a positive self-concept and a positive attitude toward good food, it is important for parents to help their children remember that they are good kids. What they *do* may sometimes be unacceptable; but what they *are*, on the inside, are normal, healthy, growing, fine human beings.

[a]L. L. Birch and M. Deysher, Caloric compensation and sensory specific satiety: Evidence for self-regulation of food intake by young children, *Appetite* 7 (1986): 323–331.
[b]L. L. Birch, D. W. Marlin, and J. Rotter, Eating as the "means" activity in a contingency: Effects on young children's food preference, *Child Development* 55 (1984): 431–439.
[c]E. M. Satter, *Child of Mine: Feeding with Love and Good Sense* (Palo Alto, Calif.: Bull Publishing, 1983).
[d]N. R. Beyer and P. M. Morris, Food attitudes and snacking patterns of young children, *Journal of Nutrition Education* 6 (1974): 100–103.
[e]Adapted with permission from E. N. Whitney and E. M. N. Hamilton, *Understanding Nutrition*, 4th ed. (St. Paul, Minn.: West, 1987).
[f]M. E. Breckenridge, Food attitudes of five- to twelve-year- old children, *Journal of the American Dietetic Association* 35 (1959): 704–709.
[g]B. K. Phillips and K. K. Kolasa, Vegetable preferences of preschoolers in day care, *Journal of Nutrition Education* 12 (1980): 192–195.
[h]L. L. Birch and D. W. Marlin, I don't like it; I never tried it: Effects of exposure on two-year-old children's food preferences, *Appetite* 3 (1982): 353–360, as cited in Manipulation of children's eating preferences, *Nutrition Reviews* 44 (1986): 327–328.
[i]L. L. Birch, Effects of peer models' food choices and eating behaviors on preschoolers' food preferences, *Child Development* 51 (1980): 489–496, as cited in Manipulation of children's eating preferences, *Nutrition Reviews* 44 (1986): 327–328.
[j]Birch, Marlin, and Rotter, 1984.
[k]L. L. Birch, S. Zimmerman, and H. Hind, The influence of social effective context on preschool children's food preferences, *Child Development* 51 (1980): 856–861.
[l]S. L. King and E. S. Parham, The diet-stress connection, *Journal of Home Economics*, Fall 1981, pp. 25–28.

Food Allergies and Sensitivities

Adverse reactions to foods can threaten children's nutritional health to varying extents depending on their severity and duration and on the classes of foods they involve. Diagnosis is often elusive. Many food aversions are labeled allergies when they are not; and some real allergies go undetected. Adverse reactions that are only temporary may lead to permanant avoidance of foods, to the detriment of a child's health; conversely, true allergies and sensitivities that go undetected can cause chronic illness.

The term *food allergy* is used loosely, even by many physicians, as a catchall term for any unexplained adverse reaction to foods. Thus, a parent whose child has any kind of discomfort after eating—stomachache, headache, pain, rapid pulse rate, nausea, wheezing, hives, bronchial irritation, cough, or any other—may conclude that an allergy is responsible when in fact something

allergy: an immune reaction to a foreign substance (such as some components of food) in which antibodies are produced. Allergies may be **symptomatic** or **asymptomatic**.

else is the cause. Only careful, skilled testing can distinguish the many possibilities.

Possibilities other than allergy, some of which were already mentioned in Chapter 4, include reactions to bacterial toxins; reactions to the chemicals in foods such as monosodium glutamate or the natural laxative in prunes; digestive tract disorders such as obstructions or injuries; enzyme deficiencies such as inborn errors of metabolism or lactose intolerance; and even psychological aversions.

Allergies The prevalence of food allergies is highest in the first several years of life and tends to decline with age.[41] A true food allergy occurs when a large molecule, most commonly a protein, enters the system. (Recall that large molecules of food are normally dismantled in the digestive tract to smaller ones that are absorbed without problem.) The body's immune system reacts to a food protein or other large molecule as it does to other antigens—by producing antibodies or other defensive agents.

The term allergy has two components—antibodies and symptoms. A person may produce antibodies *without* having any symptoms (known as asymptomatic allergy) or may produce antibodies *and* have symptoms (known as symptomatic allergy). Symptoms without antibody production are *not* due to allergy.

Depending on its location in the body, the allergic reaction causes different symptoms. In the digestive tract, it causes nausea or vomiting; in the skin, it causes rashes; and in the nasal passages and lungs, it causes inflammation or asthma. A generalized, all-systems reaction is anaphylactic shock.

Allergic reactions to food occur with different timings, simply classified as immediate and delayed. In both, the interaction of the antigen with the immune system is immediate, but the appearance of symptoms may come within minutes or after several (up to 24) hours.[42] Diagnosis of an immediate allergic reaction is easy because symptoms correlate closely with the eating of the offending food. Diagnosis of delayed reactions is more difficult, because the symptoms may not appear until a day after the offending food is eaten; by this time, many other foods will have been eaten, too, complicating the picture.

The foods that most often cause immediate allergic reactions are listed in Table 5–5. According to one investigator, 91 percent of adverse reactions in children are caused by only four major foods—nuts (43 percent), eggs (21 percent), milk (18 percent), and soy (9 percent).[43] Allergic reactions to single foods are common. Reactions to multiple foods are the exception, not the rule.

A number of tests and food challenges are required to identify a true food allergy. A simple elimination diet that enables a person to avoid the offending food is the preferred test diet.[44] This requires the initiation of a diet with the suspected food eliminated for a week or two. If the symptoms do not disappear, the suspected food is not guilty. If symptoms resolve, the food is reintroduced into the diet in small quantities. If there is a reaction, the food is eliminated for a month or two, and then reintroduced. Unless the reaction is severe, food challenges are performed at regular intervals until the food is either tolerated or clearly never will be. A large majority of allergic reactions resolve themselves.[45] Allergies are not always diagnosed by these time-consuming, laborious methods, however. A number of unreliable tests, such as cytotoxic testing, are available that offer people quick, unfounded results.[46]

antigen: a substance foreign to the body that elicits the formation of antibodies or an inflammation reaction from immune system cells. Food antigens are usually glycoproteins (large proteins with glucose molecules attached).

antibody: a large protein that is produced in response to an antigen, and that inactivates the antigen.

anaphylactic (an-AFF-ill-LAC-tic) **shock:** a whole-body allergic reaction to an offending substance. Symptoms: abdominal pain, nausea, vomiting, diarrhea, inflamed nasal membranes, chest pain, hives, swelling, low blood pressure.

cytotoxic testing: an unreliable allergy test. One test tube of blood is taken from an individual and the white blood cells are mixed with plasma and sterile water and placed on microscope slides. Each slide is coated with a dried extract of a particular food. If the cells collapse, disintegrate, or change shape, the individual is supposedly allergic to that food. No controlled experiments show that white cells shrink or change shape when exposed to foods to which a person is allergic.

Table 5–5 Foods That Most Often Cause Allergies

Nuts	Peanuts
Eggs	Chicken
Milk	Fish
Soybeans	Shellfish
Wheat	Mollusks

Source: R. H. Buckley and D. Metcalfe, Food allergy, *Journal of the American Medical Association* 248 (1982): 2627–2631.

celiac disease: a sensitivity to gliadin, a fraction of the wheat protein gluten, that causes flattening of intestinal villi and generalized malabsorption; also called **gluten-sensitive enteropathy** or **celiac sprue.**

milk allergy: an abnormal immunologic reaction to cow's milk proteins; beta-lactoglobulin and casein are the most common cow's milk allergens.

milk intolerance: the experience of subjective symptoms, such as gastrointestinal discomfort, after consuming milk. It can be due to lactose, or to other substances in milk in people capable of efficient digestion of lactose.

lactose intolerance: the experience of gastrointestinal symptoms; gas, abdominal cramping, nausea, and/or watery stools after ingestion of lactose (either in milk, in other dairy foods, or as purified sugar). The terms *tolerance* and *intolerance* refer to the symptomatic response to a defined dose of lactose and are not interchangeable with **lactase deficiency.** Lactase deficiency or lactase nonpersistence is determined by a biopsy of the intestinal mucosa or indirectly by methods such as the lactose-tolerance test or breath-hydrogen test.

congenital lactase deficiency: a rare, life-threatening condition due to a genetic enzyme defect that manifests itself at birth. When the infant with this inborn error of metabolism receives milk or milk-based formula, symptoms of diarrhea, flatulence, and a lack of weight gain occur.

secondary lactase deficiency: a transient or temporary state of lactase activity in previously lactase-persistent individuals following injury to the small intestinal mucosa.

Celiac disease About 1 in 3000 U.S. children is afflicted with a type of food sensitivity known as celiac disease, or gluten sensitive enteropathy.[47] These children are sensitive to gluten, a protein in barley, rye, oats, and wheat. Treatment consists of feeding the child a gluten-free diet, from which these foods are omitted. Such treatment is easier described than administered, since barley, rye, oats, and wheat are common in many foods. Rice, corn, and potatoes are well tolerated by children on a gluten-free diet. Rice cereal is frequently the first food introduced to infants because it contains almost no gluten and causes few allergic reactions. Children can outgrow celiac disease, but it may reappear in adulthood.

Milk intolerance and lactose intolerance Milk intolerance in children is a confusing issue for parents and health care professionals alike. Even the meaning of the term itself is confusing, implying different things to different people. Children with nonspecific problems such as skin rash, diarrhea, vomiting, or persistent nasal congestion are often labeled milk intolerant. Milk intolerance in infants due to milk toxicity was discussed in Chapter 4.

Lactose intolerance may be due to a genetically predetermined, age-related decrease in lactase activity, called primary lactase deficiency, resulting in low lactase activity usually by about five or six years of age. Because low intestinal lactase is not an abnormal state, nor actually a deficiency, the World Health Organization has suggested that the term *primary lactase deficiency* be replaced with *lactase nonpersistence*.[48] About 70 percent of the world's population is lactase nonpersistent, the incidence ranging from 1 or 2 percent among Scandinavians to about 100 percent among Asians.[49]

Two other types of lactase deficiency exist. One is congenital lactase deficiency, a rare, life-threatening condition due to an enzyme defect present at birth. The other is secondary lactase deficiency, a temporary state of low lactase activity following injury to the small intestine from protein malnutrition or gastrointestinal infection.

Adjusting the diet Parents are advised to watch for signs of food dislikes and take them seriously: "Dislike of a food may be only a whim or fancy, but it should be regarded as significant until proven otherwise."[50] For a parent to demand that a child eat a specific food is to create unnecessary, often harmful conflict. Although many cases of suspected allergies and intolerances turn out to be minor and temporary, real adverse reactions do occur. Do not prejudge, in any case. Test.

When parents stop serving a suspected food to their child, they risk feeding the child an unbalanced diet that could lead to nutrient deficiencies. Whenever a food is excluded from the diet, care must be taken to include other foods that offer the same nutrients as the omitted food contains. Milk is often perceived as an offending food and all too casually omitted from a child's diet. Continued restriction of milk in the child's diet without appropriate substitutions can result in energy, protein, calcium, vitamin A, vitamin D, and riboflavin deficiencies. It is critical that nutritionally comparable milk substitutes be introduced.

Sometimes milk allergy can be treated by elimination of the offending milk protein from the diet for a period of time, followed by gradual reintroduction. During the elimination time, possible substitutes for milk are boiled milk (milk protein is altered with cooking), goat's milk, soy milk (although soy is also a common allergen), yogurt, and cheeses. Liquid or powdered milk can be cooked into foods such as custards, soups, and casseroles.

The child who is lactose intolerant can usually handle small amounts of milk periodically throughout the day—up to half a glass each time, especially if offered with other foods. Fermented milk products such as yogurt offer the same nutrients as milk but with a lower lactose content.

As a last resort, the milk's nutrients may be offered in supplement form. Chapter 1 discusses calcium supplements for adults, but the factors bearing on the choice apply equally to children, and Figure 5–3 offers a decision tree for choosing a milk substitute.

Nutrition at School

While parents are doing what they can to establish favorable eating behaviors during the transition from infancy to childhood, other factors are entering the picture. During preschool or grade school, children encounter foods prepared and served by outsiders. The U.S. government funds several programs to provide nutritious, high-quality meals for children at school. (School lunches in Canada are administered locally and therefore vary from area to area.) School lunches are designed to meet certain requirements. They must include specified servings of milk, protein-rich foods (meat, poultry, fish, cheese, eggs, legumes, or peanut butter), vegetables, fruits, and breads or other grain foods. The design is intended to provide at least a third of the RDA for each of the nutrients. The U.S. school lunch pattern is split into several patterns to provide for the needs of different ages (see Table 5–6).

Parents rely on the school lunch program to meet a significant part of their children's nutrient needs on school days. Indeed, students participating in the school lunch program have higher intakes of food energy and nutrients than students who do not. Because children do not always like what they are served, school lunch programs attempt to offer children both what they want and what will nourish them. In response to children's differing needs and tastes, the best programs:

▶ Present a variety of offerings and allow children to choose what they are served.

▶ Vary portion sizes so that little children can take little servings.

Figure 5–3 Choosing a Milk Substitute

[a]You can buy milk already treated or add the enzyme (LactAid) yourself. Enzyme treatment may not reduce lactose content sufficiently to relieve symptoms, and you may have to try the other alternatives.

Source: Adapted from E. N. Whitney and C. B. Cataldo, *Understanding Normal and Clinical Nutrition* (St. Paul, Minn.: West, 1983), pp. 559–568.

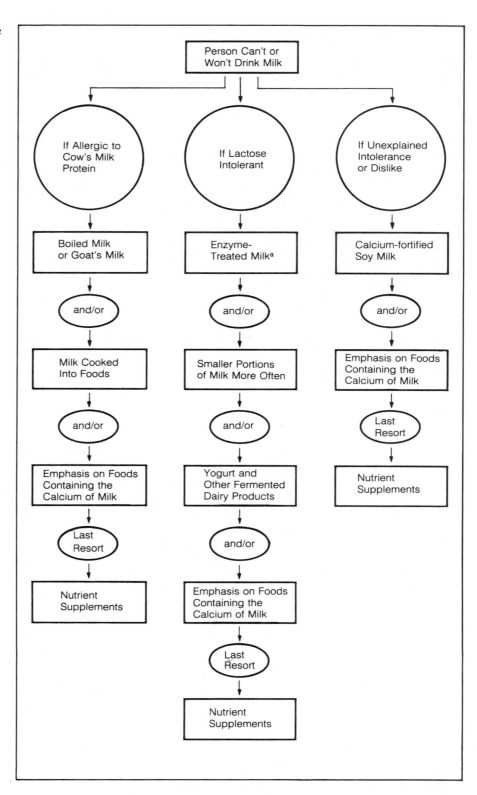

▶ Involve students (in secondary schools) in the planning of menus.

▶ Schedule lunches so that children can eat when they are hungry and can have enough time to eat well.

Many schools are taking steps toward making the lunches more consistent with today's ideals of healthful food. Schools offer low-fat or nonfat milk instead of whole milk. To help the schools economize, programs permit children to select what they will eat, so that there will be less plate waste. Many schools offer salad bars, potato bars, and taco bars, providing students an opportunity to create their own meals from a selection of nutritious foods.

Whether to eat the school's lunch is not the only choice facing children in the school. Some children bring lunch from home, others rely on vending machines. Many health professionals and parents would like to eliminate the sale of confections as snacks in schools, but because vending machines are an important source of income for the schools' extracurricular activities, so far such efforts have met with little success. Most progress has been made by way of individual, voluntary initiatives. Experiments have shown that children choose more nutritious snacks if they are offered side by side with sugary foods. When apples are made available in vending machines, children choose

Table 5–6   School Lunch Patterns for Different Ages

| Food Group | Preschool | | Grades | | |
	Ages 1 to 2	Ages 3 to 4	K to 3	4 to 6	7 to 12
Meat or meat alternate					
1 serving					
Lean meat, poultry, or fish	1 oz	1½ oz	1½ oz	2 oz	3 oz
Cheese	1 oz	1½ oz	1½ oz	2 oz	3 oz
Large egg(s)	1	1½	1½	2	3
Cooked dry beans or peas	½ c	¾ c	¾ c	1 c	1½ c
Peanut butter	2 tbsp	3 tbsp	3 tbsp	4 tbsp	6 tbsp
Vegetable and/or fruit					
2 or more servings, both to total	½ c	½ c	½ c	¾ c	¾ c
Bread or bread alternate					
Servings[a]	5 per week	8 per week	8 per week	8 per week	10 per week
Milk					
1 serving of fluid milk	¾ c	¾ c	1 c	1 c	1 c

[a]A serving is 1 slice of whole-grain or enriched bread; a whole-grain or enriched biscuit, roll, muffin, and so on; or ½ c cooked pasta or other cereal grain such as bulgur or grits.

Source: School lunch patterns: Ready, set, go! *School Food Service Journal* 34 (August 1980): 31.

chocolate bars less often. When milk is made available, soft drink use drops considerably.

Coincident with the school lunch program is a program of nutrition education and training (NET program) in all the public schools. Originally allocated 50 cents per year per child, this program was cut in 1980 to 9 cents per child, but program administrators are highly motivated and have been ingenious and creative in accomplishing the program's highest-priority objectives.[51]

Few elementary education curricula include a nutrition course. At best, children are taught the basic Four Food Groups Plan. Creative methods for teaching nutrition to children can center on the use of stories, puppets, and games. For classes with computers, a number of nutrition education programs are available beginning at the preschool level. One way in which children can learn about nutrition, sometimes with only small expense to the school, is to take field trips to nearby food operations facilities. Among the possible places to visit are those listed in the margin. At the very least, children can go to the depots where the school food comes in and to the kitchens where it is prepared. Knowledgeable teachers can then use the questions that arise as opportunities to teach nutrition. Children need not only to be fed well, but to learn enough about nutrition to become able to make healthy food choices when the choices become theirs to make.

On the average, children in the United States spend as much time watching television as they do attending school.[52] Little wonder that television viewing has become associated with a variety of child and teen behaviors. Television's influence is evident in dental health and childhood obesity, and is discussed in Focal Points 3 and 5.

Children can learn from:

▶ Bakeries.
▶ Mills.
▶ Dairy farms.
▶ Milk-bottling plants.
▶ Farmers markets.
▶ Vegetable farms and fields.
▶ Food-processing plants.
▶ Fast-food places.
▶ Institutional kitchens.
▶ Supermarkets.
▶ Convenience stores.
▶ Neighborhood gardens.
▶ Natural-food stores.
▶ Food salvage banks.

Tomorrow's Adults

The task of parents and health care professionals is not simply to keep children healthy. They need to look ahead and put forth efforts to create future healthy adults. Many adult diseases develop out of personal habits and styles of living that take root in childhood. Among behavior patterns children can pick up are cigarette smoking, lack of exercise, and dietary habits that lead to obesity, elevated cholesterol, and hypertension. These behaviors—behaviors that are initiated in childhood and carried into adulthood—contribute the major risk factors of today's major killers of adults, coronary heart disease and other diseases. The task, then, is to facilitate the child's optimal physical, mental, emotional, and social growth and development. A foundation for a lifetime of health begins with the development of positive behaviors for nutrition, exercise, work, play, and personal interactions. By adopting a healthy lifestyle early in life, a child may establish beneficial habits that have a good chance of persisting throughout life.

Eating habits help determine whether development takes place in a positive or negative direction. The childhood years may be a parent's last chance to influence these habits. In addition to providing healthy foods, parents need to foster the development of children's preferences for them.

Prevention of Obesity

To prevent obesity, train preschool children to "eat thin." Teach children to eat slowly, to pause and enjoy their table companions, and to stop eating when they are full. Stamp out the "clean your plate" dictum for all time, and in its place learn to serve smaller portions that can be followed by additional servings, if needed. Encourage physical activity on a daily basis to promote strong skeletal and muscular development and to establish habits that will undergird good health throughout life.

The child who is already obese needs careful handling. As in pregnancy, weight loss may easily impair growth in children.[53] J. L. Knittle, who has worked with obese children, recommends that they be fed so as to maintain a constant weight while they grow taller. The object is to restrict the multiplication of fat cells while promoting normal lean body development. Thus, children can "grow out" of their obesity (see Focal Point 5).

Prevention of Cardiovascular Disease

Primary prevention of cardiovascular disease is a pediatric task. The symptoms of atherosclerosis present themselves in adulthood, but fatty streaks and fibrous plaques are evident early in life. The gradual accumulation of lipids along the inner walls of the arteries is a lifelong process influenced by several factors. An elevated plasma cholesterol level is one major factor. In populations where the incidence of adult coronary artery disease is high, the children have average to high levels of plasma cholesterol. In contrast, where the incidence is low, the cholesterol level of the children is low to average.[54] In the United States, children have higher cholesterol levels than children in other populations where atherosclerosis is less widespread.

Many experts seem to agree that the risk of adult heart disease will be lessened if a diet low in fat, saturated fat, and cholesterol, with polyunsaturated fat replacing some of the saturated fat, is implemented early in life. The American Heart Association recommends prudent modification of diet in healthy children over the age of two.[55] The dietary recommendations are:

1. The diet should be nutritionally adequate, consisting of a variety of foods.
2. The energy intake should be based on growth rate, activity level, and subcutaneous fat so as to maintain desirable body weight.
3. The total fat intake should be approximately 30 percent of kcalories, with 10 percent or less from saturated fat, about 10 percent from monounsaturated fat, and less than 10 percent from polyunsaturated fat. The emphasis should be on reduction of total fat and saturated fat rather than on increasing polyunsaturated fat.
4. The daily cholesterol intake should be approximately 100 milligrams cholesterol per 1000 kcalories, and should not exceed 300 milligrams.
5. Protein intake should be about 15 percent of kcalories, derived from varied sources.

6. Carbohydrate intake should be about 55 percent of kcalories, derived primarily from complex carbohydrate sources to provide necessary vitamins and minerals.

7. High-salt processed foods, sodium-containing condiments, and added salt at the table should be limited.

The proposed diet, designed for a healthy child, is adequate in all essential nutrients. It provides lean meats, poultry, fish, and vegetable sources of protein; fruits and vegetables; whole grains; and low-fat dairy products. This dietary effort to moderate consumption of fat, cholesterol, sodium, and sugar in children appears to be safe; growth and development are not affected.[56]

However, not all children are healthy and receive adequate nourishment regularly. For these reasons, some members of the pediatric health profession oppose the adoption of a prudent-type diet for children. They caution that while the intentions are good, such dietary restrictions may compound nutrient deficiencies in deprived children. One physician warns, "If parents get too zealous, such diets might stunt a child's growth."[57] Perhaps dietary restrictions are not needed for all children.

The American Academy of Pediatrics adds qualifications to the dietary recommendations for children.[58] Childhood obesity must not be overlooked as a source of elevated cholesterol levels. A large majority of children with elevated cholesterol levels are obese. Early treatment of obesity, maintenance of ideal weight, and regular exercise will modify cholesterol levels and benefit cardiac health. Children can be identified as "high risk" by examining family histories. Children of parents with elevated cholesterol levels are almost three times as likely to have cholesterol levels in the 95th percentile as children in the general population. Once a child is identified as being at risk, at least two cholesterol measurements should be taken to confirm the diagnosis. Finally, the committee warns parents to avoid extremes; follow the prudent diet with moderation.

Nutritional screening of children is outlined in Appendix A.

Routine screening of all children can determine what conditions are likely to develop, but family histories are the primary method of identifying "high-risk" children. The blood-lipid profiles of children whose fathers were diagnosed with coronary artery disease closely resembled the blood-lipid profiles of the fathers.[59] As soon as children are identified as "high risk," appropriate dietary and medical intervention can be implemented.

Thus, it would be advisable to feed the child of a parent with high blood pressure a diet relatively low in salt; the child of a parent with diabetes a diet low in sugar and high in complex carbohydrates; and the child of a parent with coronary artery disease a diet low in fat—especially saturated fat—and possibly low in cholesterol. In all these situations, the greatest success is likely to be achieved if the whole family, and not just the child, follows the diet rules.

Prevention of Osteoporosis

Like atherosclerosis, osteoporosis is an adult disease that may reflect a person's childhood dietary habits. Milk consumption is encouraged throughout childhood, primarily to provide the calcium needed for skeletal growth, but the benefits of young people's consuming calcium-rich foods reach far into the future. Frequent and adequate milk consumption throughout life maximizes growth of bone (within genetic limits, of course).[60] Bones grow not only in length, but also in density; bone density is the best defense against osteoporotic fractures. High bone density maintains skeletal integrity and defends against bone loss in later life.

Prevention of Dental Caries

The care and nourishment of children's teeth is important from before they first erupt, and become children's own responsibility as they learn to wield the toothbrush at about the age of three or so. Attention to their eating habits and dental hygiene beginning in childhood can lay the foundation for good dental health throughout life. The relationships of nutrition and diet to dental health were the subjects of Focal Point 3.

It may be difficult to convince a young person to invest in tomorrow's health, but there is little question that prevention is the best treatment of obesity, atherosclerosis, osteoporosis, and dental caries. No doubt, developing healthful habits is easier than changing poor habits later.

Chapter 5 Notes

1. D. Sinclair, *Human Growth after Birth*, 4th ed. (New York: Oxford University Press, 1985), pp. 23–50.

2. Sinclair, 1985, pp. 102–122.

3. H. E. Sauberlich, J. H. Skala, and R. P. Dowdy, *Laboratory Tests for the Assessment of Nutritional Status* (Boca Raton, Fla.: CRC Press, 1979), pp. 92–103.

4. S. E. Morris, *The Normal Acquisition of Oral Feeding Skills: Implications for Assessment and Treatment* (New York: Therapeutic Media, 1982).

5. Food and Nutrition Board, Committee on Dietary Allowances, *Recommended Dietary Allowances*, 9th ed. (Washington, D.C.: National Academy of Sciences, 1980), pp. 39–54.

6. The Nutrition Monitoring Division, Human Nutrition Information Service, Nationwide Food Consumption Survey, *Nutrition Today*, November/December 1986, pp. 31–33.

7. J. L. Brown, Hunger in the United States, *Scientific American* 256 (1987): 37–41.

8. Brown, 1987.

9. M. Leung and coauthors, Dietary intakes of preschoolers, *Journal of the American Dietetic Association* 84 (1984): 551–554.

10. *Iron Nutrition Revisited—Infancy, Childhood, Adolescence*, Report of the 82nd Ross Conference on Pediatric Research, (Columbus, Ohio: Ross Laboratories, 1981), p. 1.

11. Summary of a report on assessment of the iron nutritional status of the United States population, *American Journal of Clinical Nutrition* 42 (1985): 1318–1330.

12. N. R. Raper, J. C. Rosenthal, and C. E. Woteki, Estimates of available iron in diets of individuals 1 year old and older in the Nationwide Food Consumption Survey, *Journal of the American Dietetic Association* 84 (1984): 783–787.

13. P. G. Taylor and coauthors, Daily physiological iron requirements in children, *Journal of the American Dietetic Association* 88 (1988): 454–458.

14. Raper, Rosenthal, and Woteki, 1984.

15. P. R. Dallman, M. A. Siimes, and A. Stekel, Iron deficiency in infancy and childhood, *American Journal of Clinical Nutrition* 33 (1980): 86–118.

16. M. W. Breskin and coauthors, Supplement use: Vitamin intakes and biochemical indexes in 40- to 108-month-old children, *Journal of the American Dietetic Association* 85 (1985): 49–56.

17. Committee on Nutrition, American Academy of Pediatrics, Vitamin and mineral supplement needs in normal children in the United States, *Pediatrics* 66 (1980): 1015–1021.

18. W. B. Deichmann and H. W. Gerarde, *Toxicology of Drugs and Chemicals* (New York: Academic Press, 1969), pp. 333–334.

19. Committee on Nutrition, American Academy of Pediatrics, *Pediatric Nutrition Handbook* 2nd ed., ed. G. B. Forbes and C. W. Woodruff (Elk Grove, Ill.: American Academy of Pediatrics, 1985), pp. 170–173.

20. K. M. Hambridge and coauthors, Low levels of zinc in hair, anorexia, poor growth, and hypogeusia in children, *Pediatric Research* 6 (1972): 868–874; C. Xue-Cun and coauthors, Low levels of zinc in hair and blood, pica, anorexia, and poor growth in Chinese preschool children, *American Journal of Clinical Nutrition* 42 (1985): 694–700.

21. D. M. Tucker and H. H. Sandstead, Body iron stores and cortical arousal, in *Iron Deficiency: Brain Biochemistry and Behavior,* ed. E. Pollitt and R. L. Leibel (New York: Raven Press, 1982), pp. 161–182.

22. T. E. Webb and F. A. Oski, Iron deficiency anemia and scholastic achievement in young adolescents, *Journal of Pediatrics* 82 (1973): 827–830; T. E. Webb and F. A. Oski, Behavioral status of young adolescents with iron deficiency anemia, *Journal of Special Education* 8 (1974): 153–156.

23. Y. H. Neggers and K. R. Stitt, Effects of high lead intake in children, *Journal of the American Dietetic Association* 86 (1986): 938–940.

24. Neggers and Stitt, 1986

25. Neggers and Stitt, 1986.

26. W. S. Watson and coauthors, Food iron and lead absorption in humans, *American Journal of Clinical Nutrition* 44 (1986): 248–256.

27. K. Mahaffey and coauthors, Blood lead levels and dietary calcium intake in 1- to 11-year-old children: The Second National Health and Nutrition Examination Survey, 1976 to 1980, *Pediatrics* 78 (1986): 257–262.

28. F. L. Cerklewski and R. M. Forbes, Influence of dietary zinc and lead toxicity in the rat, *Journal of Nutrition* 106 (1976): 689–696, as cited in Neggers and Stitt, 1986.

29. M. E. Markowitz and J. F. Rosen, Zinc and copper metabolism in $CaNa_2EDTA$-treated children with plumbism (abstract), *Pediatric Research* 15 (1981): 635.

30. E. Pollitt, R. Leibel, and D. Greenfield, Brief fasting, stress and cognition in children, *American Journal of Clinical Nutrition* 34 (1981): 1526–1533.

31. Pollitt, Leibel, and Greenfield, 1981.

32. M. Kiester, Relation of mid-morning feeding to behavior of nursery school children, *Journal of the American Dietetic Association* 26 (1950): 25–29, as cited in E. Pollitt, M. Gersovitz, and M. Gargiulo, Educational benefits of the United States School Feeding Program: A critical review of the literature, *American Journal of Public Health* 68 (1978): 477–481.

33. *Diagnostic and Statistical Manual (DSM III),* 3rd ed. (Washington, D.C.: American Psychiatric Association, 1980), p. 41.

34. National Advisory Committee on Hyperkinesis and Food Additives, *Final Report to the Nutrition Foundation,* (New York: Nutrition Foundation, Inc., 1980).

35. National Advisory Committee, 1980; National Institutes of Health Consensus Development Panel, National Institutes of Health, Consensus development conference statement: Defined diets and childhood hyperactivity, *American Journal of Clinical Nutrition* 37 (1983): 161–165.

36. National Institutes of Health, Defined diets and childhood hyperactivity, *Journal of the American Medical Association* 248 (1982): 290–292.

37. L. Eisenberg, Clinical use of stimulant drugs in children, *Pediatrics* 49 (1972): 709–715.

38. M. L. Arbeit and coauthors, Caffeine intakes of children from a biracial population: The Bogalusa Heart Study, *Journal of the American Dietetic Association* 88 (1988): 466–471.

39. J. L. Rapoport and coauthors, Behavioral effects of caffeine in children, *Archives of General Psychiatry* 41 (1984): 1073–1079.

40. T. A. Morck, S. R. Lynch, and J. D. Cook, Inhibition of food iron absorption by coffee, *American Journal of Clinical Nutrition* 37 (1983): 416–420.

41. S. A. Bock, The natural history of adverse reactions to food in young children, address presented at the 70th Annual Meeting of the American Dietetic Association, Atlanta, Georgia, 19 October 1987.

42. S. L. Taylor, Food allergy—the enigma and some potential solutions, *Journal of Food Protection* 43 (1980): 300–306.

43. C. D. May, Food allergy: Perspective, principles, practical management, *Nutrition Today,* November/December 1980, pp. 28–31.

44. Bock, 1987.

45. Bock, 1987.

46. R. C. Thompson, The flaw in cytotoxic testing: There's no proof it works, *FDA Consumer,* October 1984, pp. 34–36.

47. *Baby Foods,* A Report by the American Council on Science and Health (Summit, N.J.: American Council on Science and Health, 1987).

48. World Health Organization sponsored workshop on "Lactose Malabsorption," Moscow, Russia, 10–11 June 1985, as cited in National Dairy Council, Nutritional implications of lactose and lactase activity, *Dairy Council Digest* 56 (1985): 25–30.

49. A. D. Newcomer, Lactase deficiency, *Contemporary Nutrition* 4 (1979): 1–2.

50. V. J. Fontana and F. Moreno-Pagan, Allergy and diet, in *Modern Nutrition in Health and Disease,* 6th ed., ed. R. S. Goodhart and M. E. Shils, (Philadelphia: Lea and Febiger, 1980), pp. 1071–1081.

51. H. R. Armstrong and D. B. Root, Managing a lean NET program, *Community Nutritionist* 2 (1983): 8–10.

52. W. H. Dietz and S. L. Gortmaker, Do we fatten our children at the television set? Obesity and television viewing in children and adolescents, *Pediatrics* 75 (1985): 807–812.

53. W. H. Dietz and R. Hartung, Changes in height velocity of obese preadolescents during weight reduction, *American Journal of Diseases of Children* 139 (1985): 705–707.

54. Task Force Committee of the Nutrition Committee and the Cardiovascular Disease in the Young Council of the American Heart Association, Diet in the healthy child, *Circulation/American Heart Association Report* 67 (1983): 1411A–1414A.

55. Task Force Committee of the Nutrition Committee and the Cardiovascular Disease in the Young Council of the American Heart Association, 1983.

56. C. J. Glueck, Pediatric primary prevention of atherosclerosis, *New England Journal of Medicine* 314 (1986): 175–177.

57. R. E. Olson, M.D., professor of pharmacology and medicine, as quoted in Low-cholesterol diet 'not for everyone,' *Modern Medicine,* August 1986, p. 13.

58. Committee on Nutrition, American Academy of Pediatrics, Toward a prudent diet for children, *Pediatrics* 71 (1983): 78–80.

59. J. L. Lee, R. M. Lauer, and W. R. Clarke, Lipoproteins in the progeny of young men with coronary artery disease: Children with increased risk, *Pediatrics* 78 (1986): 330–337.

60. R. B. Sandler and coauthors, Postmenopausal bone density and milk consumption in childhood and adolescence, *American Journal of Clinical Nutrition* 42 (1985): 270–274.

▶ *Focal Point 5*

Childhood Obesity

What causes obesity? To put it quite simply: obesity results from an excess of food energy eaten over energy expended. And yet, obesity is not a simple problem to solve. Its underlying causes are complex, its effects far-reaching, and its treatment difficult.

Obesity is the most prevalent and serious nutrition problem in the United States. The best solution to this national health problem is prevention.

Prevention depends on our understanding of how and when obesity arises. Simple questions to ask are: At what age can obesity be predicted? When does it truly set in and persist? It seems that the critical period of development with ramifications on adult obesity occurs during the first five years of life.[1] It can be *predicted* as early as age two for girls and three for boys.[2] Actual obesity, however, usually begins to *set in* between the ages of six and nine. Estimates of its incidence among our nation's youth range from 5 to 25 percent. A large majority (80 percent) of overweight children remain overweight into adulthood. Additional obesity sets in among adults, so that two-thirds of obese adults were actually normal-weight children.[3]

Researchers studying the growth patterns of children from one month to 16 years identified trends that could predict obesity.[4] An infant's level of obesity increases during the first year and then decreases. At about age six, another increase in obesity, termed adiposity rebound, occurs and continues into adolescence. A relationship is seen between the age of rebound and later obesity. Obese one-year-olds with an early rebound (before 5 1/2 years of age) tend to remain obese; obese 1-year-olds with a normal (6 years of age) or delayed (7 years of age) rebound eventually join the average group; nonobese 1-year-olds with an early rebound reach the higher percentiles by adolescence; nonobese 1-year-olds with a normal or delayed rebound remain in the low-to-average weight range.

adiposity rebound: the onset of the second period of rapid growth in body fat.

Overweight infants most often grow into children who are no longer heavy in relation to their height; they are not destined to become obese adults. Almost 80 percent of obese infants lose their obesity in childhood.[5] The early high-risk period for the onset of obesity, then, is not infancy, but the early childhood years. Most obese infants do not become obese children; many obese children do become obese adults. The earlier the onset of obesity, the greater the likelihood of spontaneous resolution with age; obesity of later onset has a higher risk of persistence.[6] One study found that children who were overweight as toddlers were even more overweight as teenagers.[7] Wherever obesity has shown signs of truly setting in, in children, prevention efforts need to be instituted promptly. Assessment is important in identifying those in need of intervention.

Appendix A provides a discussion of assessment, including forms, indexes, tables, and graphs.

obesity: excessive body fatness.

percentile: one of 100 equal divisions of data. For example, if a value, such as a person's test score, is higher than that of 75% of the rest of the population, then it is at the 75th percentile in the range of test scores. A person whose weight is at the 75th percentile weighs more than 75% of the population being used for comparison.

The simplest way to define obesity is as excessive body fatness. But then we must ask, excessive compared with what standard? Beyond the point at which a person can live a healthy life? Beyond the population's average? Beyond what is considered beautiful by fashion designers and movie directors?

How is obesity identified? Most commonly, it is defined by body weight. Researchers study the distribution of weight in a population and set the definition of obesity at a standard weight for height and age. If obesity is defined as above the 95th percentile, then we label 5 percent of the population "obese." Likewise, if we defined the cutoff at 50 percent, then half of us would be obese. The definition arbitrarily determines obesity. We have no well-defined biological basis to establish the cutoff point between "normal" and "obese." Researchers generally agree that the cutoff percentile defining obesity in children is 95. The criterion for "overweight," then, lies between "normal" and "obese." While arbitrary, these points do mark a level that is associated with increased morbidity.

Causes of Obesity

As stated in the introductory remarks, obesity is the result of an energy intake in excess of energy expenditure. Therefore, the causes of obesity are those that increase kcaloric intake, decrease kcaloric expenditure, or otherwise disturb the balance of this energy budget. Many possible causes have been explored, most not proven. Quite likely, more than one cause operates in most instances, and different sets of causes may operate in different individuals. The following sections describe the many areas in which research is currently proceeding in the attempt to understand the root causes of obesity.

Fat-Cell Hypothesis

The fat-cell hypothesis has two major premises. First, overfeeding in early life causes the production of an excess number of fat cells. Second, this excess alters the mechanisms of fat storage and release in adipose tissue in such a way as to predispose the individual to obesity.[8]

hyperplasia: see definition on page 61.

hypertrophy: see definition on page 61.

The hypothesis contends that obesity begins to develop during critical periods of cellular growth. Fat cells first grow by increasing their numbers (hyperplasia). If excess energy is consumed during this time, the number of cells increases, and a number is reached at some time before adulthood that remains fairly constant throughout life. After this number is reached, cells then grow in size (hypertrophy), but no longer increase in number: subsequent weight gains and losses result in changes in cell size only. Thus, the onset of obesity in childhood is considered to be primarily hyperplastic, reflecting an increased number of fat cells, whereas adult-onset obesity is considered to be hypertrophic, a result of existing fat cells becoming overfilled.

Findings support this distinction between juvenile- and adult-onset obesity, but there is always "overlap" in both directions. Studies have confirmed that obese children do have a greater number of fat cells than nonobese children. The fat cells are also larger. The fat-cell size measurements of obese children become similar to those of adults even before the children enter their teen years.[9] It is most likely that an obese child whose number of fat cells equals or exceeds that of the average adult will remain obese. Those with the greatest number of fat cells are least likely to lose weight successfully. However, a chubby child whose number of fat cells is within the normal range (whose obesity, in other words, is hypertrophic) will more likely outgrow the "baby fat."

Thus, the time of cell number determination is critical and the number arrived at is considered irreversible. Recent studies, however, indicate that cell growth and development do not necessarily follow the simple pattern implied by this theory.

Adipocyte development   One study approached the question of how obesity arises by first studying the normal development of adipose tissues in normal-weight infants.[10] The researchers took samples of fat from beneath the skin (subcutaneous fat biopsies) and determined both the cell size and number of cells. They also determined total body fat, based on whole-body counting of potassium. They repeated these procedures and measures over time in order to determine the ways in which both cell size and cell number change in normal-weight infants. The results from this study show that normal expansion of fat depots in the first year of life is due almost exclusively to fat cell size enlargement. Fat-cell number, however, remains unchanged. During the next six months (the first half of the second year), no further increase in fat-cell size takes place, but a significant increase is noted in cell number. The size of fat cells, in fact, does not change significantly from the age of 18 months all the way to adulthood: in normal 18-month-old infants it is no different from that of normal 8-year-old children or normal 22-year-old females. On the other hand, fat-cell number at 18 months is much lower than that of a normal-weight 8-year-old child (one-half) and the still higher number of a nonobese 22-year old adult (one-fourth). Cell multiplication begins when adipocytes are filled to a size similar to that of normal adults. That is, when cells reach a "peak" size, more fat cells are produced.

Another study found it important to determine how and at what age obese children deviate from normal fat-cell development and at what age they exceed nonobese adult values. Adipocyte size and number were measured (using methods similar to those described in the previous study) several times in nonobese and obese infants, children, and adolescents.[11] Before age two, all infants were nonobese. From age six months to one year, cell size increased until it reached adult levels. Then it decreased slightly until age two. By age two, children were identified as obese based on weight-for-height measures. In the comparison between nonobese and obese children at age two, the researchers found that the adipocytes of the obese children had become significantly larger; they remained at the size normal for adults instead of shrinking, as those of the nonobese children had done. This difference persisted throughout all ages studied; that is, obese children's fat cells were larger and continued increasing in number from age two onwards. Cell size did not change in obese children from ages 2 through 16, but increased again after age 17.

In nonobese children, cells did not change in size from age two until early adolescence; then they reached the adult size. No increases in cell number occurred until after age ten. (In contrast, as mentioned, obese children's fat cells showed significant increases in number throughout the growing years.)

It is important to take notice of whether studies were conducted on normal-weight infants or obese infants.

In summary, the normal course of events is as follows. From six months to one year, increments in fat depots are primarily due to increases in cell size. During the next year, cell size decreases and cell number slightly increases. Fat depots remain fairly inactive until age ten, when both number and size again increase. In contrast, obese children's fat cells attain adult sizes by age two and then show increases in cell number continuously thereafter as illustrated in Figure FP5–1.

The researchers only counted and measured cells that had already begun to fill with fat and thus were clearly identifiable as adipocytes. Investigators differ on the question of whether and how to count preadipocytes; it is hard to tell whether a cell with no fat in it is destined to become an adipocyte or some other kind of cell. The method, with this limitation, seems to make a real distinction between nonobese and obese children's cell differentiation: whether a cell is called preadipocyte is less important than whether it fills with fat. Obese children's cells do, nonobese children's do not.[12]

This study reveals two time intervals that appear critical in adipose cell development. One is before age two, and the other during the adolescent growth spurt. These periods may prove to have important consequences for the onset and persistence of obesity.

Critical periods   The theory that the number of fat cells becomes fixed at a critical point in time, and thereafter sets a person's tendency to be normal weight or obese, has been considered and debated without confirmation over the past 20 years. It has theoretical appeal because it agrees with other findings about critical periods. However, it has drawbacks because it does not seem to concur with some research findings.

A parallel between malnutrition and obesity becomes evident when considering critical periods of cell development. When a child is malnourished

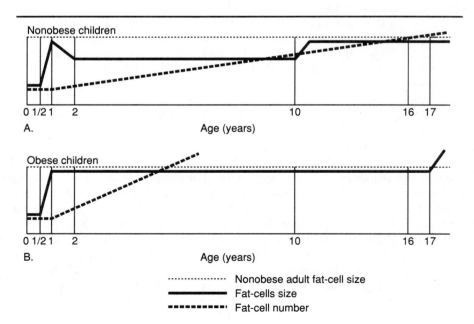

Figure FP5–1   Fat-Cell Development
Fat-cell size and number increase differently in obese and nonobese children.

during cell multiplication, cell number is permanently reduced and growth is stunted forever. The child cannot "catch up" when adequately refed. However, if the child is malnourished during cell size enlargement, growth of cells and the child's overall growth will catch up when the child is properly fed; no number increase is needed. Likewise, if factors encourage cell multiplication, obesity will result without hope of treatment. However, if it is the cell size enlargement that is altered, obesity becomes a treatable disease. By manipulating nutrition during early childhood, the parent (or other caretaker) can control cell number. Even if the range of that cell number is genetically determined, at least it could be kept to the lower end. Such dietary manipulation at critical times during the development of rats has altered the expression of their obesity within genetic limits.

While we are unable to determine exactly when critical periods begin and end, times of exceptionally rapid cell growth have been identified. Three peak periods for the development of obesity in children are late infancy, early childhood (age six), and adolescence.[13]

Adipose enzymes   If we accept that fat-cell number and size are the determining factors in weight regulation, then we must ask what mechanisms in turn determine fat-cell number and size. One obvious place to look is to the lipoprotein lipase enzyme system. Lipoprotein lipase is a membrane-bound enzyme, characteristic of fat cells, that breaks down circulating triglycerides for storage in the adipocytes. When lipoprotein lipase activity is high, more fat is stored.[14] Its activity is altered by dietary changes. For example, in fasting, lipoprotein lipase activity decreases in adipose tissue; fatty acids are not stored, but instead are used to meet energy demands. High-carbohydrate diets, on the other hand, increase adipose lipoprotein lipase activity. Obese people who have lost weight tend to have higher lipoprotein lipase activity than when they were maintaining their weight.[15] Unfortunately, their fat cells seem to be more efficient at saving energy than is normal.

Set Point

Many internal physiological variables, such as blood glucose, blood pH, and body temperature, remain fairly stable under a variety of environmental conditions. Constant monitoring of the body's internal status and delicate changes maintain these variables within certain limits. The stability of such complex systems as the human body may depend on set-point regulators. These regulators maintain variables at specified values.

Research on the regulation of body weight has been influenced by this set-point concept. Researchers propose that each individual body has a set biological weight determined by genetic and environmental factors, a "set point." However, unlike body temperature, the range of body weight in human beings is large. For example, a reasonable weight for an adult woman, 5 feet 4 inches tall, is about 120 pounds. Yet it is easy to find women of that same height who weigh less than 100 pounds and others who weigh more than 200 pounds. Such large variation does not seem consistent with a tightly regulated set-point system. Such is the picture when we look at the population. A look at individuals reveals another pattern. The range of one individual's body weight remains fairly small over periods of time.

set point: the biological weight above which the body tends to lose weight and below which it tends to gain weight.

It is thought that the body sends out signals to establish, regulate, and maintain the set point.[16] Yet these set-point regulators do more than maintain a constant body weight; they *defend* that body weight when it is challenged. People who have lost 25 percent of their body weight by restricting their dietary intake return to their normal weights when allowed to eat as they please. Similarly, people who increase their energy intake and gain 15 to 25 percent of their body weight return to their normal weight when allowed to eat as usual. This tenacious defense of body weight is unfortunate for obese people. It deters them from losing weight and encourages regaining of any weight that is successfully lost.

In using set-point regulation to explain obesity, researchers have asked several questions. How is set-point regulated? Regulation occurs in two ways. Weight loss triggers signals to increase food intake and reduce kcaloric expenditure. Weight gain triggers the opposite—reduced food intake and increased kcaloric expenditure. These changes in kcaloric expenditure may be due in part to activity level. However, the real difference is seen in an altered metabolism that becomes either more efficient with or more wasteful of its energy.

Another question asked is what mechanisms are involved in determining and regulating the set point. No one mechanism holds the answer. A body's set point could operate in many different ways. One of the ways is by fat cells; another is by inherited enzyme deficiencies; another way is by central nervous system sensitivities; another might be by the thermogenesis of brown fat.

If this theory is valid, it explains why many obese persons find it so hard to lose weight; perhaps their obesity should be accepted as normal. One proponent of the set point states, "Thus, if we view obese individuals as differing not in how they regulate body weight but rather in terms of the set point each is prepared to defend, we might better understand why [some people] remain at essentially the same body weight, without so much as trying, while others remain obese no matter how hard they try to change."[17] The theory is still controversial; even if it is valid, it is not yet possible to determine a person's set point independent of body weight—it can only be estimated from a person's weight over time. For example, a person who has weighed within a few pounds of 150 over the past several years is considered to have a set point of 150.

Genetics

We know very little about the heritability of human obesity. Genetic influences may help determine fat-cell number and size, regulate the efficiency of metabolic processes, and establish the sensitivity of the central nervous system to nutrient deprivation and repletion. Research on these possibilities is progressing.

monozygotic: originating from a single fertilized ovum; identical twins.

dizygotic: originating from two fertilized ova; fraternal twins.

Genetic studies involve observations of familial resemblances, twins, and adoptees. Familial resemblance studies strongly support the impression that obesity runs in families, but they cannot distinguish between genetic and environmental explanations for this tendency. Twin studies use estimates of heritability based on differences between the intrapair similarities of monozygotic and dizygotic twins. Adoption studies seem ideal in resolving the genetic-versus-environmental question, yet results of studies are frequently inconclusive.

Familial resemblance   The observation that obesity tends to run in families has stimulated debate over genetic versus environmental factors. No doubt, both genes and environment play a role, and interesting "family" factors emerge. When one parent is obese, the chances of infantile obesity's persisting are greater (40 percent) than when neither parent is obese (7 percent). If both parents are obese, the chances become quite likely (80 percent).[18] Similarities of "fatness" between people can be seen the longer they live together. Even the family dog shares the family's fatness profile.

A study of preschool children found strong relationships between parent and child body measurements. Both mothers' and fathers' weight for height measurements correlated with the children's weight-for-height, although mothers' measurements correlated more closely.[19]

Such family relationships are useful in the screening of children at risk for obesity. In addition, the degree of parental fatness can help in predicting the eventual severity of the child's obesity. Most important, in obese families, treatment should involve all family members.

Twin studies   Results from twin studies do suggest a genetic potential for obesity.[20] In fact, the genetic impact on fatness appears to be at least as strong as that seen in schizophrenia, alcoholism, and coronary heart disease. The concordance rate for weight of monozygotic twins is approximately twice as high as that for dizygotic twins. The influence of heredity on obesity appears to increase late in childhood, remaining high and fairly stable throughout adulthood.

Adoption studies   Adoption studies provide a natural experiment for contrasting the effects of heredity and environment. They assume that similarities between adopted children and their biological parents are genetically determined, while resemblances with adoptive parents must be environmental. Results from adoption studies usually demonstrate a significant similarity in obesity incidence between biological parents and their natural children, but not between adoptive parents and their adopted children.[21] The time of adoption is variable and may be an important factor considering the effects of early nutrition on the later development of obesity.

It is probably safe to say that fatness is not primarily inherited—at least not in the inflexible sense that blue eyes are inherited. Genetic influence appears to play an important role in determining obesity, but its expression is also influenced by environmental factors. Truly powerful genetic determinants of obesity governing metabolic pathways, such as the Prader-Willi syndrome, account for only a small percentage of obesity in human beings.

Prader-Willi syndrome: a debilitating hereditary disorder marked by childhood-onset obesity, mental retardation, small stature, small extremities, and a propensity toward diabetes.

Energy Balance and Metabolism

Several studies have reported that the energy intake of obese children is actually no greater than their normal-weight peers. Rather than answering any questions, such findings stimulate the search for explanations.

One explanation relies on the wide fluctuation in appetite that children experience. Children's appetites change daily, as do their energy intakes. The maximum daily intake for a child may be two to three times the minimum intake for that same child at any given age. Furthermore, the quantity of food eaten may not be reflected in the child's growth. So, if a study unknowingly compared an obese child's minimum kcaloric intake with a lean child's maximum kcaloric intake, it might reveal no difference. Or it might even seem to show that lean children ate more than obese ones.

Results that seem to imply that lean children eat more than obese ones may reflect the method of assessing kcaloric intake more than the reality of how much of what is eaten. For example, data based on recall interviews are of questionable reliability. Obese people will defensively minimize their food intake on self-report.

One study directly observed the eating and exercise habits of four families, each with an obese and nonobese brother within two years of each other in age. It made measurements weekly, for four to five months.[22] While findings from such a small sample are limited, the strengths of the method used make the results noteworthy. The obese boys consumed significantly more kcalories than did their nonobese brothers. Observers noted that, at home, the mothers tended to serve their obese sons larger amounts of food and that the nonobese boys left more food on their plates. At school lunch, the obese boys either purchased more food or bartered, begged, and bullied food from other children.

These results are in contrast to other studies indicating that obese children eat no more than lean children. Even the most basic question about childhood obesity—do obese children eat more than nonobese children?—has yet to be satisfactorily answered.

In one study of children, no correlation between individual energy intake and degree of fatness was apparent.[23] A relationship between energy intake and social class, however, was apparent, with the privileged-class diet providing less energy than that of the other social classes. The difference in kcaloric density of the diets was evident in the children's fatness. The lower social class had four times as many obese children as the upper social class. However, the energy intake of the children within a social class did not differ; that is, obese children had the same energy intake as their normal weight and lean peers.

Therefore, it seems appropriate to examine the diet of the social and cultural groups in which a child lives. The kcaloric density of the diet may overwhelm the regulating mechanisms of predisposed children. Obesity develops in these children even when they eat no differently than their peers.

Many obese people would like to believe they are overweight due to a "slow metabolism." Actually, metabolic disturbances account for a small percentage of childhood obesity. In fact, the basal metabolic rate (BMR) in obese people is often equal to or greater than the BMR in nonobese people. Because lean body mass is a primary determinant of the metabolic rate, and lean body mass as well as fat is increased in childhood obesity, the increased rate is easily explained.

On the other side of the energy balance scale is physical activity. Obese boys have been found to be far less active than their normal-weight brothers inside the home, slightly less active outside the home, and equally active on the school playground.[24] The biggest differences noted have been that obese boys spent more time sitting and standing and less time running. This picture changed dramatically when these activity measurements were converted from time spent into actual kcalorie expenditure. The kcalorie expenditure of obese boys at rest was greater than that of their nonobese brothers; being bigger, they required more kcalories just to maintain their weight. They also needed more kcalories to support their activity, of course: during activity, their kcalorie expenditure tripled as compared to their siblings' twofold increase.

Societal and Psychological Factors

Physical inactivity may be the most important environmental factor contributing to obesity. In the case of children, it may in turn be television that contributes most to physical inactivity. On the average, children in the United States spend as much time watching television as they do attending school. Little wonder that television viewing has become associated with a variety of child and teen behaviors. Several effects of watching television could contribute to obesity. First, television viewing requires no energy beyond the resting metabolic rate. Second, it replaces time spent in more vigorous activities. Third, watching television correlates with between-meal snacking, eating the kcalorically dense foods most heavily advertised on children's programs, and influencing family food purchases. The foods advertised on television tend not to be natural, whole, nutrient-dense foods, but rather the more processed, packaged foods that tend to be higher in fat, sugar, and kcalories, and lower in nutrients. Nonnutritious foods appear not only in commercials, but also within the television programs themselves. Children may miss the message that eating and drinking high-kcalorie foods will effect weight gain when they see television stars indulging in such behavior and remaining thin.

One study examined the data from the National Health and Nutrition Examination Survey (HANES) to determine whether obesity was associated with increased television watching.[25] Two cross-sectional samples and one longitudinal sample of children and adolescents in the United States were used. The findings reflect that children who watched more television had a greater prevalence of obesity (triceps fatfold at or above the 85th percentile) and superobesity (triceps fatfold at or above the 95th percentile) than children watching less television. In addition, evidence supported a dose-response relationship between obesity and time spent watching television. The prevalence of obesity increased by 2 percent for each additional hour of television viewed. This relationship between television and obesity held strong when control variables such as prior obesity and socioeconomic class were considered.

Food satisfies physical hunger and the biological need for energy and nutrients. Yet this simple function of food is often overshadowed by the role food plays in comforting people psychologically or connecting them with others socially. Food satisfies emotional hunger for some people.

The comfort function of food manifests itself in a particular pattern of obesity that reveals no family history of obesity. Described as a reactive obesity, it is an emotional overeating. It begins when a normal-weight child enters adolescence and grows fatter when a specific stressful event occurs. This may be a divorce, a cross-country move, or rejection by a friend. Oftentimes a look through the family photo album will alert a counselor to a major development in the young teen's life.

A **dose-response** relationship shows a correlation of increasing doses of one variable (in this case, television watching) with responses (in this case, obesity) such that the conclusion can be drawn that the more kids watch television, the more obese they are. It is stronger than a simple yes-no response (one group watches television and is obese; the other does not and is thin) because the correlation appears at all points along a continuum.

Eating Habits

One of the ways we learn is by observing the behavior of family members. Young children look to their parents and older siblings as role models in acquiring values, beliefs, and behavior patterns. Much of what we learn as youngsters persists into adulthood. This socialization process can be seen at the family dining table. Mealtime behavior is quite different for fatter and thinner children and their mothers.[26] For thinner children, mealtime provides social interaction as well as food. Fatter children and their mothers frequently have less social interactions during a meal. Obese parents also tend to overfeed their children and lack interest in physical activities. Passing this combination of overeating and underexercising on to another generation perpetuates familial obesity.

Patterns can be seen in the relationship between a child's degree of obesity and mother-child interactions.[27] Mothers of thinner children respond to their children more frequently with encouragement and approval. Mothers of fatter children provide fewer suggestions for performing a task, even when the children request assistance. In general, they offer less guidance and feedback. These observations, noted during playtime and mealtime, are consistent with opinions that obese children receive inappropriate or inconsistent responses to their expressions of need.[28] These are not limited to food-related situations, but involve all areas of daily life. This inconsistency in a family situation appears to have the power to precipitate eating disorders and weaken the child's ability to deal with problems.

This study did not report the degree of fatness of the mothers.[29] If the mother was obese, then perhaps, like the child, she too has an inability to deal with problems. She would be less able to help the child and to teach coping skills if they were lacking in herself.

Obesity seems to be a uniquely human phenomenon. Most animals in the wild or those fed standard rations do not overeat or become obese even when food is plentiful. This suggests that obesity is the result of psychological, cultural, and social influences. Animals do not face the many culinary challenges people encounter regularly. If they did, would they get fat? The possibility has been tested using laboratory rats.

Rats that had maintained normal weight eating lab chow were offered cookies, chocolate, salami, cheese, marshmallows, bananas, and peanut butter. Even though they still had the option of eating lab chow, the animals preferred the "supermarket diet" and gained more than 2 1/2 times as much weight as the controls.[30] Apparently, the animals found the supermarket foods more palatable than their accustomed meals, and so increased their food intake. The "supermarket diet" combined the three characteristics thought to be most effective in producing obesity—sweetness, greasiness, and variety—and it worked. The question was answered: special diets can make free-eating animals obese.

This experiment and others like it have demonstrated that the natural preference of both animals and human beings is for energy-dense foods. They are programmed to store energy. This was a useful mechanism during the evolutionary history of humankind when food was scarce and the food supply was unreliable. The body had to be prepared to survive times of famine. It relied on fat stores to get through those times. This same survival mechanism is detrimental in today's developed world because food scarcities rarely occur. In fact, this society surrounds us with abundant food and limits our physical exercise. Even those of us with only a mild susceptibility to obesity are bound to gain excess weight if we do not actively work to prevent it. Animals, equipped to store energy for the same reasons, become obese for the same reasons when they are placed in lab situations.

Another important consideration may be not what or how much children eat, but rather *how* they eat. Indeed, obese children do eat differently than their normal-weight peers. They take less time to complete a meal and, even more strikingly, they differ in their rates of kcalorie consumption. Obese boys eat twice as many kcalories per minute as their normal-weight siblings.[31] In general, obese children take more bites per minute and chew fewer times per bite than nonobese children.[32]

Whether an infant is breastfed and the age of introduction to solid foods are two other feeding habits that have been examined as possible links to obesity.[33] Most often, breastfed infants receive solid foods later than formula-fed infants. In fact, the longer a child is breastfed, the later solids are introduced (another dose-response relationship). The assumption that an early introduction of solids will lead to obesity has a physiological basis. Infants regulate their intake by volume, not by kcaloric density. A full stomach is a fine mechanism for monitoring breast milk or formula intake, but less adequate in regulating solid foods because they pack more kcalories per unit volume. Many solid foods offered to infants are more kcalorically dense than breast milk or formula.[34] In contrast to these theories and assumptions, studies do not support the hypothesis that early introduction of solids and duration of breastfeeding are related to obesity.[35]

Effects of Obesity

The single most important problem for obese children is the potential of becoming obese adults with all the social, economic, and medical ramifications. They have other problems, though, arising from differences in their growth, physical health, and psychological development.

On Growth

Obese children develop a characteristic set of physical traits. They begin puberty earlier and are taller than their peers, although they stop growing at a shorter height.[36] They develop greater bone and muscle mass, possibly because their skeletons respond to the demand of having to carry more weight—not only fat, but also fat-free weight. This causes them to appear "stocky" even when they lose any excess fat. They have a faster BMR, apparently due to their abundant lean body mass.

Factors seem to affect both fatness and maturity so that a relationship between obesity and maturation is evident, although not clearly understood. Early-maturing females are not only shorter than their peers, but fatter as well.[37] By age 30, they have accumulated 30 percent more fat. Such evidence of the inverse relationship between age of menarche and fatness in women is apparent throughout their lives.

On Physical Health

Obese infants do not have a higher mortality rate than normal-weight infants, but they are more likely to have respiratory infections and other illnesses. Like obese adults, obese children display an atherogenic profile—high total serum cholesterol, high serum triglycerides, high low-density lipoprotein (LDL) cholesterol and very-low-density lipoprotein (VLDL) cholesterol. These signs indicate that atherosclerosis is beginning to develop. Obese children also tend to have high blood pressure; in fact, obesity is the leading cause of pediatric hypertension.[38]

For all these reasons, prevention of excessive weight gain in childhood is important. It serves as an effective intervention in cardiovascular disease; atherosclerosis may be reversible with proper diet and exercise. Obese adolescents at high risk for the development of coronary heart disease can reduce that risk with exercise and moderate dietary restriction.[39] Weight reduction prior to or—at the latest—during adolescence is critical to forestalling this lifelong disease.

On Psychological Health

Obesity often causes psychological problems. People frequently react to others' body shapes and send signals that collectively create a "body concept." This body concept becomes incorporated into the person's total self-concept and behavior patterns.

Obese children have many of the same characteristics as minorities; they, too, are victims of prejudice. Many suffer discrimination by adults and rejection by their peers. They are teased and called names. They often have poor self-images, a sense of failure, and a passive approach to life. Television shows, which are a major influence in children's lives, frequently portray the fat person as the bumbling misfit.

The meaning body shape has for children is illustrated by some research in which children were asked to assign adjectives ascribing various behavior and personality traits to silhouettes representing extreme endomorph, mesomorph, and ectomorph body types.[40] Their responses revealed that they associated a common stereotype with each body image. They described the mesomorph favorably; they saw the endomorph in a socially unfavorable light; and they gave personally unfavorable adjectives to the ectomorph. These stereotypes were not related to the body type of the child assigning the description; overweight children themselves share the negative view of fat children. The general consensus is that obese children were children that they "did not like so well." No doubt, childhood obesity creates heartaches. Many children in this study were reasonably accurate in their perception of their own body shape. Children clearly preferred to look like the mesomorph image. In general, children believe thin children have more friends and are better looking and smarter than fat children. In fact, a common belief among obese people is that thin people have no problems.

W. H. Sheldon's classification of body types:

▶ Mesomorphic: having a husky, muscular body type.

▶ Endomorphic: having a heavy, rounded body build, often with a marked tendency to become fat.

▶ Ectomorphic: characterized by a light body build with slight muscular development.

Parents of obese children sometimes are overprotective. The children may not learn to trust their own impulses, becoming passive, demanding, frustrated, and dependent. Parental relationships that do not provide appropriate responses may give the child a feeling of being extra special, of needing to be bigger and better. Unfortunately, with such unrealistic goals, frustration is often encountered and is relieved through overeating—and so, a cycle begins.

Personality problems may also arise from the other physical changes that accompany obesity. Puberty comes earlier. For some young teens, staying fat is a way to avoid sexuality. They may overeat to postpone dealing with sexual feelings that accompany puberty. What effect a shortened childhood, or being one of the first in the class to begin the transition, has on a child is difficult to determine. The teen years are a time of finding a place in the social system. With that comes the overwhelming importance of what you look like, who your friends are, and what activities you are involved in. They are not easy years for most teens; obese teens have an added obstacle in their path.

Psychological reasons may or may not explain obesity, but obesity can cause psychological distress. Some part of treatment must focus on this distress; the counselor should at least be sensitive to it.

Treatment

With such a wide array of possible contributing causes, it is little wonder that a successful treatment for obesity has yet to be found. Medical science has worked wonders in preventing or curing many of even the most serious childhood diseases. Yet obesity remains without a surefire remedy. Once excess fat has been stored, it is stubbornly difficult to remove. As one authority on obesity noted, "If 'cure' from obesity is defined as reduction to ideal weight and maintenance of that weight for five years, then a person is more likely to recover from many forms of cancer than from obesity."[41]

Professionals need to recognize that obesity is indeed an obstinate disorder, and that each person's circumstances are unique. Not everyone is motivated to lose weight, and instilling motivation is difficult, if not impossible. Not all persons will lose weight even with strict adherence to a program, and those that do may not keep the weight off. Professionals and clients alike meet with frustration in treating obesity.

Parents and professionals need to realize that pressures on children to conform to the image presented by our society—"fat is ugly" and "thin is in"—create problems. Although not always easy to accomplish, a relaxed, nonjudgmental attitude toward the child, whatever the child's weight, will assure the best emotional growth potential. The child's individual needs must be considered and incorporated into treatment. Treatment also needs to consider the many aspects of the problem and possible solutions. An integrated approach involving diet, exercise, behavioral changes, and psychological support is recommended.

When evaluating obesity, fatness needs to be seen in light of the total needs of the child. Excess weight may only be a side effect of a psychosocial problem. In many cases, parents are part of the problem and the solution. Their ability to understand and follow through with a treatment is as critical to success as the involvement of the child. Because many treatment programs have a high rate of failure, it is important to ask if the consequences of failing at a weight loss attempt are worse than being overweight. Other questions to consider include: When is intervention most appropriate? Will the problem resolve itself without intervention? What are the child's needs and wants?

Before implementing a treatment program for a child, a caretaker must assess the medical, social, and economic risks of obesity. These must be balanced against the potential benefit of success and the possible harm of failure.

Diet

The only way to lose body fat is to establish a negative energy balance. Almost all of the causes of obesity respond to some degree to a combination of diet and exercise.

The initial goal for obese children is not to lose weight, but rather to stop gaining weight. Continued growth in height will then accomplish the desired change in weight for height. Treatment should begin with this conservative approach before other more drastic measures are taken.

The diet plan for weight reduction is easy to formulate; carrying it through to accomplish a permanent weight loss, however, is more difficult. Whether the goal is to treat or prevent obesity, the concept to teach is controlled eating. Children need to learn to eat foods that supply essential nutrients without consuming excess kcalories. Family meals should reflect kcalorie control in the foods selected and in the method of preparation.

Some physicians recommend a prudent diet to prevent and treat obesity. A prudent diet encourages normal weight gain without inhibiting growth or increasing the incidence of disease. By adopting the taste preferences and eating habits associated with a prudent diet, the child learns to select foods that prevent the deleterious effects on blood-lipid profile and blood pressure of a high-kcalorie, high-fat, high-salt diet.

Children are oftentimes unsuccessful in maintaining new eating habits and weight loss. The best we can hope for when children follow a specified diet program is that they will either lose a small amount of weight (less than ten pounds) or maintain their weight without a gain.

Diet therapy involves dietary counseling at intervals throughout various amounts of time. If the counseling is intense and effective, then short-term success may be seen. For the most part, dietary counseling is ineffective in the long run.

Physical Activity

Whether physical inactivity is a cause or a consequence of obesity, obese people are usually less physically active than their thinner peers.[42] They do not eagerly respond to the suggestion that they get more exercise. Their reluctance to exercise stems from a variety of experiences. The added weight and bulk of their bodies increases the effort required to perform activities, making some exercises uncomfortable or even painful. They may be self-conscious about the size of their bodies or have had embarrassing moments that discourage them

The prudent diet was developed by the American Heart Association for use with adults, but has been tested successfully and is recommended by some physicians for children over the age of 2.

Prudent Diet:

▶ 12% protein.
▶ 30% fat.
▶ 58% carbohydrate.

Eat More:

▶ Nonfat milk.
▶ Fish and poultry.
▶ Fruit.
▶ Vegetables.
▶ Whole grains.

Eat Less:

▶ Whole milk.
▶ Red meat and eggs.
▶ Sugar.
▶ Salt.
▶ Fat.

from exercising where others can watch. Needless to say, after years of avoiding exercise, many do not perform well at athletic activities. The many benefits of exercise are well known, but often are not incentive enough to motivate obese persons, especially children.[43] A large majority will quit exercise programs.

One key to a successful program is to begin at a level that is attainable and enjoyable, gradually increasing the intensity, duration, and frequency of exercise. Even though a short, slow-paced walk may have limited physical benefits, the psychological effects will be positive. The person is actively doing something constructive toward attacking obesity.

Social Support

Social factors play a key role in influencing people. Support or lack of support from family and friends can help or hinder a person's recovery process. The long-term nature of a social system offers the potential for a lasting effect. Two social-support systems have been studied in obesity treatment for children: parental involvement and school programs.

Parental involvement   Just as parents may have a critical role in the development of their child's obesity, so too can their involvement in a treatment program be significant. Programs that involve parents in treatment report greater weight losses. When parents are not involved, obesity treatment programs are less successful. Because obesity in parents and children tends to be positively correlated, both benefit from a weight-loss program.

Parental attitudes about food greatly influence their children's eating behavior. Unaware that they are teaching their children, parents pass on lessons at the dinner table, on television trays, and in drive-through restaurants. Parents who have battled aginst being overweight themselves and failed may model for their children the behaviors that have led them to failure—eating too much, dieting inappropriately, exercising too little. Those who have fears about their offspring's being overweight may teach their children fears that are unproductive.

Many childhood obesity treatment programs do include parents. Some provide specific instructions, while others allow passive observation. In general, the parent's role is to:

► Provide a nutritionally adequate diet.
► Serve food under pleasant conditions.
► Allow the child to eat according to need.
► Allow the child to eat without being nagged or cajoled.
► Encourage the child to enjoy nutritious foods.
► Encourage the child to exercise.

One program was designed to assess three methods of parental involvement in the treatment of obese adolescents (12 to 16 years old).[44] The groups were: Mother-Child Separately—children and mothers attended separate groups; Mother-Child Together—children and mothers met together in the

Benefits of exercise:

► Increases energy expenditure.
► Enhances the thermogenesis produced by eating.
► Increases metabolic rate.
► Lowers blood pressure.
► Changes blood-lipid levels.
► Increases self-esteem.
► Improves coronary efficiency.
► Suppresses appetite.

same group; and Child Alone— children met in groups and mothers were not involved. All children received the same treatment; the only difference was parental involvement. The program involved behavior modification, nutrition education, exercise instruction, and social support. The Mother-Child Separately group lost more weight during treatment than did the other two groups. This group also maintained the loss for a year, compared with gains in the other two groups. While parental involvement can have an effect on weight loss, the kind of involvement is as critical as its presence or absence.

Parental involvement had a powerful effect on the child's weight loss, yet there was no relation between changes in children's weight and changes in mother's weight. Perhaps this was because not all mothers needed to lose weight or no effort was made to encourage mothers to lose weight. A trend was seen in obese mothers losing more weight than nonobese mothers, but this was not significant. Nor did it seem to matter which group the mother was in.

School programs   The school can play a three-part role in treating childhood obesity, by way of the foods served, the exercise program, and the classroom teaching. The school cafeteria can offer lunches that not only meet the nutrient needs of children, but are also low in kcalories. Nutrient-dense snacks can replace empty-kcalorie ones.

In physical education class, the emphasis should be on lifelong activities. Physical activities that can be done alone and at any age with minimal equipment are most valuable in adulthood. An instructor who instills motivation and enthusiasm for athletics serves students well.

In the classroom, nutrition education can affect eating behaviors. Teachers may want to include lessons on:

► Body fatness.
► Relative kcalorie value of foods.
► Relative kcalorie value of activities.
► Nutrient density.
► Energy balance.
► Benefits of exercise.
► Changing needs throughout the life cycle.
► Food sources and variety.
► Cooking.
► Learning to enjoy tastes of new foods.

The public school system offers many opportunities to attack the problem of obesity.[45] It can reach a large number of children, the treatment can be continuous, and it can be offered at minimal cost. The setting is also conducive to nutrition education, an important facet of treatment. Perhaps most importantly, a broad base of social support can be established. School personnel, family, and peers can offer an obese child the reinforcement needed to continue efforts in a weight-loss program.

One school-based program using behavior modification, nutrition education, and physical activity involved such a social network.[46] A positive social environment was created in which the child received support from parents, a nurse's aide, teachers, peers, lunchroom personnel, and school administrators. These people received information on the child's treatment program and were instructed in ways of providing emotional support. The results showed a significant weight loss in contrast to the steady gains noted in the three years prior to treatment. Children not included in the program continued to gain weight relative to their heights, clearly headed for obesity as adults.

Behavioral Therapy

Behavior modification techniques have shown modest success when used to control obesity in children. In contrast to traditional weight-loss programs that focus on *what* to eat, behavioral programs focus also on *how* to eat. These techniques involve changing learned habits that lead a child to eat excessively. Several principles are involved.

Self-monitoring   The child keeps a careful record of food eaten and physical activity. This procedure provides baseline information and heightens awareness of dietary patterns such as portion sizes and snack times. In some cases, the procedure itself favorably alters the behavior.

Stimulus control   Stimulus control limits problems by keeping high-kcalorie foods out of the house. By eliminating the cues that trigger the desire to eat, children can learn skills in modifying eating behavior. They are encouraged to eat at scheduled times and to avoid other activities (such as watching television) while eating.

Stimulus-control procedures:

▶ Do not bring high-kcalorie foods into the home.
▶ Remove serving dishes from the table.
▶ Eat meals at the dining table only at set times.
▶ Leave some food on the plate.
▶ Use smaller plates.
▶ Eat slowly.

Family involvement   Family involvement is crucial to the successs of treatment programs for childhood obesity. Family members can provide emotional support and reinforcement for adhering to a diet and exercise program.

Reinforcement   Items are given to reward attaining goals. It is most effective to use small, tangible items and to reward frequently at the attainment of small goals.

Cognitive restructuring   This practice encourages positive, realistic thinking in place of illogical and self-defeating thoughts. Cognitive restructuring has three major components. The first, success rehearsal, mentally prepares a child for handling new or difficult situations. By role-playing and rehearsing high-risk situations, a child can learn to anticipate possible setbacks and appropriate coping strategies. The second component minimizes self-disappointment by recognizing failings and renewing plans to do better. Rather than overindulging after having "blown it," a person can simply return to the program without feelings of guilt. The third component teaches children how to handle teasing and criticism about their weight and how to identify their positive characteristics. Learning to cope with size and appearance and to increase self-esteem is a part of growing up for children of all shapes and sizes. Like other children, the overweight child needs to grow and mature in a positive environment.

Harmful Treatments

While drugs are occasionally used to treat adult obesity, they should not be used to manage obesity in children. The possible side effects and potential for abuse make drug therapy a dangerous route for treating growing children.

Severe energy restriction (less than 1000 to 1200 kcalories per day) must also be avoided, especially in the first few years of life. The growth of the child can be compromised with inadequate nutrients and energy. The aim of a restrictive diet is to have the child maintain weight while "outgrowing" obesity.

Weight loss without exercise can also have a negative effect on body composition, especially if the weight is regained. A person who diets without exercising loses both lean and fat tissue. If the person then gains weight without exercising, more fat than lean is gained. Fat tissue is less active metabolically than lean tissue, and so the person's daily energy expenditure is less. Each time a person loses weight and regains it without exercising, that person's metabolism requires fewer kcalories. If the person eats the same amount as before the last diet, the person will not maintain, but will gain weight. This is one explanation for the ratchet effect of dieting and underlies the importance of exercise as part of a weight-loss plan.

ratchet effect: the effect of repeated rounds of dieting; the person rebounds to a higher weight (and higher body fat content) at the end of each round.

Obesity is prevalent in our society. Its far-reaching effects make the need to remedy it urgent. Yet the wide and varied spectrum of interacting factors causing obesity makes solutions difficult. The prevention and treatment of obesity is frequently unsuccessful. Perhaps as research continues and our understanding of obesity becomes clearer, the answers will become more evident, the treatment more successful.

Focal Point 5 Notes

1. J. L. Knittle, Obesity in childhood: A problem in adipose tissue cellular development, *Journal of Pediatrics* 81 (1972): 1048–1059.
2. K. J. Morgan, M. E. Zabik, and G. A. Leveille, Food consumption and weight/height ratios of children, *Agricultural Experiment Station Research Report* 459 (1984): 1–12.
3. W. H. Dietz, Jr., Childhood obesity: Susceptibility, cause, and management, *Journal of Pediatrics* 103 (1983): 676–686.
4. M. F. Rolland-Cachera and coauthors, Adiposity rebound in children: A simple indicator for predicting obesity, *American Journal of Clinical Nutrition* 39 (1984): 129–135.
5. Morgan, Zabik, and Leveille, 1984.
6. Dietz, 1983.
7. C. L. Shear and coauthors, Secular trends of obesity in early life: The Bogalusa Heart Study, *American Journal of Public Health* 78 (1988): 75–77.
8. J. Kirtland and M. I. Gurr, Adipose cellularity: A review, *International Journal of Obesity* 3 (1979): 15–55.
9. Knittle, 1972.
10. A. Hager and coauthors, Body fat and adipose tissue cellularity in infants: A longitudinal study, *Metabolism* 26 (1977): 607–613.
11. J. L. Knittle and coauthors, The growth of adipose tissue in children and adolescents, *Journal of Clinical Investigation* 63 (1979): 239–246.
12. Knittle and coauthors, 1979.
13. M. Winick, Childhood obesity, *Nutrition Today*, May/June 1974, pp. 6–12.
14. M. R. McMinn, Mechanisms of energy balance in obesity, *Behavioral Neuroscience* 98 (1984): 375–393.
15. McMinn, 1984.
16. R. E. Keesey, A set-point analysis of the regulation of body weight, in *Obesity,* ed. A. J. Stunkard (Philadelphia: W. B. Saunders Company, 1980), pp. 144–165.
17. Keesey, 1980.
18. Winick, 1974.
19. R. E. Patterson and coauthors, Factors related to obesity in preschool children, *Journal of the American Dietetic Association* 86 (1986): 1376–1381.
20. A. J. Stunkard, T. T. Foch, and Z. Hrubec, A twin study of human obesity, *Journal of the American Medical Association* 256 (1986): 51–54.
21. A. J. Stunkard and coauthors, An adoption study of human obesity, *New England Journal of Medicine* 314 (1986): 193–198.
22. M. Waxman and A. J. Stunkard, Caloric intake and expenditure of obese boys, *Journal of Pediatrics* 96 (1980): 187–193.
23. M. F. Rolland-Cachera and F. Bellisle, No correlation between adiposity and food intake: Why are working class children fatter?, *American Journal of Clinical Nutrition* 44 (1986): 779–787.
24. Waxman and Stunkard, 1980.

25. W. H. Dietz, Jr., and S. L. Gortmaker, Do we fatten our children at the television set? Obesity and television viewing in children and adolescents, *Pediatrics* 75 (1985): 807–812.

26. L. L. Birch and coauthors, Mother-child interaction patterns and the degree of fatness in children, *Journal of Nutrition Education* 13 (1981): 17–21.

27. Birch and coauthors, 1981.

28. H. Bruch, Family transactions in eating disorders, *Comprehensive Psychiatry* 12 (1971): 238–248.

29. Birch and coauthors, 1981.

30. A. Sclafani and D. Springer, Dietary obesity in adult rats: Similarities to hypothalamic and human obesity syndromes, *Physiology and Behavior* 17 (1976): 461–471.

31. Waxman and Stunkard, 1980.

32. R. S. Drabman, D. Hammer, and G. J. Jarvie, Eating rates of elementary school children, *Journal of Nutrition Education* 9 (1977): 80–82.

33. J. H. Himes, Infant feeding practices and obesity, *Journal of the American Dietetic Association* 75 (1979): 122–125.

34. Himes, 1979.

35. P. G. Wolman, Feeding practices in infancy and prevalence of obesity in preschool children, *Journal of the American Dietetic Association* 84 (1984): 436–438; S. Dubois, D. E. Hill, G. H. Beaton, An examination of factors believed to be associated with infantile obesity, *American Journal of Clinical Nutrition* 32 (1979): 1997–2004; D. L. Yeung and coauthors, Infant fatness and feeding practices: A longitudinal assessment, *Journal of the American Dietetic Association* 79 (1981): 531–535; R. E. Patterson and coauthors, Factors related to obesity in preschool children, *Journal of the American Dietetic Association* 86 (1986): 1376–1381.

36. J. L. Knittle and coauthors, Childhood obesity, in *Textbook of Pediatric Nutrition*, ed. R. M. Suskind (New York: Raven Press, 1981), pp. 415–434.

37. S. M. Garn and coauthors, Maturational timing as a factor in female fatness and obesity, *American Journal of Clinical Nutrition* 43 (1986): 879–883.

38. L. K. Rames and coauthors, Normal blood pressures and the evaluation of sustained blood pressure elevation in children: The Muscatine Study, *Pediatrics* 61 (1978): 245–251.

39. M. D. Becque and coauthors, Coronary risk incidence of obese adolescents: Reduction by exercise plus diet intervention, *Pediatrics* 81 (1988) 605–612.

40. J. R. Staffieri, A study of social stereotype of body image in children, *Journal of Personality and Social Psychology* 7 (1967): 101–104.

41. K. D. Brownell, Ph.D.

42. Shear and coauthors, 1988.

43. K. D. Brownell and A. J. Stunkard, Physical activity in the development and control of obesity, in *Obesity* ed. A. J. Stunkard (Philadelphia: W. B. Saunders Co., 1980).

44. K. D. Brownell, J. H. Kelman, and A. J. Stunkard, Treatment of obese children with and without their mothers: Changes in weight and blood pressure, *Pediatrics* 71 (1983): 515–523.

45. C. C. Seltzer and J. Mayer, An effective weight control program in a public school system, *American Journal of Public Health* 60 (1970): 679–689.

46. K. D. Brownell and F. S. Kaye, A school-based behavior modification, nutrition education, and physical activity program for obese children, *American Journal of Clinical Nutrition* 35 (1982): 277–282.

Adolescence: Changing Times

6

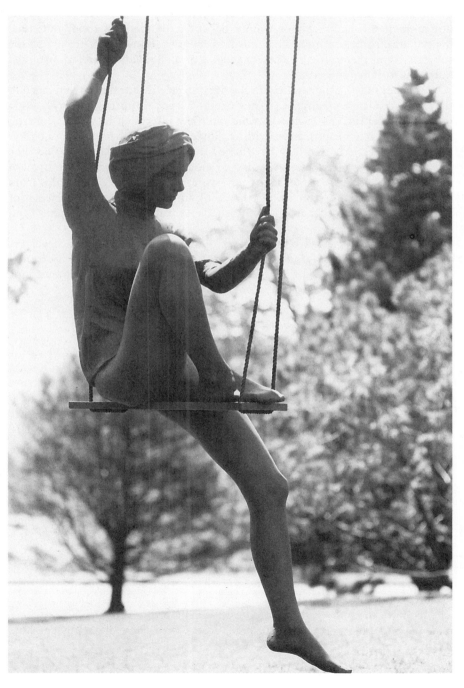

259

Girl on a Swing by Richard Fleischner.

The teen years are a time of change—the child is becoming an adult. Changes are evident in the physical body, emotional maturity, and intellectual achievements. As expected, nutrient needs are high during this time of growth, and the challenge to make sure that nutrient intakes match the needs continues.

One element of great importance in the transition from child to teen is that teens make many more choices for themselves than they did as children. Teens are not fed; they eat. They are not sent out to play; they choose whether to invest their energy seriously in sports. Therefore the person concerned with the nutrition of teenagers cannot simply deliver it to them as food, but must instead inspire motivation. That means becoming knowledgeable about the subjects teens themselves are interested in, and showing the relationship of nutrition to those subjects.

Another major element, new in the life of teens, is that they are engaged in the effort to define themselves. They are all wrapped up in their own body images and self-images. Some become intensely interested in weight control, even to the point of obsession with it. Some become concerned about their complexions, especially if they have acne (or even one pimple). Many become interested in physical fitness, and some develop self-images as athletes. In all of their interests, they are susceptible to pressures from the media, and also from their peers, as well as from adults they look up to. Thus a whole new set of topics appear in this chapter—topics such as eating disorders, acne, and athletics.

A few teenage girls face pregnancies, while their own nutrition needs for growth are still high and difficult to meet. A section of this chapter is devoted to their special needs, and the Focal Point that follows investigates questions related to the use of alcohol, tobacco, and other drugs.

Growth and Development

The rate of growth, which has been fairly steady throughout childhood, rises abruptly and dramatically with the onset of adolescence. The adolescent growth spurt is genetically controlled, with its intensity and duration mediated by hormones. For females, the spurt begins between the ages of 10 1/2 and 11 years and peaks around age 12; for males, the spurt begins between the ages of 12 1/2 and 13 years and peaks around age 14.[1] The duration is between 2 and 2 1/2 years. Of course, wide variations are seen for individuals.

The early stage of adolescent growth is linear; the child "shoots up." Males add approximately eight inches in height during the growth spurt; females, six inches. Skeletal growth ceases with the closure of the epiphyses. The later stage of the spurt is lateral; the child "fills out." Males add approximately 45 pounds to their weight; females, about 35 pounds.[2]

Many changes in body shape and posture become evident during adolescence. The first areas to accelerate growth are the feet and hands, then the calves and forearms, followed by the hips and chest, and then the shoulders.[3] The trunk of the body is the last to go through a growth spurt. This sequence of development takes teenagers through an awkward phase of having large and ungainly limbs compared with the rest of the body.

epiphyses: the end segments of long bones that contain a thin area of active bone growth; this growth eventually stops, after which no further significant growth can occur.

Before puberty, the differences between male and female body composition are minimal. Sex differences in the skeletal system, lean body mass, and fat stores become apparent during the adolescent spurt.[4] In males, the shoulders grow substantially. In females, the pelvis becomes wide, shallow, and spacious in preparation for childbearing. During the growth spurt, males increase their lean body mass more than females.

Just prior to the adolescent growth spurt, body fat begins to increase.[5] During the male growth spurt, total body fat decreases. Females have no such decrease and, in fact, lay down additional fat. Additional fat deposition dramatically alters body shape. Why females deposit fat in specific locations is unknown, although the fat in the breasts does protect the mammary glands and provide energy for future gestation and lactation needs.

Hormones control the secondary sex changes experienced by both males and females. The earliest sign of puberty in males is the growth of the testicles and penis.[6] Changes in the larynx, skin, and hair distribution follow. The earliest internal sign of puberty for females is growth of the ovaries.[7] Externally, the breasts enlarge and pubic hair appears. Menarche occurs after the peak of growth in height and corresponds with maximum growth deceleration.[8] With growth slowing rapidly, a female can expect to grow perhaps an additional three inches in height after menarche.

menarche: definition appears on page 16.

Growth is reflected not only in the changing size of the body, but in the relative proportions of the body's water, fat, and lean tissues. The greatest change in body composition in females during the adolescent growth spurt is seen in the ratio of lean body weight to fat. Of course, the total amount of body fat varies with females of different sizes, but the percentage of body weight as fat (22 percent) and the ratio of lean body weight to fat (3 to 1) at menarche appear always to fall within a specific range.

Researchers have attempted to define the relationship between growth and menarche, suggesting that a minimum amount of body fat is required for the onset of menses.[9] Not all studies support the hypothesis that menarche depends on a minimal amount of body fat. One study found no relationship between body size or composition and the onset of sexual maturity in female adolescents who had been undernourished as young children.[10] These adolescents were much smaller than their well-nourished peers even at the same stage of sexual development.

Throughout childhood, hemoglobin and red blood cells steadily increase. During the adolescent growth spurt, hemoglobin concentration and red blood cell number rise considerably; no corresponding spurt occurs in the number of white blood cells.[11] The heart muscle grows markedly, resulting in a rise in blood pressure and a fall in heart rate.

Mean hemoglobin values for adolescents:

▶ 10 yr: 13.0 g/100 ml.

▶ 12 yr: 13.4 g/100 ml.

▶ >14 yr: 13.9 g/100 ml (females).
     15.8 g/100 ml (males).

Development during the adolescent period depends not only on the individual's present nutrition status, but also on previous nutrient intake. Several studies have examined the impact of undernutrition in early childhood on adolescent growth. A follow-up study of adolescent females who had suffered varying degrees of undernutrition during early childhood revealed that undernutrition in early life diminished eventual body size.[12] Malnourished children are shorter and lighter than their well-nourished peers at the end of the adolescent growth spurt. But undernourished children add more to their height during their growth spurt than do well-nourished children; weight gains are comparable. In other words, adolescence serves as a catch-up period to

Mean hematocrit values for adolescents:

▶ 10 yr: 39.0%.

▶ 12 yr: 39.6%.

▶ >14 yr: 42.0% (females).
     47.0% (males).

regain some growth losses due to undernutrition in the early years. A possible explanation for the greater increment in height seen in females could be delayed menarche. Menarche is delayed by two years in females undernourished as children.[13] With delayed menarche, epiphyseal fusion is delayed, and this allows for a longer period of rapid growth. Delayed sexual maturation is also reported in males undernourished as children. Their attainment of sexual maturity is postponed by up to three years.

Biochemical values shift from "normal" child values to "normal" adult values during adolescence. Some biochemical measurements parallel the growth pattern, rising with the growth velocity, and serve as useful indicators of physical maturity.[14] When assessing adolescent growth and nutrient status, the health care provider must consider many changes and individual variations that occur during this time. For example, the stage of sexual maturation affects assessment of adolescent serum zinc concentrations. Males and females who have reached adult sexual maturity have higher serum zinc concentrations than adolescents at less mature stages.[15]

Nutrient Needs and Eating Patterns

The rapid growth that occurs during adolescence is reflected in the high nutrient needs of this period. In general, *total* nutrient needs are greater during adolescence than at any other time of life, with the exception of pregnancy and lactation. Nutrient and food energy deficiencies during this time can retard growth and delay sexual maturation.

Chronological age provides an inappropriate timetable for measuring development and stating requirements. Growth would be preferable. Yet, because it is easy to keep track of age and it works in a general way, age is most often used in establishing guidelines. The RDA split the teen years into four-year blocks, on the assumption that the physical changes that occur during those periods are similar for most adolescents. The amount of change in each nutrient need during adolescent growth varies with each individual. Needs depend on the age of puberty onset, the velocity of growth, and the length of time required to complete the maturation process.

Energy-Yielding Nutrients

Protein RDA
11–14 yr: 45 g (males).
46 g (females).
15–18 yr: 56 g (males).
46 g (females).

The body requires energy and protein for metabolic processes, physical activity, and growth. When compared on a per-kilogram-body-weight basis, the energy and protein allowances for adolescents are lower than for younger age groups. However, when total values for the average individual are compared, energy and protein allowances for adolescents are greater than for any other age group. Caution is offered that the energy recommendations for the adolescent years may not be appropriate for all individuals. Activity, growth, and tendency toward obesity must be considered in determining the appropriate energy allowance for each individual.

Vitamins

Recommended allowances for vitamins are based on body weight and growth needs. The RDA for most vitamins increase with age and body weight (see RDA table on the inside front cover). Several of the nutrient recommendations for adolescents are the same as those for adults. One exception is vitamin D. The special role of vitamin D in skeletal growth is reflected in a higher RDA during the adolescent growing years (10 μg) than in adulthood (5 μg).

Minerals

A look at the RDA table reveals that the RDA for magnesium, zinc, and iodine rise from low values for children to high values at adolescence and remain there for adults. For calcium and phosphorus, the RDA reach a peak during the adolescent years and return to preadolescent values for adults.

Calcium needs are high during adolescence. Milk consumption is encouraged during adolescence, primarily to provide the calcium needed for skeletal growth. The benefits of young people's consuming calcium-rich foods today reach far into the future. Frequent and adequate milk consumption prior to and during adolescence supports the attainment of optimal bone density (within genetic limits, of course).[16] Bones grow not only in length, but also in density during the adolescent growth spurt. High bone density achieved in early life is the major defense against osteoporotic fractures in later life. It may be difficult to convince a young person to invest in tomorrow's health, but there is little question that prevention is the best treatment of osteoporosis.

Calcium
1980 RDA: 1200 mg (11-18 yr).

Iron needs are also high during adolescence. Iron status is most affected during four times of life: in infancy, during growth spurts, during the female reproductive years, and in pregnancy.[17] All adolescents are in growth spurts, and half of them are females in their reproductive years. During periods of growth, blood volume and muscle mass are increased, thus increasing the iron need for hemoglobin and myoglobin synthesis. The RDA for iron during adolescence is the same for males and females. Females have greater iron losses from menstruation, while males have greater needs to build and maintain a larger blood volume and muscle mass.[18] For females, the high values at adolescence remain high for adults. For adult males, they return to preadolescent values.

Iron
1980 RDA: 18 mg (11–18 yr).
1987 RDI: 12 mg (10–17 yr males).
15 mg (10–50 yr females).

Eating Patterns and Nutrient Intakes

Perhaps the safest generalization that can be made about adolescent eating patterns is that no one pattern exists. At any given time on any given day, a teenager may be skipping a meal, eating a snack, preparing a meal, or consuming food prepared by a parent or restaurant.

Meals and snacks Using 24-hour food records, one study examined the meal and snack patterns of adolescents and offered a glimpse of what might be considered typical of teenage eating patterns.[19] Approximately one-third of the adolescents skipped breakfast. Not too surprisingly, breads and cereals were the popular breakfast foods and milk the most common beverage consumed by those students who did eat breakfast. Students who omitted breakfast had lower total nutrient and food energy intakes for the whole day than those who did eat breakfast. These differences were even greater than the intake quantities of the breakfast meals, indicating that the breakfast eaters made better food choices and consumed more energy throughout the day. Breakfast skippers did not compensate for lost nutrients and energy at other eating times.

Almost 75 percent of the students ate lunches scored as "good"—that is, meals that provided adequate protein, vitamins, and minerals. Most of the lunch-eating students ate food brought from home or purchased from the school cafeteria. The most popular lunch food was a sandwich.

Almost all of the adolescents ate an evening meal at home or at the home of a friend or relative. These evening meals contributed significantly to daily intakes of nutrients and provided more than one-third of the total food energy. Most evening meals included foods such as cheese, meat, eggs, potatoes, bread, and pasta. The beverage of choice was a soft drink.

Most of the adolescents ate one or more snacks, providing approximately one-third of the daily food energy intake. On the average, the snacks were lower in nutrients than the meals. However, the snacks were not always "empty kcalories," but did contribute to daily nutrient intakes. Typical snack foods such as carbonated beverages, candies, desserts, and chips were popular, but many teenagers selected breads, cereals, meats, and milk products for snacks.

Independence is especially valued during the teen years, and food selection is one way to express it. Half of the breakfast eaters prepared their own meals, and one-third of the adolescents either prepared their evening meals or selected from restaurant menus (see Practical Point: Fast Food). However, independence has its price: adolescents who prepared their own meals consumed less of several nutrients than those who ate parent-prepared meals.

In this study, males met the RDA for all nutrients except iron; females met the RDA for all nutrients except iron, calcium, and vitamin A. These inadequacies are frequently reported in nutrient intake studies of teenagers.[20] In addition, various studies have reported dietary inadequacies of vitamin B_6, zinc, folacin, iodine, vitamin D, and magnesium prevalent among adolescent girls.[21] The gender difference in diet adequacy primarily reflects the males' consuming larger quantities of food.

Another study took a closer look at adolescent beverage consumption patterns using a 24-hour recall and two-day diet records.[22] Similar to the findings from the previous study, this study found that milk is more likely to be consumed with a meal (especially breakfast) than as a snack. Most adolescents drink milk, but males drink larger quantities than females. Fruit juice is consumed primarily at breakfast. Soft drinks are likely to be consumed with lunch, supper, or snacks.

The study then asked what impact soft drinks had on the nutrient intakes of adolescents. The greatest impact was found for calcium intake, which varied inversely with soft-drink consumption. For males, high soft-drink users met almost 90 percent of the calcium RDA, whereas female high soft-drink users met only approximately two-thirds of the RDA.

In addition to displacing milk (and therefore calcium intake), some researchers are concerned that soft drinks may threaten bone integrity in

Fast Food

Teenagers eat many meals away from home, quite often fast-food fare. They find the convenience and relative low cost of fast foods accommodating to their lifestyles. Fast foods do not necessarily mean total abandonment of nutrition. They have an acceptable place in a teenager's diet provided such meals do not dominate the diet and that their shortcomings are compensated for at other meals. A fast-food meal once a week or so has little impact on a teenager's overall diet. Teenagers who consume fast-food meals frequently, however, are wise to vary their menu selections and pay close attention to their other meal selections.

One shortcoming of a fast-food meal is its high energy content. A typical lunch of a hamburger, french fries, and a chocolate milk shake provides 860 kcalories, many of them (37 percent) from fats. Fast foods can be extraordinarily high in fat because most of the items either contain meat, are fried, or are made with whole milk. Many fast-food establishments list the kcalorie, fat, and cholesterol contents of their products, allowing customers to choose meals compatible with their needs. Teenagers wanting to limit their energy intakes should select lower-kcalorie menu items, eliminate high-kcalorie toppings such as mayonnaise and salad dressing, choose fewer items, or limit energy intake at other meals.

Active teenagers may be able to afford a kcalorically-expensive fast-food meal provided they receive substantial percentages of their recommended intakes for several nutrients. Such is the case for the hamburger, french fries, and milk shake fast-food meal which contributes its share of protein, thiamin, riboflavin, niacin, vitamin B_{12}, calcium, and iron to a day's intake. As is true of most fast-food meals, however, this one falls short in its contribution to a day's intake of fiber, vitamin A, folacin, and vitamin C. Teenagers wanting to eat fast-food meals can compensate for their lack of these vitamins and fiber by eating a large salad, several fruits, and a generous serving of dark green vegetables at other meals and snacks during the day. Snacks rich in the nutrients that are missing from meals can bring an inadequate diet up to par.

Snacks are a part of the teenage lifestyle. They fit in nicely when socializing, studying, working, playing, and relaxing. Because they are a part of the daily food intake, snacks need to provide nutrients. To get extra iron into the day's intake, a teenager might snack on bran muffins, hard-boiled eggs, or crackers with peanut butter. Calcium is available from yogurt, cheese, and ice cream (if the kcalories can be afforded). Good vitamin A snack ideas include carrot and broccoli pieces, apricots, peaches, and cheddar cheese.

another way—by inhibiting calcium absorption with their high phosphorus content.[23] Manufacturers add phosphoric acid to colas and root beers and phosphate salts to powdered beverage mixes. The combination of a low calcium intake with a high phosphorus intake alters the calcium-to-phosphorus ratio, which may influence calcium absorption. Researchers debate the ideal calcium-to-phosphorus ratio and have suggested ratios between 2 to 1 and 1 to 2.[24] The consensus seems to be that as long as calcium intake is adequate, its absorption will not be inhibited by a high phosphorus intake.

Supplement use   In addition to food and beverages, supplements offer nutrients to a few adolescents. Approximately 10 percent of adolescents report taking vitamin and mineral supplements.[25] These adolescents are more likely to take single-nutrient supplements than multivitamin and mineral preparations.

Teenage Pregnancy

The teen years are a time of sexual awareness. Young people are experiencing new changes in their bodies and relationships with others. The number of females having sexual intercourse increases from less than 20 percent to 55 percent between the ages of 15 and 19.[26] Percentages for males are slightly higher. With this sexual activity comes the responsibility of contraception. Teenagers who do practice contraception most often use oral contraceptives.[27]

The impact of oral contraceptive use on nutrient status is discussed in Chapter 1.

Health and Nutrition Implications

Nine out of ten sexually active teenagers who do not use contraception become pregnant within a year. The birthrate among teenagers in the United States is higher than that in most developed countries, as shown in Figure 6–1.[28] Even though it has declined in all countries in the last decade, teenage pregnancy continues to be a major problem in the United States.[29] One out of every ten teenage girls becomes pregnant each year. Of these approximately 1 million teens, more than half give birth.[30] Putting it another way, one out of five women bears a child before reaching her 20th birthday.[31]

The timing of adolescent growth and sexual maturation varies greatly among teenagers, but, in general, females attain physiological maturity about four years after menarche.[32] Pregnancy before the end of these four years, while the mother is still growing, presents serious threats to health. The demands of pregnancy compete with those of growth, placing the young female at high risk for pregnancy complications.

Perhaps the greatest risk of a teenage pregnancy is death of the infant. The infant mortality rate for mothers under age 20 is high, with mothers under 15 having the highest rate of all age groups.[33] A closer look at infant mortality reveals that the risks to infants of young mothers are greatest during the first month of life. Problems that arise shortly after birth reflect gestational problems.

The complications of premature birth are discussed in Chapters 2 and 4.

When reviewing infant mortality rates, researchers must consider the role of premature, low-birthweight infants, for these infants have the highest risk of mortality. The percentage of low-birthweight infants is greater for teenage mothers than for any other age group.[34] In fact, premature birth is the most critical aspect of teenage pregnancy because of its associated risk of mortality.

Figure 6–1   Birthrates among Adolescents
The national birthrates per 1000 women aged 15–19 as reported in 1980 are shown in
rank order. Pregnancy rates were only available for one-third of the nations listed here
but, in general, seemed to follow a similar ranking. As you can see, the United States has
a higher pregnancy rate than all but a few developed countries.

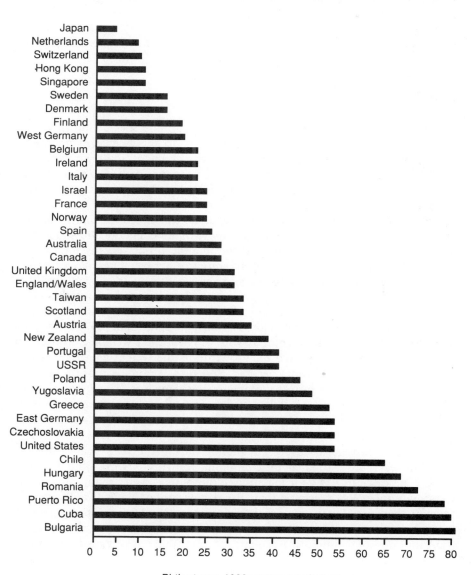

Birthrate per 1000 women aged 15-19 years

Source: Adapted from E. F. Jones and coauthors, *Teenage Pregnancy in Industrialized
Countries: A Study sponsored by the Alan Guttmacher Institute* (New Haven: Yale University
Press, 1986), pp. 251–255.

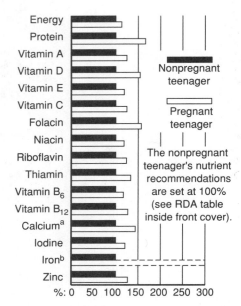

Energy
Protein
Vitamin A
Vitamin D
Vitamin E
Vitamin C
Folacin
Niacin
Riboflavin
Thiamin
Vitamin B6
Vitamin B12
Calcium^a
Iodine
Iron^b
Zinc

%: 0   50 100 150 200 250 300

■ Nonpregnant teenager

□ Pregnant teenager

The nonpregnant teenager's nutrient recommendations are set at 100% (see RDA table inside front cover).

^aRecommended intakes of phosphorous and magnesium change similarly.

^bThe pregnant woman may need to take an iron supplement—the pregnant woman needs the RDA of 18 mg of iron, as shown here, only if her iron nutrition has been optimal prior to pregnancy—a rare case. Usually her iron needs cannot be met by ordinary diets, and she requires a supplement.

Figure 6–2   Nutrient Needs of Pregnant and Nonpregnant Teenage Girls Compared
These values derive from adding the increment of recommended nutrients for the pregnant adult woman to the RDA for females 15 to 18 years of age.

In contrast to the above statistics, maternal mortality is *lowest* for mothers under age 20.[35] However, maternal illness is especially common in teenage pregnancies, with the rates for preeclampsia and eclampsia 50 percent higher than for older women. Other complications common to teenage pregnancy are iron-deficiency anemia and prolonged labor, which may reflect poor diets and inadequate prenatal care. Only about half of all teenage mothers receive prenatal care in the first trimester of pregnancy.[36] A note of interest from the research on teenage pregnancy: women giving birth before the age of 18 have a low risk of breast cancer.[37] The risk of breast cancer increases as age at first birth increases.

Nutrient Needs and Weight Gain

Unfortunately, due to limited research, not much more specific information is available on the nutrient needs of the pregnant adolescent. Estimates are usually made by adding the increment for the pregnant adult woman to the RDA for the nonpregnant teenager 15 to 18 years of age.[38] The estimate may overstate some nutrient needs due to physiological changes that occur during pregnancy.

Figure 6–2 shows that a teenage pregnant girl's needs for many nutrients increase above prepregnant levels much more than her energy allowance does. This raises the question of how to determine the proper energy intake for a pregnant teenage girl. The best way is to monitor her weight gain over time. A young teenage mother (13 to 16 years of age) needs to gain approximately 30 to 35 pounds in order to deliver an infant of optimum birthweight. When compared with older adolescent and adult mothers (17 to 25 years of age) with the same prepregnant weight and pregnancy weight gain (24 pounds), the younger mothers have smaller newborns.[39] Their total weight gain needs to equal the weight gain expected for growth plus the weight gain required for pregnancy. Young adolescents need to gain 6 to 9 pounds more than older females in order to give birth to infants of the same size. This greater weight gain helps to offset the unfulfilled weight growth of adolescence. Reduced physical activity of the pregnant teenager may reduce her energy needs compared with those of her nonpregnant peers.

Like the nutrient needs of pregnancy during the teen years, those of lactating teens are estimated by combining teen needs with adult lactation needs. The calcium RDA for lactating adolescents is 1600 milligrams. When lactating adolescents consume their usual diet containing 900 milligrams of calcium, they lose 10 percent of their bone minerals by 16 weeks postpartum.[40] In contrast, lactating adolescents consuming a diet that meets their calcium RDA lose no bone minerals. Adequate calcium intake is obviously important to preventing bone loss during lactation in adolescents.

Support Needs

The plight of a pregnant teenager is often compounded by a multitude of social and economic problems. Most are from low-income families. Oftentimes, they have several children during their teen years, which further increases their pregnancy risks.

Pregnant teenagers often find themselves isolated, without resources or access to prenatal care. They urgently need programs addressed to all their problems, including medical attention, nutrition guidance, and emotional support. Continued schooling is most important to their future.

Many communities offer programs such as San Francisco's Teenage Pregnancy and Parenting Project (TAPP) to improve the health of adolescent mothers and their infants.[41] The goals of TAPP are to keep pregnant teenagers enrolled in school, reduce the rate of subsequent unwanted pregnancies, and encourage father and family involvement. The program's success is evident in not only meeting these goals, but in the above-average birthweight of infants born to mothers involved with TAPP.

In addition to local programs, the federal WIC program provides nutrition supplementation and education to eligible teenagers. Chapter 2's discussion of maternal nutrition highlighted the positive effects participation in WIC has on infant birthweight. Compared with similar, but non-WIC, participants, WIC mothers have fewer low-birthweight infants, and the average birthweight of their infants is higher.[42] These benefits are even greater for teenagers than for others in the WIC program.

Counseling the pregnant teenager is a challenge. It is extremely important to establish rapport. Teenagers typically turn a deaf ear to lectures. Empathy and support are critical. Open-ended questions will encourage the young woman to talk about herself. Once she has told you something of herself, use this information to employ nutrition counseling. For example, if she tells you she eats meals away from home, provide her with tips on how to get the most nutrients for the money she spends. If she enjoys snacking, provide her with ideas for nutritious snacks. Show her respect and support her good judgment whenever possible. Do whatever you can to help her see how eating well will benefit herself and her infant. She will look and feel better throughout the pregnancy, and her infant will have a better chance of being born healthy and staying that way.

Eating Disorders

To teenagers, growing means getting taller and heavier. For many female teenagers, this is not a welcome occurrence. They do not want to grow bigger; they become dissatisfied with their appearances. Adolescence is a time of increased concern for body image, anyway, and peer pressure and media pressure make it worse. Fear of obesity is prevalent even among those who are at or below normal weight. The result of being "terrified about being overweight" and "preoccupied with the thought of having fat on their body" is frequent dieting. In fact, one survey of females (ages 14 to 18) reported that over 70 percent had dieted to lose weight; almost 40 percent were dieting at the time of the survey.[43]

Obesity is discussed in Focal Point 5.

Most women see themselves as one-fourth larger than they actually are.[44] The more inaccurately they perceive their body size, the worse they feel about themselves. Quite often female adolescents diet to lose weight even when they are within or below the average range for body weight.[45] Such a goal is neither healthy nor obtainable for most teenagers. Females 15 to 17 years of age consume an average of 350 kcalories less than the RDA. Distorted attitudes and self-perceptions can lead to such eating disorders as compulsive over-eating, anorexia nervosa, or bulimia.

Anorexia nervosa or bulimia affects an estimated 1 million teenagers.[46] Specific causes of these eating disorders still baffle clinicians. Some speculate that society's excessive pressure to be thin is to blame, others point to neurological links with depression and impulsive behaviors or other biological malfunctions, and still others believe it to be the result of an inability to cope. Their point of agreement is that the cause is most likely multifactorial—sociocultural, neurochemical, and psychological—and that treatment requires a multidisciplinary approach. The nutrition component of treatment requires both intervention and education.[47]

Anorexia Nervosa

anorexia nervosa: a disorder involving compulsive self-starvation and extreme weight loss, not explainable by disease, most common in adolescent females.

an = not
orexis = appetite
nervos = of nervous origin

Anorexia nervosa is characterized by extreme weight loss, distorted body image, and preoccupation with food coupled with an intense fear of becoming obese.[48] This pathological fear of gaining weight leads to unusual eating patterns, malnutrition, and excessive weight loss.[49] Most victims of anorexia nervosa are white females from middle- or upper-class families. Males account for less than 10 percent of the cases.[50] Most often the saga begins when a teenager who either is overweight, or perceives herself to be overweight, begins a weight-loss regimen. Oftentimes she receives encouragement and praise from friends and family members. Her efforts to lose weight are heroic and include a severe kcalorie-restricted diet and excessive physical activity. A person with anorexia nervosa would consider it a normal day's workout to swim 96 laps at the pool, run five miles, attend an aerobic dance class, and do body-building exercises.[51]

The physical consequences of anorexia nervosa are similar to those of starvation. They include diminished norepinephrine synthesis, elevated growth hormone concentrations, defective temperature regulation, and lowered basal metabolic rate.[52] In addition, estrogen concentrations are depressed, and this contributes to the amenorrhea and osteoporosis common in female anorectics. In males, serum testosterone concentrations are low, depressing sexual desire.[53] One study found medical problems such as cardiovascular abnormalities, hypothermia, renal dysfunction, and electrolyte imbalance present in over half the adolescents with anorexia and in almost one-fourth of those with bulimia.[54]

A typical psychological profile of a female with anorexia includes depression, early developmental failure, and family dysfunction.[55] For these reasons, treatment usually involves parents to ensure appropriate family interactions subsequent to treatment.[56] A teenager with anorexia strives for perfection and control over her life, finds fat disgusting and thin admirable, and believes gaining weight means being out of control. For a teenager in a growth phase, gaining weight is normal. Thus, part of recovery for the teenager with anorexia is an understanding of growth and its relationship to food.[57] For some teenagers with mild anorexia nervosa, this is all that is necessary to elicit a positive response. Those with strong resistance to treatment and severe weight loss require hospitalization.

As mentioned earlier, the specific causes of anorexia are difficult to define because they are often interwoven and the symptoms manifest themselves in a variety of physical and psychological ways. Treatment must therefore artfully combine medical and dietary intervention to initiate and sustain weight gain with psychological techniques to resolve personal and family problems. Teams of physicians, nurses, psychiatrists, family psychologists, and dietitians work together to treat clients with anorexia nervosa.

Part of treatment involves recognition of the power struggle between therapists and clients.[58] When treatment programs try to manage their clients' eating regimens by counting kcalories and checking food trays, they are heading for failure. Instead, clients are encouraged to maintain control over their lives by designing healthy diet plans.[59]

Bulimia

Bulimia is a distinct eating disorder that shares some characteristics with anorexia nervosa. Like the person with anorexia, the teenager with bulimia spends much time thinking about her body weight and food. Her preoccupation with food manifests itself in secretive binge-eating episodes followed by self-induced vomiting, fasting, or the use of laxatives and diuretics.[60] Such behaviors typically begin in late adolescence after a long series of various unsuccessful weight-reduction diets. People with bulimia commonly follow a pattern of restrictive dieting interspersed with bulimic behaviors and experience weight fluctuations of ten pounds gained and lost—up and down—over short periods of time.

A person with bulimia is difficult to identify; she hides her secret well. To the world outside, she is bright, successful, near normal weight, without obvious psychological problems.[61] Internally, her self-image is one of being too fat; her fears are of being unable to stop eating and of getting fatter; her ultimate ambition is to be slim.

In an attempt to attain the thin ideal, the person with bulimia severely restricts food intake, especially "forbidden" sweet treats. When she can no longer resist the temptation, she loses control and begins to binge. The average binge takes her about an hour, and she consumes about 3400 kcalories.[62] Binge episodes most often occur secretly, followed by guilt, depression, and self-condemnation. With the guilt comes a renewed compulsion to lose weight—by either starving or purging.

Purging involves inducing vomiting (either manually or with emetic drugs), or using enemas, laxatives, or diuretics. Not all people with bulimia purge. Those who do believe they have found the ideal solution to their weight problem—that purging will help to eliminate the fattening effect of the excess food eaten as well as the guilt associated with the overindulgence in food. For them, it serves to cleanse both the body and the soul. But in "cleansing" the body, a person loses water and minerals, incurring dehydration and electrolyte imbalances, which can lead to fatigue, seizures, muscle cramps, and irregular heartbeats, and, over the long term, to decreased bone density and osteoporosis. Table 6–1 lists other physical consequences of purging. Even more severe than the physical consequences of bulimia are the associated behavioral and psychological problems.[63] The rates of alcohol, marijuana, and cigarette use

bulimia: a disorder involving recurring binge eating, most common in women. Bulimia followed by purging is referred to as **bulimarexia nervosa.**

binge eating: rapid consumption of a large quantity of food.

Table 6–1   Consequences of Purging

In general:
   Electrolyte imbalances

Specifically:
   Diuretic use causes:
      Hypokalemia
   Emetic use causes:
      Poisoning
      Cardiac arrest
   Laxative use causes:
      Rectal bleeding
      Hypokalemia
   Vomiting causes:
      Damage to the esophagus and stomach
      Swelling of the salivary glands
      Recession of the gums
      Erosion of tooth enamel
      Skin rashes
      Broken blood vessels on the face
      Aspiration pneumonia

Source: Adapted from D. B. Herzog and P. M. Copeland, Eating disorders, *New England Journal of Medicine* 313 (1985): 295–303; D. Farley, Eating disorders: When thinness becomes an obsession, *FDA Consumer*, May 1986, pp. 20–23.

and of depression among bulimics are high.[64] For these reasons, a mental health professional should be one of the members on the multidisciplinary treatment team.

The goal of a dietary plan to treat bulimia is to help clients gain control and establish regular eating patterns.[65] Initial dietary management requires a structured eating plan with little flexibility. Such a plan prevents the client from making decisions and reduces anxiety about eating. Binge foods are avoided at first and gradually reintroduced in moderate amounts.

These eating disorders illustrate how a desired end (in this case, weight loss) can alter a person's eating habits and food choices, and therefore nutrition status. Teenagers are willing to go to considerable trouble and expense, at the risk of jeopardizing their health, to achieve their perception of physical beauty. A similar effort (although usually to a lesser degree and with fewer ill consequences) is made by the teenager in search of a remedy for acne.

Acne

acne: a chronic inflammation of the skin's follicles and oil-producing glands that involves the accumulation of sebum inside the ducts that surround hairs, usually associated with adolescence.

Many a teenager would pay dearly for the remedy for acne. Many approaches have been suggested and tried with varying success in individual cases. While advances are being made that offer hope for the treatment of acne in the future, there is as yet no surefire way to get rid of it.

Some teenagers hopefully believe that if they stop eating certain foods and drinking certain beverages, they can prevent acne. Among foods charged with aggravating acne are chocolate, cola beverages, fatty or greasy foods, milk, nuts, sugar, and foods or salt containing iodine. None of these foods has proven to worsen acne.[66] Of course, with the exception of milk, most teenagers would suffer no harm if these foods were limited in their diets. Such a dietary practice may actually benefit their nutrient status and health.

Not all dietary practices attempting to treat acne are innocuous. Misinformed teenagers taking vitamin A supplements may create problems greater than acne. Vitamin A supplements taken internally have no beneficial effect on acne, but can cause the symptoms of vitamin A toxicity. The belief that vitamin A cures acne arises from the knowledge that it is needed for the health of the skin. Similar claims have been made for zinc because of its roles in skin maintenance and retinol-binding protein synthesis. As with other nutrients, however, vitamin A and zinc promote health when enough is supplied; more than enough actually causes harm.

retinol-binding protein: the vitamin A-carrying protein.

Dermatologists sometimes treat cystic acne with medicines related to vitamin A but chemically different from over-the-counter supplements. Isotretinoin (13-*cis*-retinoic acid) is available in soft gelatin capsules for oral administration under the trade name Accutane. Its mechanism of action is not completely understood, although it seems to inhibit sebaceous gland function and keratinization. Accutane is responsible for a number of adverse effects, including serious birth defects in infants of women using it during pregnancy. As mentioned in Chapter 1, an effective form of contraception is advised beginning one month before and continuing until one month after Accutane's use.

Another vitamin A relative, tretinoin (retinoic acid), is available for the topical treatment of acne under the trade name Retin-A. Retin-A seems to affect the follicular epithelial cells, decreasing their cohesiveness and increasing their turnover.

retinoic acid: the acid form of vitamin A.

No one knows why some people get acne while others do not, but heredity is one factor. In addition, the hormones of adolescence increase the activity of the sebaceous glands in the skin (see Figure 6–3).[67] Even though it is true that the skin of a person with acne is oily, the diet's fat and oil content is not at fault. Because stress worsens acne, and because adolescents easily develop guilt feelings over what they eat, perhaps the best nutrition advice is to dispense with food-related guilt. The guidelines for the acne-plagued teenager, as for anyone, are to eat nutritious foods in abundance and to enjoy sweet treats in moderation as a harmless pleasure.

Miniglossary of Acne Terms

blackhead: an open lesion with an accumulation of the natural, dark pigments of the skin (not dirt) in the opening.

cyst: an enlarged, deep pimple.

sebaceous gland: the oil-secreting gland of the skin.

sebum: the skin's natural mixture of oils and waxes that help keep skin and hair moist.

whitehead: a pimple caused by the plugging of oil-gland ducts with shed material from the duct lining.

Figure 6–3   Acne

The skin's natural oil, sebum, is made in deep sebaceous glands and is supposed to flow out through the tiny ducts around the hairs to the skin surface. In acne, the oily secretions exceed the skin's clearance capacity.

Inside each of the ducts is a skinlike lining that regularly sheds cells. These cells mix with the oil and then are pushed to the surface of the skin. When acne develops, they stick together, forming a plug that blocks the duct. The duct enlarges, allowing oil and the skin-surface bacteria to leak into the surrounding skin. The oil and bacterial enzymes are irritating and cause redness, swelling, pus formation—and the beginning of a whitehead, or pimple. A cyst may form, or the skin may open above the plug, revealing an accumulation of dark skin pigments just below the surface—a blackhead.

Note that acne is not caused by the skin bacteria, although once the process has begun, they make it worse. Also note that the color of a blackhead is caused by skin pigments, not by dirt. Squeezing or picking at the lesions of acne in an attempt to remove their contents can cause more scars than the acne.

Among the over-the-counter acne treatments, preparations that contain benzoyl peroxide are safe and effective. Careful washing helps remove skin-surface bacteria and oil and keeps the oil ducts open; surface treatment with antibiotics also helps control the bacteria. A cream or gel containing retinoic acid can help: retinoic acid loosens the plugs that form in the ducts, allowing the oil to flow again so that the ducts will not burst. Care is necessary because the acid may burn the skin and even cause pimples to form, making the acne look worse rather than better at first.

Stress, with its accompanying hormonal secretions, clearly worsens acne. Vacations from school pressures help to bring acne relief. The sun, the beach, and swimming also help, perhaps because they are relaxing, and also because the sun's rays kill bacteria and water cleanses the skin.

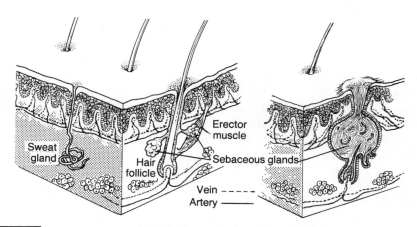

Adapted from *Acne*, a pamphlet available from the National Institute of Allergy and Infectious Diseases, Bethesda, MD 20205, NIH Publication no. 80-188, May 1980; *Stubborn and Vexing, That's Acne*, a pamphlet available from the Food and Drug Administration, 5600 Fishers Lane, Rockville, MD 20857, HHS Publication no. (FDA) 80-3107, May 1980.

Fitness for Teens

Fitness is important throughout life. Each chapter has extolled its virtues, recommending regular exercise prior to pregnancy, during pregnancy, and during lactation, and recommending regular outdoor play in infancy and childhood. The teen years are the time when outdoor play transits to sports for many and sedentary indoor life for many more. In the teen years, exercise should become a habit as regular as eating, practiced in a way that will bring optimal benefits. Regular, frequent exercise does much to promote both physical and mental health and prevent obesity and the degenerative conditions of later life, such as osteoporosis and heart disease.

As mentioned at the start, teens choose whether to exercise. Some become seriously interested in athletics. The person who wants to provide nutrition and fitness education for teenagers should speak their language on this important topic.

Fitness expert Dr. George Sheehan says that, "We are all athletes, it's just that some of us are in training and others are not." He means that the human body—any human body—can adapt to intense, prolonged exercise by developing a greater and greater capacity for it. All that is required is the appropriate training, supported by appropriate nutrition. Teens who admire the image of the athlete should be encouraged to see themselves this way—as people with bodies that will respond to athletic training. Accordingly, the following sections are devoted to the special nutrition needs of bodies during exercise.

An athlete is defined here as anyone who participates in any kind of competitive sport, exercises on a regular, frequent basis, or is serious about improving fitness and health through exercise. Thus, in this discussion, athletes include world-class Olympians, college basketball players, high school football players, members of the Little League team, and all individuals who spend at least 30 minutes a day, three days a week or more, running, walking, swimming, cycling, rowing boats, dancing, or engaging in any other activity that makes the heart beat fast and the muscles work hard for most of that time. Athletes all along this spectrum reap the benefits that come with sound nutrition.

The two major contributors to athletic achievement are heredity and training, while nutrition and psychological preparation play lesser but important parts. Heredity sets the ultimate potential; training permits realization of the potential; and nutrition supports training by supplying the fuels, the building materials, and the metabolic regulators the muscles demand.

Many sports nutrition experts agree that the diet most athletes need is simply an ordinary balanced diet, consisting of a variety of nutrient-dense foods and ample fluids. This is a simple enough nutrition prescription for the athlete, and is easy to follow, provided that athletes and their coaches are informed as to exactly what constitutes sound nutrition and a balanced diet. The discussion that follows emphasizes energy nutrients for the athlete, vitamins and minerals most essential to athletic performance, fluid needs, and the foods that provide these nutrients and promote good health. Along the way, it explores some misconceptions relevant to the topics at hand.

Energy and Fuels in Exercise

The body receives usable energy from food in the form of three classes of compounds—carbohydrates, lipids, and proteins. The first two of these give rise to glucose and fatty acids, which are normally the body's preferred energy sources, although amino acids from protein can be used if necessary. In the absence of food, the body draws glucose and fatty acids from its own stores of carbohydrate (glycogen) and lipids (body fat)—and, if necessary, from its protein tissues. Figure 6–4 shows the pathways of metabolism by which glucose and fatty acids yield their energy for the body's use.

The principal form into which energy from glucose and fatty acids is transferred and made available to do work within cells is the compound ATP (adenosine triphosphate). The muscles' own supply of ATP lasts only for about two minutes; thereafter, various body reserves must be drawn upon.

The sources of additional ATP available to muscles are shown in Figure 6–4. One is PC (phosphocreatine), available within the muscles themselves, for about 30 seconds' worth of energy. The synthesis of ATP from PC is not dependent on a person's eating food and does not require oxygen.

Other sources of ATP are glycogen, fatty acids, and if necessary, amino acids. Their usefulness as fuel depends partly on whether oxygen is available for their breakdown. Figure 6–4 shows that anaerobic metabolism yields a little ATP, and that aerobic metabolism yields much more ATP. Normally, exercise metabolism of any duration beyond about two minutes requires that the muscles receive oxygen and the two main muscle fuels—glucose and fatty acids. The oxygen comes from the lungs, which pass it to the blood, which carries it to the muscles. The glucose originates mainly from the glycogen stores within the muscle itself; some comes from the liver, via the blood. The fatty acids come partly from fat stores within the muscles, but mostly from the body's fat tissues, delivered by the blood.

Let us consider each of these sources in turn, beginning with glycogen. If glycogen can be broken down aerobically all the way to carbon dioxide and water, it can yield abundant ATP. If it cannot be (if insufficient oxygen is available to permit breakdown below the dotted line in Figure 6–4), then it must stop at pyruvate and take an alternative path to lactic acid (part B of Figure 6–4). Lactic acid is an important, quickly available source of ATP, but when it accumulates in the muscles and blood, temporary fatigue occurs. (A strategy for dealing with lactic acid buildup is to relax the muscles at every opportunity so that the blood can carry it away.) Lactic acid yields a relatively small quantity of ATP compared with the ATP generated when glycogen or fat breakdown occurs in the presence of oxygen.

Fatty acids can only be broken down aerobically. As long as oxygen is available, fatty acids can serve as an inexhaustible source of abundant ATP. But the other ATP sources have to stand behind them to permit exercise to continue during bursts of intensive activity, when oxygen supply momentarily fails to meet demand.

Protein stores can also be used for energy. Some amino acids can be broken down to pyruvate and hence be used anaerobically like glucose if need be. Other amino acids can be broken down to acetyl CoA and require oxygen, as fatty acids do, to be used as fuel.

ATP: adenosine triphosphate; the major form of immediately available energy in the body.

PC: phosphocreatine; a high energy compound stored in the muscle and used to regenerate ATP.

anaerobic: not requiring oxygen.

aerobic: requiring oxygen.

lactic acid: a product of anaerobic glucose metabolism.

Normally, during exercise, all fuels are in use to varying degrees from moment to moment, depending on their availability, on the availability of oxygen, on the duration and intensity of the exercise, and on local conditions within the muscle. The ATP-PC energy system fuels short (less than 30 seconds), intense bursts of physical activity such as lifting heavy weights or short sprints. The pyruvate-lactic acid conversion comes into play during exercise that is slightly less intense and of longer duration (1/2 to 3 minutes). Energy generated from the lactic acid system fuels bursts of activities such as running or cycling at maximal speed for a half mile or so. Trained muscles tolerate more and produce less lactic acid than untrained muscles, and so can exercise at high intensities somewhat longer than untrained muscles.[68]

Of the two major fuels, glycogen and fatty acids, only glycogen can be used anaerobically. The better the body is at supplying oxygen to its muscles, and the better the muscles are at using it, the less glycogen will have to be used this way and the longer it will last. Beyond three minutes, glycogen and fatty acids are used in a mixture, although glycogen use may predominate early and fatty acid use later (see the table in Figure 6–4).

Body protein stores are used for energy to some extent during all muscular activity, but will be used to a greater extent if the other fuels are in short supply. They are an inefficient fuel, and their use results in the loss of structural, enzymatic, and hormonal proteins from the tissues from which they are taken. The following sections describe the energy fuels in greater detail.

Carbohydrate   The body stores carbohydrate as glycogen, most of it in the muscle. The liver contains a smaller amount (less than a pound) of glycogen, which it breaks apart into glucose and releases into the bloodstream when the body needs it. During exercise, the muscles pick up and use the glucose donated by the liver, along with glucose from their own private glycogen stores. The more glycogen stored, the longer the stores will last during exercise. Compared to fat, the carbohydrate stores of the body are limited.

Body glycogen is closely related to the carbohydrate content of the diet. How much carbohydrate the athlete eats determines how much glycogen is stored, and influences the rate at which glycogen is used in any given exercise.[69] The rate at which an athlete uses glucose also depends partly on the duration of the exercise and partly on its intensity.

Exercise intensity is expressed as a proportion of an individual's maximum aerobic capacity or oxygen consumption (percent VO_2 max). At rest or at intensities below 50 percent of maximum aerobic capacity, the primary fuel is fat, while muscle glycogen use is minimal. As exercise *intensity* rises above 70 percent of maximum oxygen consumption (the average intensity of most athletic events), *glycogen* becomes the primary fuel.[70] As exercise *duration* continues to increase, and intensity lessens, *fat* becomes the preferred fuel, but only to a point. The endurance athlete continues to use glycogen, and will eventually run out of it.

Fatigue is the inevitable consequence of glycogen depletion, and sets in earlier when the muscle glycogen stores are small. Glycogen depletion does not limit short-term, intense exercise, but it has a profound effect on performance during endurance exercise. Glycogen use is rapid at the beginning of intense

VO_2 **max:** the maximum volume of oxygen that a person can consume during a minute of heavy work; a measure of cardiovascular and muscular fitness. Also called **MOC (maximum oxygen consumption).**

Figure 6–4 Food, Fuels, and Exercise

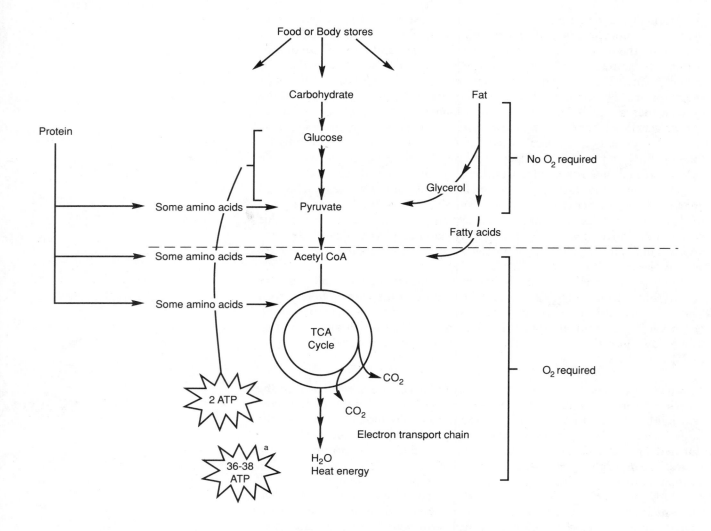

A. The Central Metabolic Pathway That Generates Energy (ATP).The two main fuels for exercise, carbohydrate (glucose, from food or body glycogen stores) and fat (fatty acids, from food or bodyfat stores), are broken down by separate pathways to a common intermediate, acetyl CoA, and then by a common pathway to carbon dioxide and water. In the process, energy is released, and some is used to make the compound ATP (adenosine triphosphate), which serves in all cells as a source of readily available energy. Some of the earlier steps in glucose breakdown yield ATP without oxygen's involvement (they are anaerobic), but the later ones, including all of the steps by which fat is broken down, require oxygen (they are aerobic). These later, aerobic steps yield by far the most ATP and so are the most important for endurance exercise.

[a]Each glucose yields 38-40 ATP as explained in E.N. Whitney, and E.M.N. Hamilton, Appendix C in *Understanding Nutrition*, 4th ed. (St. Paul, Minn: West , 1987).

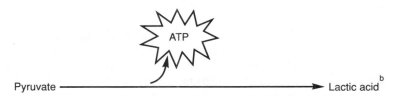

Pyruvate ⟶ Lactic acid[b]

B. Alternative Way of Generating ATP If Oxygen is Not Available. If oxygen is not available, then pyruvate cannot be converted to acetyl CoA. It can, however, be converted to lactic acid, producing a small amount of ATP. In muscle, lactic acid can break down no further. While the muscles are working, lactic acid accumulates, causing burning pain and fatigue. When the muscles relax, lactic acid drains away and is carried by the blood to the liver. When oxygen becomes available again, the liver converts the lactic acid back to glucose. Then the glucose may travel back to the muscles to serve again as fuel.

[b] When O_2 is again available, an ATP is consumed to regenerate pyruvate so that it can be completely broken down to yield much more ATP.

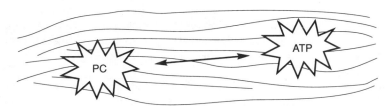

C. ATP Use in Muscle. ATP is available instantaneously and is the muscles' immediate energy source—that is, the one they actually use when they are working. A temporary nearby storage form of ATP's energy is PC (phosphocreatine); limited amounts are made from ATP and held in readiness near working muscle fibers. PC's energy can be transferred back into ATP at a moment's notice when the ATP supply runs short. ATP can thus be derived from three sources—the central pathway from food or body stores (A), lactic acid (B), or PC. The accompanying table compares the timing with which these different energy sources are used under different conditions.

Characteristics of the Body's Energy Systems

Energy System	Performance Time	Oxygen Needed	Exercise Intensity	Activity Example
ATP-PC (immediate availability)	Less than 30 seconds	No	Extreme	100-yard dash, shot put
ATP from anaerobic/ carbohydrate (lactic acid)	30 seconds to 3 minutes	No	Very high	1/4-mile run at maximal speed
ATP from aerobic/ carbohydrate	3 minutes to 20 minutes	Yes	High	Cross-country skiing, distance swimming or running
ATP from aerobic / fat	More than 20 minutes	Yes	Moderate	Distance running or jogging

Source: Adapted in part from M. H. Williams, Human energy, in *Nutritional Aspects of Human Physical and Athletic Performance*, 2nd ed. (Springfield, Ill. : Charles C. Thomas, 1985), pp. 21–57, E. L. Fox, Sports activities and the energy continuum, in *Sports Physiology*, 2nd ed. (New York : W. B. Saunders Company, 1984), pp. 26–39.

respiratory exchange ratio (R value): the ratio of carbon dioxide production to oxygen consumption and an indicator of the type of fuel being utilized. At rest, the R value is 0.85, which indicates that 50 to 60 percent of the energy for metabolism is fat derived, the remainder is carbohydrate derived. During exercise, as intensity increases, the R value rises, indicating greater carbohydrate utilization.

glycogen supercompensation: a technique of exercising, followed by eating a high-carbohydrate diet, that enables muscles to store glycogen beyond their normal capacity; also called **glycogen loading**.

exercise.[71] As exercise continues, glycogen use slows down. The body begins to rely more on fat for fuel, conserving the remaining glycogen supply. If exercise continues long enough and at a high enough intensity, glycogen will run out almost completely. Muscle glycogen depletion occurs within about 90 to 120 minutes when exercise intensity averages 70 percent of aerobic capacity.

It has long been known that the composition of the diet affects fuel availability during exercise. A classic study in 1939 compared fuel usage during exercise among runners who had consumed three different diets.[72] Researchers determined fuel utilization by observing the respiratory exchange ratio (R value). The R value rises as carbohydrate utilization during exercise increases.[73] The study participants consumed either a normal diet (55 percent carbohydrate), a high-carbohydrate diet (83 percent carbohydrate), or a high-fat diet (94 percent fat) for several days before exercising. The study was one of the first to demonstrate the importance of carbohydrate in supporting long-duration exercise, as Figure 6–5 shows.

Thus, ample stores of glycogen enhance an athlete's endurance.[74] The greater the muscle glycogen stores, the longer the athlete is able to perform at a sustained high intensity. Athletes who want to perform well in long-duration events, then, are wise to maintain their glycogen stores with a high-carbohydrate diet.

"If some is good, more may be better" is an adage that may be true for glycogen, at least up to a point. Muscle glycogen supercompensation has been demonstrated by studying the thigh muscles of individuals who had exercised one leg heavily to deplete glycogen stores. When this regimen was followed by a high-carbohydrate diet for several days, glycogen repletion was rapid and exceeded normal levels. This supercompensation of glycogen occurred only in the exercised muscles. The highest concentrations of muscle glycogen were obtained when depletion was followed by a low-carbohydrate diet for several days and then by a high-carbohydrate diet. This procedure was, until recently, the strategy followed by endurance athletes wishing to prolong performance at a given intensity. Extreme manipulation of an individual's diet can be dangerous, however, and is not recommended. Later research indicates that exhaustive exercise followed by a high-carbohydrate diet has the same glycogen supercompensation effect as a low-carbohydrate diet followed by a high-carbohydrate diet.[75] Researchers speculate that muscle glycogen super-compensation occurs partially because a high-carbohydrate diet following exhaustive exercise increases insulin sensitivity, which, in turn, enhances glucose transport into the glycogen-depleted muscle cells.[76]

When researchers compare the effect of simple versus complex carbohydrates on muscle glycogen synthesis after strenuous exercise, some interesting results emerge.[77] During the first 24 hours after exercise, the type of carbohydrate an individual eats makes no difference in muscle glycogen concentration. After 48 hours, however, muscle glycogen concentrations are significantly higher in runners who ingest complex carbohydrates. Such is the basis for recommendations that the athlete or active person consume a large proportion of kcalories from complex carbohydrates (50 to 55 percent) and additional kcalories from simple carbohydrates (to bring the total to 60 percent or more).[78] Athletes who wish to pack their muscles with extra glycogen can try for a diet that is even higher in carbohydrate, up to 80 percent for a few days before competition. Whole, minimally processed foods are most beneficial:

Figure 6–5   The Effect of Diet on Physical Endurance
A high-carbohydrate diet can triple an athlete's endurance.

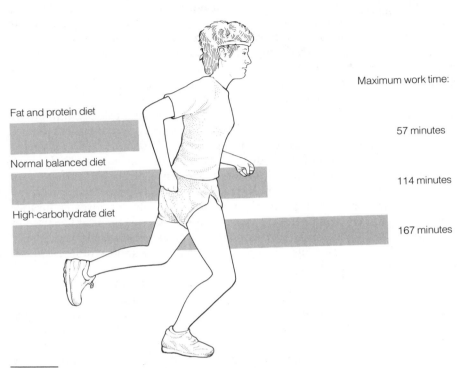

Maximum work time:

Fat and protein diet

57 minutes

Normal balanced diet

114 minutes

High-carbohydrate diet

167 minutes

Source: Data from P. Astrand, Something old and something new . . . very new, *Nutrition Today,* June 1968, pp. 9–11.

they provide the carbohydrate the athlete needs as well as protein, vitamins and minerals; are low in sugar, salt, and fat; and are protective against disease. The food groups that donate the most carbohydrate are grains/starchy vegetables, fruits, and milk. The athlete who relies on whole foods for complex carbohydrates and to meet energy needs should have no trouble meeting other nutrient needs as well. A later section discusses the athlete's diet in more detail.

Fat   Body fat is an important metabolic fuel for exercise and is a virtually unlimited source of energy for the human body. Fat is available as fuel to the muscles in two forms: as free fatty acids (FFA) transported from fat stores, and as triglyceride stores within the muscles themselves. As with carbohydrate, the availability and utilization of fat as a fuel for the muscles is somewhat conditional. As already discussed, diet influences fuel preference, but even more influential is exercise intensity. Unlike carbohydrate, which can be metabolized with oxygen via the TCA cycle or without oxygen via the lactic acid system, fat metabolism absolutely requires oxygen. Accordingly, at low or moderate exercise intensities (less than 70 percent of maximal aerobic capacity), when oxygen is plentiful, fat is a major fuel source. As exercise intensity increases, the energy contribution of fat diminishes, and carbohydrate-derived energy dominates.[79] Researchers have examined methods of increasing FFA availability.[80] The logic was that greater FFA availability might slow down glycogen depletion during exercise. Athletes consumed a high-fat, low-carbohydrate diet in the effort to increase FFA utilization, but could not sustain intensity because the glycogen stores were low and were rapidly depleted.[81] In short, the high-fat diet does enhance FFA utilization, but not athletic performance. Furthermore, such a diet is a risk factor for heart disease and other conditions, and so is best avoided for health's sake.

An alternative to using a high-fat diet to increase FFA availability is to ingest caffeine prior to exercise. Moderate caffeine consumption (2 milligrams per pound of body weight, or two to three cups of coffee) one hour before exercise improves endurance and makes the work seem easier.[82] Caffeine facilitates the utilization of the body's fat stores, thus sparing muscle glycogen during exercise. Caffeine ingestion is not without risk either. Caffeine is a stimulant and a diuretic. Its use as an ergogenic aid may pose hazards to some individuals who are particularly sensitive to it, or who perform endurance exercise in a hot environment. Caffeine-containing beverages should be used in moderation and in *addition* to other fluids, not as a substitute for them.[83] Caffeine is banned as an illegal drug for international and olympic competition, and urine is tested for it.

The use of FFA by muscles depends partly on how much is available in the blood. Eating a high-fat diet and ingesting caffeine are dietary means of enhancing fat utilization—a desirable goal because this will improve endurance by sparing glycogen. However, as mentioned, a high-fat diet is incompatible with optimal health, and caffeine ingestion is inappropriate at times. Fortunately, the athlete has another advantage to draw on: conditioning. With endurance training, muscles develop a greater capacity for FFA oxidation.[84] The physically conditioned athlete can therefore rely on fat for energy at higher exercise intensities, and in doing so, conserve limited glycogen stores. Enhanced fat metabolism is critical to the endurance athlete's performance.

Protein   As with carbohydrate and fat, changes in protein metabolism during exercise appear to be related to diet, glycogen stores, physical conditioning, and exercise intensity and duration. During exercise of moderate intensity, protein metabolism is greater in glycogen-depleted individuals than in those who are not glycogen depleted.[85] Thus, carbohydrate appears to exert a protein-sparing effect during exercise.

Protein contributes about 15 percent of total energy fuel consumed whether a person is resting or exercising.[86] However, the larger total energy cost of exercise imposes a larger total protein contribution than during rest.[87] Nevertheless, the protein content of diets in developed countries is ample. If athletes meet their increased energy needs by selecting and consuming nutrient-dense foods, they will easily meet their protein needs as well.

Years ago, protein was thought to be a major fuel source for muscular work. This thought gave rise to the misconception that athletes require protein supplementation. Despite later proof that protein is not a major fuel source during exercise, many athletes continue to place protein on a performance pedestal by using expensive, unnecessary protein supplements. Even in the face

ergogenic: term used to imply "energy giving;" no food or nutrient is ergogenic. *ergo* = work

of new evidence that exercise induces more changes in protein metabolism than previously thought, protein supplementation still appears to be unnecessary for the healthy athlete.[88] For a variety of reasons, protein supplementation may actually impair performance in endurance events.

Athletes may also take protein supplements in the false hope that since muscles are made of protein, eating extra protein will build bigger muscles. Of course, muscle work builds muscle; protein supplements do not, and athletes do not need them. Food energy spares body protein; protein and carbohydrate serve this purpose equally well, and carbohydrate is safer. A balanced diet supplies enough protein, so protein or amino acid supplements are not needed by normal, healthy people, even vegetarian athletes.

Furthermore, protein supplements are expensive and less well digested than protein-rich food; when used as a total replacement for food, they are often dangerous. The "liquid protein" diet, advocated some years ago for weight loss, caused deaths in some users.

That athletes use protein supplements is not a reflection on them. They are the targets of misguided coaches and trainers as well as quacks who try to convince them that they need supplements of all kinds, and that the established scientific community, and especially the nutrition community, is not up on the latest research. These tactics work; athletes spend millions of dollars on supplements each year. They do this because they have one correct piece of knowledge: nutrition makes a difference. In a world where body condition and skill are hard won, promises of performance gains in pills or potions are enticing.

In summary, carbohydrate and fat are the major fuel sources of exercise, and the degree of energy contribution by each is dependent on several factors. Training state, diet, and intensity and duration of exercise influence fuel use in physical activity. Recently, protein metabolism during exercise has gained renewed attention. Even though the athlete's protein needs may be greater than those of sedentary people, the protein content of typical diets in the United States and Canada more than suffices. Although many questions about energy sources and exercise remain, from the evidence to date, the following conclusions emerge:

▶ During activity of low intensity (less than 40 percent of maximal aerobic capacity) fat is the primary fuel.

▶ As exercise intensity increases, so does the contribution of carbohydrate as an energy source.

▶ Above 70 percent of maximal aerobic capacity, carbohydrate is the predominant fuel.[89]

▶ Muscle glycogen depletion by way of exercise, in addition to a high-carbohydrate diet, results in greater-than-normal muscle glycogen concentrations.

▶ Physical conditioning enhances the capacity for fat metabolism at greater intensities, which in turn spares limited carbohydrate stores (glycogen).

Vitamins

Most people who are interested in fitness and sport are fascinated with the vitamins and especially with how vitamins might affect performance. According to one survey, 84 percent of world-class athletes use vitamin supplements.[90] Popular belief has it that supplements have something to offer, both in health benefits and in athletic performance. Do athletes need more vitamins than other people? The answer to this question lies in the metabolic workings of the muscles in relation to each vitamin. Table 6–2 shows some exercise-related functions of vitamins and minerals. Space limits discussion of all of those listed in Table 6–2.

The B vitamins Unlike the energy nutrients, vitamins are not oxidized for energy. Without them, however, the production of energy for the body's use would be impossible. Thus, it seems logical to assume that a person who uses more energy in a day might need more of the vitamins involved in the breakdown of energy-yielding nutrients—the B vitamins. The RDA for thiamin, for example, is expressed in amounts per 1000 kcalories of food consumed because the more food the body processes, the more thiamin it needs to extract energy from the food.

To answer the question of whether athletes in training need thiamin in amounts greater than the RDA, scientists supplemented athletes with the vitamin and compared their physical performance with that of athletes eating only a regular adequate diet.[91] They found that extra thiamin conferred no benefits on performance. The thiamin in an *adequate* diet supplies all the thiamin a person needs, even for heavy work. This is because almost any kind of whole, unprocessed food supplies thiamin, and when an athlete meets energy demands with nourishing food, thiamin is sure to be plentiful. For

Table 6–2   Exercise-Related Functions of Vitamins and Minerals

Vitamin or Mineral	Function
Thiamin, riboflavin, niacin, magnesium	Energy-releasing reactions
Vitamin B_6, zinc	Building of muscle protein
Folacin, vitamin B_{12}	Building of red blood cells to carry oxygen
Vitamin C	Collagen formation for joint and other tissue integrity; hormone synthesis
Iron	Transport of oxygen in blood and in muscle tissue; energy transformation reactions
Calcium, vitamin D, vitamin A, phosphorus	Building of bone structure; muscle contractions; nerve transmissions
Sodium, potassium, chloride	Maintenance of fluid balance; transmission of nerve impulses for muscle contraction
Chromium	Assistance in insulin's energy-storage function
Magnesium	Cardiac and other muscle contraction

Note: This is just a sampling. Other vitamins and minerals play equally indispensable roles in exercise.

Source: E. M. N. Hamilton, E. N. Whitney, and F. S. Sizer, *Nutrition: Concepts and Controversies,* 4th ed. (St. Paul, Minn.: West, 1988).

thiamin, then, the answer is that athletes do not benefit from more than the RDA amount; they can get what they need from food.

The link between riboflavin and physical performance arises from its role as part of the coenzyme flavin adenine dinucleotide (FAD), central to the mitochondrial oxidative reactions of electron transport. Unlike thiamin, riboflavin requirements do not appear to increase with greater energy expenditure.[92]

To try to answer the question of whether riboflavin at levels beyond the RDA assists in athletic performance, researchers studied groups of overweight, sedentary women who began an exercise regimen in addition to weight-loss dieting.[93] One group of women consumed the RDA of riboflavin (1.2 milligrams per day), while the other group consumed slightly more (1.4 milligrams). Blood tests to evaluate riboflavin activity seemed to indicate a deficiency in the group that consumed only the RDA amounts. However, aerobic capacity of both groups increased similarly. Riboflavin intakes above the RDA did not improve physical performance, as would be expected if true riboflavin deficiency had existed. For both groups of women, however, exercise resulted in decreased urinary excretion of riboflavin suggesting a greater need for riboflavin during exercise. Questions about riboflavin requirements during exercise remain to be answered by more research.

Riboflavin is widespread in the food of developed countries, so deficiencies are almost nonexistent. People addicted to alcohol may drink rather than eat and are at risk for riboflavin deficiency, as are drug abusers who hardly eat at all. But in a society where even sweet pastries are enriched with riboflavin, and other (preferable) choices such as green leafy vegetables, milk products, and enriched and whole-grain cereals and breads abound, almost any diet based on nutritious foods provides riboflavin in amounts close to the RDA.

Vitamin B_6 is a part of over 60 enzyme systems involved in the metabolism of protein and the other energy nutrients. It functions in the breakdown of glycogen and is involved in the formation of hemoglobin. Such roles are the basis for claims that vitamin B_6 in amounts greater than the RDA promotes aerobic endurance. Thus far, research does not support these theories. Vitamin B_6 supplementation does not improve aerobic performance.[94]

To ensure that the diet is adequate in vitamin B_6, a person need only include some green leafy vegetables, meats, fish, legumes, fruits, and whole grains. These foods deliver a cargo of many needed nutrients in addition to vitamin B_6. They are whole foods, not processed, low in sugar and salt, and high in nutrients per kcalorie. Athletes who choose these foods prepare themselves, nutritionally, to win. Pills, even of megadoses of vitamin B_6, cannot compete with an optimal diet and they carry the potential for toxicity as well.

The belief that vitamin B_{12} supplementation will enhance performance stems from its role in the production of red blood cells. In anemia, a diminished number of circulating red blood cells robs the blood of its oxygen-carrying capacity, starving the cells and restricting aerobic energy metabolism. Vitamin B_{12} deficiency is only one cause of anemia. Iron and folacin deficiencies are equally destructive to performance, as are medical anemias.

Some athletes take vitamin B_{12} injections or pills prior to competition because they believe that they can enhance endurance and oxygen delivery in this way. The limited research thus far does not lend support to the concept that vitamin B_{12} injections enhance performance of the well-nourished athlete. In fact, taking *any* vitamin directly before a competition runs contrary to science. Vitamins usually function only as small parts of larger working units, usually involving proteins. A molecule of a vitamin, floating around in the blood, is simply waiting for the tissues to combine it with its appropriate enzymes or other parts so that it can do its work. This takes time—hours or days. Vitamins taken right before competition are still waiting in the blood during exercise and are useless for improving performance during that event, even if the person happened to be deficient in that vitamin. Vitamin B_{12} supplements are the appropriate treatment for a vitamin B_{12} deficiency. For a well-nourished athlete, they have not been shown to improve performance.[95]

Vitamin C   Evidence concerning the excretion of vitamin C after exercise was reported in the 1970s and early 1980s. This early work seemed to indicate that vitamin C in amounts two or three times the RDA might best serve the needs of the athlete. Since that time, the great bulk of work designed to explore this theory has disproved it—athletes perform no better when taking vitamin C supplements than when they receive the RDA amount from food.

Even so, athletes are often told by "advisors" in health-food stores to ingest huge quantities of vitamin C, measured in multiples of a gram. These amounts are clearly beyond those indicated as potentially useful, and could be harmful. Besides, if an athlete eats mostly whole foods, it is almost impossible *not* to receive two or three times the RDA for vitamin C. A person who drinks a cup of orange juice and eats a baked potato and a generous serving of broccoli in a day will receive about two times the RDA for vitamin C from the orange juice, half the RDA from the potato, and another two times the RDA from the broccoli. When shown not only the nutrient values for vitamin C, but those of the full array of vitamin and mineral values in foods such as these, athletes have been known to throw away their pills and learn to cook broccoli.

Vitamin E   Vitamin E has enjoyed many claims to fame. For the most part, these claims are exactly that, unsubstantiated claims. The relevance of vitamin E to physical performance has to do with its role as an antioxidant of polyunsaturated fatty acids. Vitamin E deficiency in animals causes anemia and limits oxidative phosphorylation.[96] Oxidation of phospholipids in the red blood cell membrane causes the anemia; the membrane weakens, the cell breaks open, and hemoglobin leaves. Such effects would no doubt hinder athletic performance, should it occur in people, but that is unlikely. Vitamin E is so widespread in foods that scientists who wish to study its deficiency effects in animals must go to some trouble to concoct a vitamin E-free diet to induce the condition. People who want to ensure an adequate intake of vitamin E need not take pills, but can enjoy some walnuts, some sesame seeds, many fruits and vegetables, and whole-wheat bread.

Vitamin supplementation for the healthy athlete appears unwarranted. Excessive amounts of vitamins can be toxic and should be avoided. The athlete's vitamin needs can be met by a balanced diet consisting of a variety of nutrient-dense foods from the four food groups.

Minerals

Like the vitamins, minerals play roles in exercise. Iron in hemoglobin and myoglobin provides oxygen to the exercising muscles. The major minerals calcium, phosphorus, and magnesium are structural components of bone. Calcium and magnesium are also indispensable for muscle contraction. Phosphorus is part of the high-energy compounds ATP and PC, already mentioned. Calcium and iron deficiencies are common. Therefore, calcium and iron stand out among minerals of importance in planning diets for athletes.

Calcium   Osteoporosis is a disease of decreased bone mass and increased susceptibility to fractures, including stress fractures incurred during exercise. The risk of developing osteoporosis increases with age, and is greater in women than in men because women's bone mass declines rapidly after menopause when estrogen secretion diminishes.[97] Estrogen replacement therapy can prevent osteoporosis in many women who have ceased to menstruate.

Although the causes of decreased bone mass are not fully understood, lower circulating estrogen concentrations appear to be causative, while an adequate lifelong calcium intake seems to be preventive. Moderate exercise is thought to be protective against bone loss, but intense exercise may be detrimental to the bone health of some young women.[98] A side effect of endurance training for some women is athletic amenorrhea, characterized by low estrogen concentrations and possibly increased calcium requirements. Considering that the food energy intakes of some amenorrheic athletes are abnormally low, and that the calcium intakes of women in the United States are also low, amenorrheic athletes may be at much greater risk for osteoporosis than other women.[99]

A recent survey of almost 200 female athletes indicates that one-third of them practice pathological eating behaviors such as using laxatives and diet pills, inducing vomiting, and binge eating—bulimia.[100] The damage is greatest for the athlete who practices these behaviors in conjunction with an abnormally low food intake—anorexia nervosa. These behaviors are harmful to bone health and general health, and they impair physical performance. As mentioned earlier, treatment of anorexia nervosa and bulimia requires a team of medical personnel, dietitians, psychologists, and family counselors for greatest efficacy, and is well beyond the scope of nutrition alone. It is safe to say, though, that women athletes who have eating disorders should be encouraged to aim for intakes of calcium between 1000 and 1500 milligrams per day to help protect their bones.[101] Should such women be unable to consume that amount from food, supplements may be appropriate. Treatment of the eating disorder should be high priority however. The practice of encouraging and teaching bulimic behavior by some coaches to keep weight down for gymnasts, wrestlers, or ballet dancers should be actively discouraged.

Iron   Iron deficiency is the most common nutrient deficiency in both developing and developed countries.[102] It is most prevalent among infants, young children, teenagers, and menstruating young women.[103] In fact, the only group with reliably adequate iron nutriture is adult men, and even they can

athletic amenorrhea: cessation of menstruation associated with strenuous athletic training.

runners' anemia: a true iron-deficiency anemia that develops in many high-mileage runners.

experience anemia if they run long distances in training. Endurance athletes, especially women, are prone to iron deficiency; the condition has been dubbed runners' anemia.[104]

In a recent nutrition study, 35 percent of women runners had diminished iron stores as indicated by serum ferritin concentrations.[105] In another study, some female high school runners were given a combination iron and vitamin C supplement, and others were given vitamin C alone.[106] All but one of the women taking the combination supplement maintained sufficient iron stores throughout the study, while 40 percent of those taking only vitamin C did not. This indicates that in high school-age female athletes, iron supplements should be useful for maintaining adequate iron status. Habitually low intakes of iron-rich foods and increased iron losses usually cause iron deficiency in young women athletes. In addition, blood losses through the gastrointestinal tract correlate with strenuous exercise, and at least some iron is lost in sweat.[107] Iron-deficiency anemia dramatically impairs physical performance by reducing the oxygen-carrying capacity of the blood and inhibiting mitochondrial enzyme function.[108] Even marginal iron deficiency without frank anemia may impair physical performance to some extent, although this effect is still under study. On the other hand, decreased iron indicators in the blood do not always accompany decreases in performance. In a 20-day study of 12 male marathon runners, hematocrit and hemoglobin measures decreased significantly, indicating marginal anemia, even though running speeds remained unchanged.[109] The below-normal hematocrit and hemoglobin measures observed in these runners are not unusual for distance runners.

Sports anemia is a condition distinct from the true iron-deficiency condition, runner's anemia. Sports anemia is characterized by a temporary decrease in hemoglobin concentration after a sudden increase in aerobic exercise.[110] The exact cause of the condition remains controversial, but it is thought that marginal iron intakes may contribute to it.[111] In addition, strenuous, aerobic exercise promotes destruction of fragile, older, red blood cells, and increases the plasma volume of the blood.[112] Sports anemia appears to be an adaptive, temporary response to endurance training. Iron-deficiency anemia requires iron-supplementation therapy; after a few weeks of training, sports anemia usually goes away by itself. The best advice about iron and iron supplements may be to individualize the recommendation. Many young menstruating women probably border on iron deficiency even without the additional iron losses incurred through exercise, and vigorous exercise worsens iron status. Especially for women and teens, then, low hematocrit and hemoglobin measures may warrant the use of supplements, along with attention to the diet, to prevent depletion of iron stores.

sports anemia: a transient condition of low hemoglobin in the blood, associated with the early stages of sports training or other strenuous activity.

Fluids

The athlete's need for water far surpasses the need for any other nutrient. Water's role in temperature regulation is of critical importance in athletes. Working muscles release some of the energy spent as heat. The heat generated during exercise is absorbed by water and eventually transported to the skin for release as sweat, cooling the body when it evaporates. Although the major route of water loss during exercise is through sweating, water is also lost through breathing, as vapor.

Evaporation of sweat is the body's cooling system during exercise in hot environments. As the humidity rises, however, sweat evaporates less readily. In the face of limited evaporation and cooling, the increasing body heat signals greater sweating; dehydration can result, and water loss beyond a 2 percent loss of body weight impairs temperature control and aerobic endurance. Water loss equal to 5 percent of body weight reduces muscular work capacity by 20 to 30 percent.[113] A dangerous rise in body heat accompanied by fluid loss through sweating sets the stage for life-threatening heat stroke.

Water loss during strenuous exercise can amount to as much as 2 to 4 liters per hour. During vigorous exercise in a hot, humid environment, thirst is an inadequate indicator of fluid need because it occurs only after significant fluid depletion.[114] Fluid replacement under these conditions requires a planned schedule. The athlete can defend against heat stroke and promote optimal performance and endurance by drinking cold water before, during, and after exercise as shown in Table 6–3. The human body cannot be conditioned to use less water. Coaches who restrict water during practice are liable for sanction by the American College of Sports Medicine. Cold water (40 to 50 degrees Fahrenheit) promotes rapid gastric emptying and prevents bloating discomfort.

Plain, cold water is the optimal fluid for athletes under most conditions. Sugar- and electrolyte-containing beverages (sports drinks) have a higher concentration of dissolved solids than the body fluids do (that is, they are hypertonic) and demand dilution in the digestive tract. This dilution steals fluid from the tissues and takes time, so the beverage is held in the stomach, away from the thirsty tissues; plain, cold water passes through the stomach unimpeded and rushes to the tissues that need it.[115]

A glucose-containing beverage may be desirable in one extreme case—that of the endurance athlete who competes in events lasting more than two hours. In this instance, once the event is well under way, a dilute solution containing 2 tablespoons of sugar or 1 cup of fruit juice in a quart of water can provide a glucose alternative to glycogen, and so forestall exhaustion. For the average weekend athlete, however, plain water holds the fluid advantage.

In an effort to provide the endurance athlete with a carbohydrate-containing drink that does not slow gastric emptying, researchers developed glucose polymer beverages. Glucose polymer beverages supply glucose in chains of three or four linked glucose units rather than singly. Research results on these beverages are mixed: some show the polymers to demand less dilution in the stomach, and others show them to slow down gastric emptying just as much as the glucose drinks do.[116]

dehydration: loss of excessive fluid and electrolytes from the body.

heat stroke: an acute and dangerous reaction to heat buildup in the body, characterized by high body temperature, loss of consciousness, low blood pressure, and possible death. **Heat exhaustion** precedes it, with warning signs of fatigue, nausea, dizziness, and stomach cramps.

hypertonic: higher osmotic pressure than body fluids.

glucose polymers: compounds that supply glucose not as single molecules, but linked in chains somewhat like starch. The object is to attract less water from the body into the digestive tract (osmotic attraction depends on the number, not the size, of particles).

Table 6–3 Schedule of Hydration before, during, and after Exercise

When to Drink	Amount of Fluid
2 hours before exercise	About 3 c
10 to 15 minutes before exercise	About 2 c
Every 10 to 20 minutes during exercise	About 1/2 c or more
After exercise	Replace each pound of body wieght lost with 2 c fluid

Source: Adapted from J. B. Marcus, ed., *Sports Nutrition* (Chicago: American Dietetic Association, 1986), p. 57.

Water losses surpass losses of electrolytes such as sodium, potassium, and chloride during exercise. Sodium helps maintain fluid volume, helps regulate the acid-base balance of the blood, and allows muscle contraction and nerve impulse transmission. Various organs and hormones tightly control sodium concentration of the blood. When the body loses sodium-containing sweat in exercise, it conserves sodium. In time, if training and sweating occur repeatedly, the athlete's body adapts by reducing the sodium contents of sweat and urine, and so excretes less sodium.

Most athletes' diets supply ample sodium, potassium, chloride, and other electrolytes to replace losses in sweat. Even if losses are high, replacement of these minerals need not occur right away during exercise; later meals that contain them are usually soon enough.

hyponatremia: low concentrations of sodium in the blood.

A caution is in order regarding fluid and electrolyte replacement for the athlete. Elite, ultraendurance athletes, such as triathletes who compete and train for many grueling hours on consecutive days in extreme high heat and humidity, can lose 5 to 10 pounds of body weight in fluid a day. If these athletes were to drink large amounts of water throughout competition, they would risk water intoxication—excess dilution of the blood, called hyponatremia. This can be dangerous; diarrhea, fatigue, and central nervous system disturbances signal the onset, and death can occur soon if treatment is delayed.[117]

water intoxication: excessively high body water contents.

Water intoxication is rare, but it is possible with excessive water consumption in athletes who sweat heavily for many consecutive days. For the few athletes at risk for water intoxication, electrolyte replacement during the activity is necessary.[118] Salt tablets are never advisable as they cause stomach distress and worsen dehydration.

Up to now, this discussion has focused on the role each nutrient plays in muscular work, while recommending for the most part that the athlete receive nutrients from food. Most athletes, and especially high school and college athletes, do not choose foods based on their nutrient needs. In a study of men athletes, only half knew even the basic nutrition facts.[119] In a study of women athletes, all of them knew the importance of calcium, but only 12 percent chose diets that would provide the RDA amount.[120] The next section is about choosing diets for athletes.

Diets for Athletes

Notice that the word *diets* in the title of this section is plural—there is no one best diet for performance, and many variations on the advice given here will support the athlete's performance superbly. However, choices must be made within a framework of two absolutely unbreakable rules. The athlete who obeys these rules can be confident that the diet is adequate.

The first absolutely unbreakable rule is to eat a nutrient-dense diet composed mostly of whole foods. The word *whole* means that foods are as close to the farm-fresh state as possible, for it is in this state that foods provide maximum vitamins and minerals for the kcalories they contain. When athletes rely heavily on processed foods that have suffered nutrient losses and are flavored with sugar and fat, nutrient status suffers. Even if these foods are fortified or enriched, manufacturers cannot replace the full array of nutrients and nonnutrients lost in processing. Consider, for example, that manufacturers mill and process the trace mineral magnesium out of foods but do not replace it—and that magnesium is essential to optimal performance. This does not mean that athletes can *never* choose a white bread, bologna, and mayonnaise sandwich for lunch, but only that they later eat a large, fresh salad or big portions of vegetables and drink a glass of milk to compensate. That way, the whole foods provide the needed nutrients; the bologna sandwich was extra.

This next bit of advice to the athlete may seem timeworn, but it is the other absolutely unbreakable rule for dietary adequacy—build the diet according to a food group plan to ensure that the vitamins and minerals are in full supply. What should be clear from the sections on the metabolic roles of vitamins and minerals in exercise is that the diet must supply each one amply for an athlete to perform, and especially for the athlete to compete. While any food group plan will do, the "basic four" plan is most familiar and therefore easiest to remember (see Appendix C).

Beyond adequacy, energy needs may be immense, and the athlete may want full glycogen stores as well. Simply stated, a diet that is high in carbohydrate, not too high in fat, and adequate in protein while meeting the athlete's energy needs works best. Even if the athlete does not compete in glycogen-depleting events, such a diet is also recommended to control weight, to provide adequate fiber, and to reduce the risk of diabetes while supplying abundant nutrients. A day's worth of food according to such a plan might look like this:

Breakfast:
- ► 1 c oatmeal.
- ► 1/4 c raisins.
- ► 1/2 c 2% lowfat milk.
- ► 2 pieces whole-wheat toast.
- ► 1 tbsp preserves.
- ► 1 c orange juice.

Lunch:
- ► cheese, lettuce, tomato, and mayonnaise sandwich on whole-wheat bread.
- ► carrot sticks (1 carrot).
- ► 1 large apple.
- ► 4 chocolate chip cookies.
- ► 1 c 2% lowfat milk.
- ► 1 Popsicle.

Dinner:
- ► 2 pieces fried chicken.
- ► 1/3 c baked beans.
- ► 1/3 c cole slaw.
- ► 1 biscuit.
- ► 1 12 oz cola.

Snack:
- ► 1 banana.
- ► 1 brownie.
- ► 1 c 2% lowfat milk.

The foods listed represent realistic choices for the adolescent, based on accessibility and eating habits of individuals in this age group. Figure 6–6 shows that most of the nutrients in these meals meet the RDA for an active adolescent. The folacin and iron intake of this day's meals would improve by including more fruits, vegetables, and legumes. Anyone would benefit by such changes, and adolescents wanting to improve their nutrition status would be wise to initiate them. This may not be a realistic option, however, for adolescents who eat away from home more often than not.

As mentioned earlier, many diet variations are suitable, as long as nutritious foods are the basis. This day's meals provide 2750 kcalories, 54 percent of them from carbohydrate, 27 percent of them from fat, and 19 percent of them from protein. Table 6–4 shows some sample diet plans for athletes who wish to increase their energy and carbohydrate intakes by using whole foods. These plans are effective only if the user chooses whole foods to provide nutrients as well as energy—extra milk for calcium and riboflavin, many vegetables for B vitamins, meat or alternates for iron and other vitamins

Figure 6–6   Dietary Analysis of a Typical Day's Meals and the Adolescent RDA Compared[a]

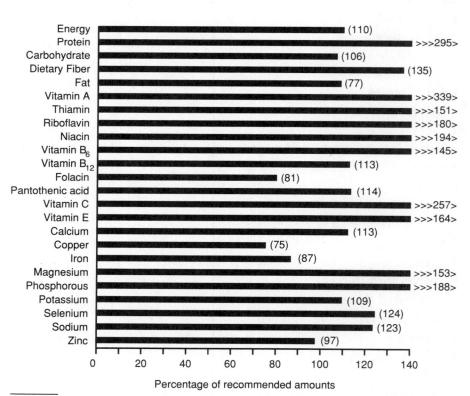

[a] The RDA used in this comparison is for an active 16-year-old female of average height (5 ft 4 in) and weight (124 lb).

Table 6–4   Diet Plans for High-kCalorie, High-Carbohydrate Intakes

Use the number of exchanges indicated, to arrive at the specified energy levels.

Exchange	3100	3900	4600
Low-fat milk	3	5	6
Vegetable	9	11	13
Fruit	9	11	15
Starchy vegetable/ grain	15	19	20
Lean meat	6	7	10
Fat	9	11	11

Note: These plans supply 55 to 60% of kcalories as carbohydrate and less than 30% as fat. To increase the carbohydrate content to over 60%, substitute 1/3-c servings of legumes for the meats. People who cannot eat these quantities of whole food may have to replace some of them with refined sugars and fats in order to meet their energy needs.

and minerals, and whole grains for magnesium, zinc, and chromium. In addition, these foods provide plenty of sodium, potassium, and chloride.

Adding more carbohydrate-rich foods is a sound and reasonable option for increasing kcalories, up to a point. The point at which it becomes unreasonable is when the kcalories needed by the individual outstrip the ability to eat the quantity of food that will provide them. At that point, the person must find ways of adding kcalories to the diet, mostly through the addition of refined sugars and even some fat. Still, this kcalorie-rich diet must be superimposed on the nutrient-rich choices for adequacy. Energy alone is not enough.

A way that an athlete may be able to eat large quantities of food is to consume it in six or eight meals each day. Large snacks of milk shakes, dried fruits, peanut butter sandwiches, or cheese and crackers can add substantial food energy and nutrients.

The Pregame Meal

No single food is known to confer specific physical benefits to athletic performance, although some kinds of foods are preferable to others. The individual athlete may eat particular foods or practice pregame rituals that convey psychological advantages. As long as these foods or rituals are harmless, they should be respected.

The recommended pregame meal is light, easy to digest, and eaten three to four hours before competition to allow time for the stomach to empty before the event. The meal or snack should contain between 300 and 1000 kcalories, although the lighter the better.[121] Table 6–5 shows some sample pregame meals. Breads, potatoes, pasta, and fruit juices—carbohydrate-rich foods, low in fat, protein, and fiber—are the basis of the pregame meal. Fiber-rich carbohydrate foods such as raw vegetables or whole grains, while usually desirable, are best avoided at the pregame meal. Fiber in the digestive tract attracts water out of the blood, and can cause stomach discomfort during performance. Some athletes prefer liquid meals that are commercially available and easily digested.

Table 6–5 Sample Pregame Meals

These foods, to be eaten three to four hours before competition, do *not* have many vitamins or minerals for the most part, and should not be overemphasized in the daily diet. The hours before competition are too late for vitamins and minerals, but the special needs for energy and fluid can be met by eating the following meals.

Food	Serving Size	Energy (kcal)	Energy Donated by Carbohydrate % of kcalories)
Sample Meal #1			
White bread	2 slices	140	74
Jam or jelly	2 tbsp	130	100
Gelatin dessert	1 c	70	97
Grape juice	1 c	165	100
Total		505	94
Sample Meal #2			
Spaghetti and tomato sauce	1 c	190	80
Roll	1	85	71
Popsicle (3 oz)	2	140	100
Limeade	1 c	100	100
Total		515	90
Sample Meal #3			
Banana	1	100	100
Sweetened dry cereal	3/4 c	115	90
Nonfat milk	1/2 c	45	53
Cranberry juice cocktail	2/3 c	109	100
Gumdrops	1 oz	100	100
Total		469	95

Note: Substitutions can be made for cereal (1 c), spaghetti (1 c), or bread (2 slices):
▶ 1 c white or flavored rice.
▶ 1 3-inch-diameter muffin (plain).
▶ 1 piece angel food cake.
▶ 3 small pancakes and syrup.
To substitute liquids (gelatin, juices, limeade), use 1 c for each: 1 c any sugar-sweetened beverage.

Source: E. M. N. Hamilton, E. N. Whitney, and F. S. Sizer, *Nutrition: Concepts and Controversies,* 4th ed. (St. Paul, Minn.: West, 1988).

In addition to causing discomfort, a meal eaten within an hour or two of competition can slow the athlete down, especially if that meal contains sugar. Research on runners shows that sugar taken directly before exercise can reduce athletic performance by 25 percent.[122] The sugary meals of Table 6–5 can enhance performance, but only if they are finished well in advance of the event; the guideline suggested above works well— finish the meal three to four hours before competition.

Athletes who want to excel will apply in their daily routines the most accurate possible nutrition knowledge, along with dedication to rigorous training. A diet that provides ample fluid and consists of a variety of nutrient-dense, whole foods in quantities to meet energy needs will enhance not only athletic performance, but overall health as well. Training and genetics being equal, it is easy to guess who would win a competition—the athlete who habitually consumes half or less of the needed nutrients, or the one who arrives at the event with a long history of full nutrient stores and well-met metabolic needs.

This text began with a discussion of the fertile years prior to conception and followed life through pregnancy, lactation, infancy, childhood, and on into adolescence. As this chapter on adolescents closes, the cycle is complete. The adolescent is physically mature and has full reproductive capability. To the extent that sound nutrition and beneficial physical activity have attended that individual's life from conception onwards, she or he is physically prepared to begin another turn of the cycle. The next chapter of this book could have been Chapter 1, a discussion on preparing for conception. May the next generation begin in the best of health.

Chapter 6 Notes

1. D. Sinclair, Growth in height and weight, in *Human Growth after Birth*, 4th ed. (New York: Oxford University Press, 1985), pp. 23–50.

2. Sinclair, 1985, pp. 23–50.

3. D. Sinclair, Changes in shape and posture, in *Human Growth after Birth*, 4th ed. (New York: Oxford University Press, 1985), pp. 123–147.

4. Sinclair, 1985, pp. 123–147.

5. D. Sinclair, Growth of tissues, in *Human Growth after Birth*, 4th ed. (New York: Oxford University Press, 1985), pp. 51–72.

6. D. Sinclair, Indices of maturity, in *Human Growth after Birth*, 4th ed. (New York: Oxford University Press, 1985), pp. 102–122.

7. Sinclair, 1985, pp. 102–122.

8. Sinclair, 1985, pp. 102–122.

9. R. E. Frisch, Fatness, menarche, and female fertility, *Perspectives in Biology and Medicine* 28 (1985): 611–633.

10. H. E. Kulin and coauthors, The effect of chronic childhood malnutrition on pubertal growth and development, *American Journal of Clinical Nutrition* 36 (1982): 527–536.

11. D. Sinclair, Growth of systems, in *Human Growth after Birth*, 4th ed. (New York: Oxford University Press, 1985), pp. 73–101.

12. K. Satyanarayana and coauthors, Effect of nutritional deprivation in early childhood on later growth—a community study without intervention, *American Journal of Clinical Nutrition* 34 (1981): 1636–1637.

13. Kulin and coauthors, 1982.

14. Sinclair, 1985, pp. 102–122.

15. P. A. Wagner and coauthors, Serum zinc concentrations in adolescents as related to sexual maturation, *Human Nutrition: Clinical Nutrition* 39C (1985): 459–462.

16. R. B. Sandler and coauthors, Postmenopausal bone density and milk consumption in childhood and adolescence, *American Journal of Clinical Nutrition* 42 (1985): 270–274.

17. Food and Nutrition Board, Committee on Dietary Allowances, *Recommended Dietary Allowances*, 9th ed. (Washington, D.C.: National Academy of Sciences, 1980), p. 138.

18. *Iron Nutriture in Adolescence*, U.S. Department of Health, Education, and Welfare, HHS Publication no. (HSA) 77-5100 (Washington, D.C.: Government Printing Office, 1977).

19. J. D. Skinner and coauthors, Appalachian adolescents' eating patterns and nutrient intakes, *Journal of the American Dietetic Association* 85 (1985): 1093–1099.

20. Nutrition Committee, Canadian Paediatric Society, Adolescent nutrition. 2. Normal nutritional requirements, *Canadian Medical Association Journal* 129 (1983): 420–422.

21. J. A. Driskell, A. J. Clark, and S. W. Moak, Longitudinal assessment of vitamin B_6 status in Southern adolescent girls, *Journal of the American Dietetic Association* 87 (1987): 307–310; P. Thompson and coauthors, Zinc status and sexual development in adolescent girls, *Journal of the American Dietetic Association* 86 (1986): 892–897; H. McCoy and coauthors, Nutrient intakes of female adolescents from eight southern states, *Journal of the Amer-*

ican Dietetic Association 84 (1984): 1453–1460; A. J. Clark, S. Mossholder, and R. Gates, Folacin status in adolescent females, *American Journal of Clinical Nutrition* 46 (1987): 302–306.

22. P. M. Guenther, Beverages in the diets of American teenagers, *Journal of the American Dietetic Association* 86 (1986): 493–499.

23. L. K. Massey, Soft drink consumption, phosphorus intake, and osteoporosis, *Journal of the American Dietetic Association* 80 (1982): 581–583.

24. Food and Nutrition Board, 1980, pp. 126–127.

25. Skinner and coauthors, 1985; J. Bowering and K. L. Clancy, Nutritional status of children and teenagers in relation to vitamin and mineral use, *Journal of the American Dietetic Association* 86 (1986): 1033–1038.

26. M. Zelnik and J. F. Kantner, Sexual and contraceptive experience of young unmarried women in the United States 1976 and 1971, *Adolescent Pregnancy and Childbearing: Findings from Research*, NIH Publication no. 81-2077 (Washington, D.C.: Government Printing Office, 1980), pp. 43–81.

27. C. A. Bachrach, Contraceptive practice among American women, 1973–1982, *Family Planning Perspectives* 16 (1984): 253–259.

28. 1985 Natality report available from USPHS, *American Journal of Public Health* 77 (1987): 1473; K. Davis, A theory of teenage pregnancy in the United States, in *Adolescent Pregnancy and Childbearing*, ed. C. S. Chilman, U.S. Depart-

ment of Health and Human Services, NIH Publication no. 81-2077, (Washington, D.C.: Government Printing Office, 1981), pp. 309–339.

29. V. Ktsanes, The teenager and the family planning experience, in *Adolescent Pregnancy and Childbearing*, ed. C. S. Chilman, U.S. Department of Health and Human Services, NIH Publication no. 81-2077, (Washington, D.C.: Government Printing Office, 1981), pp. 83–100.

30. USDA, Food and Dietary Service, U.S. Department of Health and Human Services, March of Dimes Birth Defects Foundation, *Working with the Pregnant Teenager: A Guide for Nutrition Educators* (Washington, D.C.: Government Printing Office, 1981), p. 1.

31. A. A. Campbell, Trends in teenage childbearing in the United States, in *Adolescent Pregnancy and Childbearing*, ed. C. S. Chilman, U.S. Department of Health and Human Services, NIH Publication no. 81-2077, (Washington, D.C.: Government Printing Office, 1981), pp. 3–13.

32. Sinclair, 1985, pp. 102–122.

33. J. Menken, The health and demographic consequences of adolescent pregnancy and childbearing, in *Adolescent Pregnancy and Childbearing*, ed. C. S. Chilman, U.S. Department of Health and Human Services, NIH Publication no. 81-2077, (Washington, D.C.: Government Printing Office 1981), pp. 177–205.

34. Menken, 1981.

35. Menken, 1981.

36. Menken, 1981.

37. Menken, 1981.

38. Adolescent pregnancy—counseling considerations, *Nutrition and the MD*, January 1986, p. 4.

39. A. R. Frisancho, J. Matos, and L. A. Bòllettino, Influence of growth status and placental function on birth weight of infants born to young still-growing teenagers, *American Journal of Clinical Nutrition* 40 (1984): 801–807.

40. G. M. Chan and coauthors, Effects of increased dietary calcium intake upon the calcium and bone mineral status of lactating adolescent and adult women, *American Journal of Clinical Nutrition* 46 (1987): 319–323.

41. Evaluation of the Teenage Pregnancy and Parenting (TAPP) Project, Family Service Agency of San Francisco, October 1, 1982–September 30, 1983, submitted to the Office of Adolescent Pregnancy Programs, Department of Health and Human Services, Washington, D.C. (San Francisco: Center for Population and Reproductive Health, Institute for Health Policy Studies, University of California, 1984).

42. E. T. Kennedy and M. Kotelchuk, The effect of WIC supplemental feeding on birth weight: A case-control study, *American Journal of Clinical Nutrition* 40 (1984): 579–585.

43. N. S. Moses, M. Banilivy, and F. Lifshitz, Fear of obesity among adolescent females (abstract), *American Journal of Clinical Nutrition* 43 (1986): 664.

44. J. K. Thompson, Larger than life, *Psychology Today*, April 1986, pp. 38–44.

45. N. S. Storz and W. H. Greene, Body weight, body image, and perception of fad diets in adolescent girls, *Journal of Nutrition Education*, March 1983, pp. 15–18.

46. D. Farley, Eating disorders: When thinness becomes an obsession, *FDA Consumer*, May 1986, pp. 20–23.

47. Position of the American Dietetic Association: Nutrition intervention in the treatment of anorexia nervosa and bulimia, *Journal of the American Dietetic Association* 88 (1988): 68.

48. D. B. Herzog and P. M. Copeland, Eating disorders, *New England Journal of Medicine* 313 (1985): 295–303.

49. Health and Public Policy Committee, American College of Physicians, Eating disorders: Anorexia nervosa and bulimia, *Annals of Internal Medicine* 105 (1986): 790–794.

50. Farley, 1986.

51. J. Chalmers and coauthors, Anorexia nervosa presenting as morbid exercising (letter), *Lancet* 1 (1985): 286, as cited in Anorexia nervosa presenting as morbid obesity (abstract), *Journal of the American Dietetic Association* 85 (1985): 762.

52. Herzog and Copeland, 1985; N. Vaisman and coauthors, Effect of refeeding on the basal energy metabolism and substrate utilization of adolescents with anorexia nervosa (abstract), *American Journal of Clinical Nutrition* 43 (1986): 670.

53. Herzog and Copeland, 1985.

54. B. Palla and I. F. Litt, Medical complications of eating disorders in adolescents, *Pediatrics* 81 (1988): 613–623.

55. Herzog and Copeland, 1985.

56. Y. Danziger and coauthors, Parental involvement in treatment of patients with anorexia nervosa in a pediatric day-care unit, *Pediatrics* 81 (1988): 159–162.

57. D. M. Huse and A. R. Lucas, Dietary treatment of anorexia nervosa, *Journal of the American Dietetic Association* 83 (1983): 687–690.

58. E. Sanger and T. Cassino, Eating disorders: Avoiding the power struggle, *American Journal of Nursing* 84 (1984): 31–33.

59. Huse and Lucas, 1983.

60. Herzog and Copeland, 1985.

61. Farley, 1986

62. Farley, 1986.

63. B. G. Kirkley, Bulimia: Clinical characteristics, development, and etiology, *Journal of the American Dietetic Association* 86 (1986): 468–472.

64. J. D. Killen and coauthors, Depressive symptoms and substance use among adolescent binge eaters and purgers: A defined population study, *American Journal of Public Health* 77 (1987): 1539–1541; Health and Public Policy Committee, American College of Physicians, Eating disorders: Anorexia nervosa and bulimia, *Annals of Internal Medicine* 105 (1986): 790–794.

65. M. Story, Nutrition management and dietary treatment of bulimia, *Journal of the American Dietetic Association* 86 (1986): 517–519.

66. R. M. Reisner, Acne vulgaris, *Pediatric Clinics of North America* 20 (1973): 851–864.

67. *Acne*, a pamphlet available from the National Institute of Allergy and Infectious Diseases, Bethesda, MD 20205, NIH Publication no. 80-188, May 1980; *Stubborn and Vexing, That's Acne*, a pamphlet available from the Food and Drug Administration, 5600 Fishers Lane, Rockville, MD 20857, HHS Publication no. (FDA) 80-3107, May 1980.

68. J. O. Holloszy and E. F. Coyle, Adaptations of skeletal muscle to endurance exercise and their metabolic consequences, *Journal of Applied Physiology: Respiratory, Environmental and Exercise Physiology* 56 (1984): 831–838.

69. J. P. Flatt, Dietary fat, carbohydrate balance, weight maintenance: Effects of exercise, *American Journal of Clinical Nutrition* 45 (1987): 296–306.

70. B. Essen, Intramuscular substrate utilization during prolonged exercise, *Annals of the New York Academy of Science* 301 (1977): 30–44.

71. J. Bergstrom and E. Hultman, Nutrition for maximal sports performance, *Journal of the American Medical Association* 28 (1972): 999–1006.

72. E. H. Christensen and O. Hansen, Arbeitsfahigkeit und ehrnahrung, *Skandinavisches Archiv fuer Physiologie* 8 (1939): 160–175, as cited in E. L. Fox, *Sports Physiology*, 2nd ed. (New York: W. B. Saunders Company, 1984), pp. 40–57.

73. M. H. Williams, *Nutritional Aspects of Human Physical and Athletic Performance*, 2nd ed. (Springfield, Ill.: Charles C. Thomas, 1985), pp. 20–57 and Figure 2, The Effect of Diet on Physical Endurance.

74. Bergstrom and Hultman, 1972.

75. W. M. Sherman and coauthors, Effect of exercise-diet manipulation on muscle glycogen and its subsequent utilization during performance, *International Journal of Sports Medicine* 2 (1981): 114–118.

76. L. P. Garetto and coauthors, Enhanced insulin sensitivity of skeletal muscle following exercise, Proceedings of the 5th International Symposium on Biochemistry of Exercise, in *Biochemistry of Exercise*, ed. H. G. Knuttgen (Champaign, Ill.: Human Kinetics, 1983), pp. 681–687.

77. D. L. Costill and coauthors, The role of dietary carbohydrates in muscle glycogen resynthesis after strenuous running, *American Journal of Clinical Nutrition* 34 (1981): 1831–1836.

78. The American Dietetic Association, Position paper: Nutrition for physical fitness and athletic performance for adults, *Journal of the American Dietetic Association* 87 (1987): 933–939.

79. Bergstrom and Hultman, 1972.

80. D. L. Costill and coauthors, Effects of elevated plasma FFA and insulin on muscle glycogen usage during exercise, *Journal of Applied Physiology: Respiratory, Environmental, and Exercise Physiology* 43 (1977): 695–699.

81. W. J. Evans and V. A. Hughes, Dietary carbohydrates and endurance exercise, *American Journal of Clinical Nutrition* 41: (1985): 1146–1154.

82. D. L. Costill, G. P. Dalsky, and W. J. Fink, Effects of caffeine ingestion on metabolism and exercise performance, *Medicine and Science in Sports* 10 (1978): 155–158.

83. F. T. O'Neil, M. T. Hynak-Hankinson, and J. Gorman, Research and application of current topics in sports nutrition, *Journal of the American Dietetic Association* 86 (1986): 1007–1015.

84. Essen, 1977.

85. P. W. R. Lemon and J. P. Mullin, Effect of initial muscle glycogen levels on protein catabolism during exercise, *Journal of Applied Physiology: Respiratory, Environmental, and Exercise Physiology* 48 (1980): 624–629, as cited in E. R. Buskirk, Some nutritional considerations in the conditioning of athletes, *Annual Review of Nutrition* 1 (1981): 319–350.

86. M. N. Goodman and N. B. Ruderman, Influence of muscle use on amino acid metabolism, *Exercise and Sport Sciences Reviews* 10 (1982): 1–26.

87. M. H. Williams, The role of protein in physical activity, in *Nutritional Aspects of Human Physical and Athletic Performance*, 2nd ed. (Springfield, Ill.: Charles C. Thomas, 1985), pp. 120–146.

88. P. W. R. Lemon, K. E. Yarasheski, and D. Dolny, The importance of protein for athletes, *Sports Medicine* 1 (1984): 474–484.

89. J. R. Brotherhood, Nutrition and sports performance, *Sports Medicine* 1 (1984): 350–389.

90. M. H. Williams, Use of nutritional supplements by athletes, in *Nutrition and Athletic Performance*, ed. W. Haskell, J. Scala, and J. Whitman (Palo Alto, Calif.: Bull Publishing, 1982), pp. 106–155.

91. M. H. Williams, The role of vitamins in physical activity, in *Nutritional Aspects of Human Physical and Athletic Performance*, 2nd ed. (Springfield, Ill.: Charles C. Thomas, 1985), pp. 147–185.

92. Food and Nutrition Board, Committee on Dietary Allowances, *Recommended Dietary Allowances,* 9th ed. (Washington, D.C.: National Academy of Sciences, 1980), pp. 72–124.

93. A. Belko and coauthors, Effects of exercise on riboflavin requirements: Biological validation in weight reducing women, *American Journal of Clinical Nutrition* 41 (1985): 270–277.

94. Williams, 1985.

95. V. Herbert, N. Colman, and E. Jacob, Folic acid and vitamin B_{12}, in *Modern Nutrition in Health and Disease*, 6th ed., ed. R. S. Goodhart and M. E. Shils (Philadelphia: Lea and Febiger, 1980), pp. 229–259.

96. Williams, 1985.

97. R. P. Heaney, R. R. Recker, and P. D. Saville, Menopausal changes in calcium balance performance, *Journal of Laboratory and Clinical Medicine* 92 (1978): 953–963.

98. M. E. Nelson and coauthors, Diet and bone status in amenorrheic runners, *American Journal of Clinical Nutrition* 43 (1986): 910–916.

99. B. B. Peterkin, Women's diets: 1977 and 1985, *Journal of Nutrition Education* 18 (1986): 251–257.

100. L. W. Rosen, Pathogenic weight-control behavior in female athletes, *Physician and Sportsmedicine* 14 (1986): 79–86.

101. Nelson and coauthors, 1986.

102. P. R. Dallman, M. A. Siimes, and A. Stekel, Iron deficiency in infancy and childhood, *American Journal of Clinical Nutrition* 33 (1980): 86–118.

103. Expert Scientific Working Group of the Federation of American Societies for Experimental Biology, Summary of a report on assessment of the iron nutritional status of the United States population, *American Journal of Clinical Nutrition* 42 (1985): 1318–1330.

104. R. B. Parr, L. A. Bachman, and R. A. Moss, Iron deficiency in female athletes, *Physician and Sportsmedicine* 12 (1984): 81–86.

105. P. A. Deuster and coauthors, Nutritional survey of highly trained women runners, *American Journal of Clinical Nutrition* 44 (1986): 954–962.

106. H. J. Nickerson and coauthors, Decreased iron stores in high school female runners, *American Journal of Diseases of Children* 139 (1985): 1115–1119.

107. J. G. Stewart and coauthors, Gastrointestinal blood loss and anemia in runners, *Annals of Internal Medicine* 100 (1984): 843–845; M. Brune and coauthors, Iron losses in sweat, *American Journal of Clinical Nutrition* 43 (1986): 438–443.

108. G. W. Gardner and coauthors, Physical work capacity and metabolic stress in subjects with iron-deficiency anemia, *American Journal of Clinical Nutrition* 30 (1977): 910–917.

109. R. H. Dressendorfer, C. E. Wade, and E. A. Amsterdam, Development of pseudoanemia in marathon runners during a 20-day road race, *Journal of the American Medical Association* 246 (1981): 1215–1218.

110. Parr, Bachman, and Moss, 1984.

111. American Dietetic Association, 1987.

112. Dressendorfer, Wade, and Amsterdam, 1981.

113. Bergstrom and Hultman, 1972.

114. J. E. Greenleaf and coauthors, Drinking and water balance during exercise and heat acclimation, *Journal of Applied Physiology: Respiratory, Environmental, and Exercise Physiology* 54 (1983): 414–419.

115. D. L. Costill and B. Saltin, Factors limiting gastric emptying during rest and exercise, *Journal of Applied Physiology* 37 (1974): 679–683.

116. C. Foster, Gastric-emptying characteristics of glucose polymers, in *Ross Symposium on Nutrient Utilization during Exercise*, ed. E. L. Fox (Columbus, Ohio: Ross Laboratories, 1983), pp. 80–84.

117. R. T. Frizzel and coauthors, Hyponatremia and ultramarathon running, *Journal of the American Medical Association* 255 (1986): 772–775.

118. F. T. O'Neil, M. T. Hynak-Hankinson, and J. Gorman, Research and application of current topics in sports nutrition, *Journal of the American Dietetic Association* 86 (1986): 1007–1015.

119. L. R. Shoaf, P. D. McClellan, and K. A. Birskovich, Nutrition knowledge, interests, and information sources of male athletes, *Journal of Nutrition Education* 18 (1986): 243–245.

120. M. Perron and J. Endres, Knowledge, attitudes, and dietary practices of female athletes, *Journal of the American Dietetic Association* 85 (1985): 573–576.

121. American Dietetic Association, 1987.

122. K. Keller and R. Schwarzkopf, Preexercise snacks may decrease exercise performance, *Physician and Sportsmedicine* 12 (1984): 89–91.

▶ *Focal Point 6*

Drugs, Alcohol, and Tobacco

The physical maturity and growing independence of the teen years present adolescents with a new set of responsibilities and decisions to handle. The choices they make and the consequences of their actions will impact on their lives, for better or worse. Some of these behaviors may influence their lives only for today, others can have lifelong effects. The connections between some of these behaviors and nutrition are explored in this focal point.

Drugs

The teen years are a critical time in the development of problem behaviors such as drug use. With the exception of cocaine use, illicit drug use among adolescents in this country has declined since its peak in the late 1970s.[1] Still, three of every five high school seniors report that they have at least tried an illicit drug, most commonly marijuana, amphetamines, and cocaine. This discussion focuses on the nutrition-related effects of these drugs.

Marijuana

Half of all seniors surveyed report having tried marijuana, with half of them smoking marijuana within the past 30 days.[2] Like all substances entering the body, marijuana must be processed. The active ingredients are rapidly and almost completely (90 percent) absorbed from the lungs.[3] Then, being fat soluble, these substances are packaged (most likely in lipoproteins) before being transported by the blood to the various body tissues.[4] They are processed by many tissues (not just by the liver), and they persist for several days in the body, being excreted over a period of a week or more after the smoking of a single marijuana cigarette.[5] With repeated exposure, these substances accumulate and become concentrated in body fat, the lungs, liver, reproductive organs, and the brain.[6]

Smoking a marijuana cigarette has several characteristic effects on the body, altering, among other things, the sense of taste. Among the apparent taste changes induced by marijuana is an enhanced enjoyment of eating, especially of sweets, commonly known as "the munchies." Why or how this effect occurs is not known.[7] The drug does not change blood-glucose concentrations.[8] Some investigators speculate that the hunger induced by marijuana is actually a social effect caused by the suggestibility of the group in which it is smoked.[9] The heightened appetite and food consumption effects of THC were tested in patients with anorexia nervosa without success.[10]

THC: delta-9-tetrahydrocannabinol, the active ingredient of marijuana primarily responsible for its intoxicating effects.

Prolonged use of the drug does not seem to bring about a weight gain; in one small sample (30 smokers), regular users weighed less than comparable nonsmokers by about 7 pounds.[11]

Amphetamines

amphetamine: A central nervous system stimulant.

Statistics on amphetamine use are difficult to determine. Incidence reports vary in their inclusion of over-the-counter stimulants, medically prescribed stimulants, and illicit amphetamine use. Whatever the actual numbers, the prevalence of amphetamine use appears to be declining.[12] This is due, in part, to physicians' reducing their prescriptions of amphetamines to adolescents. When amphetamine users were surveyed, almost 30 percent indicated that their first use was via a medical prescription, whereas approximately 20 percent had never received a prescription.[13]

Physicians prescribe amphetamines to treat hyperkinesis, narcolepsy, and obesity. Amphetamines raise the pulse rate and blood pressure. Their effects include increased alertness, excitation, and euphoria; insomnia; and loss of appetite.

Cocaine

Cocaine use has not followed the declining trend of other illicit drugs. Of the seniors surveyed, 17 percent reported having tried cocaine, with approximately one-third of those students using it within the past month.[14] Cocaine's properties are like those of both amphetamines and anesthetics. The drug elicits such effects as intense euphoria, restlessness, heightened self-confidence, irritability, insomnia, and loss of appetite. Weight loss is a common side effect, and cocaine abusers often meet the criteria for eating disorders.[15] Repeated use can cause rapid heart rate, irregular heartbeats, heart attacks, and even death.

Drug abusers face multiple nutrition problems:

▶ They spend money for drugs that could be spent on food.
▶ They lose interest in food during "high" times.
▶ Some drugs induce at least a temporary depression of appetite.
▶ Their lifestyle often lacks the regularity and routine that promote good eating habits.
▶ They may contract hepatitis, a liver disease common in drug abusers, which causes taste changes and loss of appetite.
▶ Their nutrient status may be altered by treatments and medicines.
▶ They often become ill with infectious diseases, which increase their need for nutrients.

During withdrawal from drugs, an important aspect of treatment is the identification and correction of nutrition problems.

Alcohol

At some point during adolescence, teenagers face a critical choice: to drink or not to drink alcohol. Even though the law forbids sale of alcohol to people under a specific age, alcohol is still available to many teenagers who seek it. Over 90 percent of high school seniors decide to try a drink; 1 in 20 reports daily consumption of alcohol.[16] The motivating factors are numerous. A person observing adolescents might glean the following reasons for drinking alcohol:

► To be popular.

► To be grown-up.

► To defy parents.

► To drown feelings of inadequacy.

For some people, drinking an alcoholic beverage is a custom that accompanies social relations. It provides them pleasure without problems. Many teenagers find that alcohol and marijuana serve similar purposes, and the pattern of substance use indicates parallel consumption, not a displacement of one by the other.[17] Some teenagers use alcohol as an escape or for support— an ineffective way to cope with problems that leads to greater problems. Dependency on alcohol or any drug has major adverse effects on the growth and development of adolescents and deserves attention, but is beyond the scope of this text.

People use alcohol to help them relax or to relieve anxiety. They think that alcohol is a stimulant because it seems to make them lively and uninhibited at first. Actually, though, the way it does this is by sedating inhibitory nerves, which are more numerous than excitatory nerves. Ultimately, it acts as a depressant, and sedates all the nerve cells.

Alcohol is an empty-kcalorie beverage and can displace needed nutrients from the diet while simultaneously altering metabolism so that even good nutrition cannot normalize it. A discussion of alcohol absorption and metabolism provides a basis for understanding the effects alcohol has on a person's body and nutrition status.[18]

To the chemist, *alcohol* refers to a class of compounds containing reactive hydroxyl (OH) groups. To most other people, *alcohol* refers to the intoxicating ingredient in beer, wine, and hard liquor (distilled spirits). The chemist's name for this particular alcohol is *ethyl alcohol*, or *ethanol*.

The alcohols affect living things profoundly, partly because they act as lipid solvents. They can dissolve the lipids out of cell membranes, destroying the cell structure and thereby killing the cells. For this reason, most alcohols are toxic.

Like the other alcohols, ethanol is toxic—but less so than some. Sufficiently diluted and taken in small enough doses, it produces euphoria, not without risk, but with a risk that some find tolerable (if the doses are low enough). Used to achieve these effects, alcohol is a drug—that is, a substance that can modify one or more of the body's functions.

From the moment ethanol enters the body in a beverage, it is treated as if it has special privileges. Unlike foods, the tiny ethanol molecules need no

drink: a dose of any alcoholic beverage that delivers 1/2 oz of pure ethanol:

► 3 to 4 oz of wine.

► 8 to 12 oz of beer.

► 1 oz hard liquor (whiskey, scotch, rum, or vodka).

ethanol: the alcohol in beer, wine, and hard liquor.

euphoria (you-FORE-ee-uh): a feeling of great well-being, which people often seek through the use of drugs such as alcohol.
eu = good
phoria = bearing

alcohol dehydrogenase: a liver enzyme that converts ethanol to **acetaldehyde** (ass-et-AL-duh-hide).

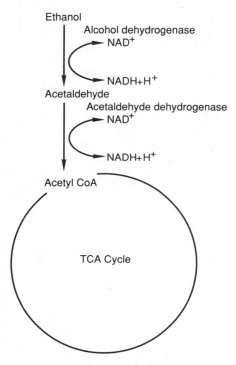

Figure FP6–1   Metabolism of Ethanol to Acetyl CoA
Alcohol dehydrogenase oxidizes ethanol to acetaldehyde within the liver. Simultaneously, this reaction reduces a molecule of the niacin coenzyme NAD^+ to NADH + H^+. A related enzyme, acetaldehyde dehydrogenase, reduces another NAD^+ to NADH + H^+, while it oxidizes acetaldehyde to acetyl CoA, the compound that enters the TCA cycle to generate energy. (All cells possess acetaldehyde dehydrogenase, so this step can take place outside the liver.)

digestion; they can quickly diffuse through the walls of an empty stomach and reach the brain within a minute, creating a feeling of euphoria almost immediately. When the stomach is full of food, the ethanol molecules have less chance of touching the walls and diffusing through, so a person does not feel the effects so quickly. Therefore, to slow ethanol absorption, a person should eat something, preferably carbohydrate snacks. High-fat snacks help, too, because they slow peristalsis.[19] The presence of food is less influential when stomach contents empty into the duodenum; intestinal absorption of alcohol is rapid, "as if it were a V.I.P. (Very Important Person)."[20]

The capillaries that surround the digestive tract merge into the veins that carry the alcohol-laden blood to the liver. Here the veins branch and rebranch into capillaries that touch every liver cell. Liver cells are the only cells in the body that can make enough alcohol dehydrogenase to oxidize ethanol at an appreciable rate. The rate of clearance is determined by the number of alcohol dehydrogenase enzyme molecules that reside in the liver. If more molecules of ethanol arrive at the liver cells than the enzymes can handle, the extra ethanol must wait. It enters the general circulation and is carried past the liver to all parts of the body, circulating again and again through the liver until enzymes are available to convert it to acetaldehyde. Prudent drinkers drink slowly, with food in their stomachs, to allow the ethanol molecules to move to the liver cells gradually enough for the enzymes to handle the load. Spacing of drinks is important, too. It takes about an hour and a half to metabolize one drink, depending on the person's body size, previous drinking experience, recent food consumption, and general health. Figure FP6–1 diagrams the primary metabolic pathway of ethanol.

That each person has a particular concentration of alcohol dehydrogenase that limits the rate of ethanol clearance explains why only time will restore sobriety. Walking will not; it makes the muscles work, but since they cannot metabolize ethanol, they do not help clear it from the blood. Drinking a cup of coffee is of no use either; caffeine is a stimulant, but it does not speed up the metabolism of ethanol.

Careful study of Figure FP6–1 reveals that ethanol metabolism uses the niacin coenzyme NAD^+, creating an accumulation of NADH + H^+. This consequence alters the body's "redox state" because NAD^+ can oxidize, and NADH + H^+ can reduce, many other body compounds. During ethanol metabolism, NAD^+ becomes unavailable for the multitude of reactions for which it is required. Consider that the metabolism of glucose, fatty acids, and amino acids all require NAD^+. For these nutrients to be completely metabolized to energy, the TCA cycle must be operating, and this also requires NAD^+. Without NAD^+, the metabolic pathways are blocked, causing metabolites to accumulate or take alternate routes. Such changes in the normal metabolism of nutrients produce altered biochemistry.

Wherever NAD^+ is converted to NADH + H^+ in ethanol metabolism, hydrogen ions accumulate, resulting in a dangerous shift of the acid-base balance toward acid. The accumulation of NADH + H^+ depresses the TCA cycle, so that pyruvate and acetyl CoA build up. The excess acetyl CoA then takes the route to the synthesis of fatty acids, and fat clogs the liver so it cannot function.[21]

The synthesis of fatty acids also accelerates as a result of the liver's exposure to ethanol. Fat accumulation can be seen in the liver after a single night of heavy drinking. Fatty liver, the first stage of liver deterioration seen in heavy drinkers, interferes with the distribution of nutrients and oxygen to the liver cells. If the condition lasts long enough, the liver cells die, and fibrous scar tissue invades the area—the second stage of liver deterioration, called fibrosis. Fibrosis is reversible with good nutrition and abstinence from alcohol, but the next (last) stage—cirrhosis—is not.

The body's altered redox state inhibits gluconeogenesis and can lead to hypoglycemia if glycogen stores are not repleted.[22] Limited glucose combined with the overabundance of acetyl CoA sets the stage for a shift into ketosis. The making of ketone bodies consumes acetyl CoA, but some ketone bodies are acids, so they push the acid-base balance further toward acid.

Figure FP6–2 illustrates the conversion of pyruvate to lactic acid when the path to acetyl CoA is blocked. The surplus of $NADH + H^+$ also favors the conversion of pyruvate to lactic acid, which serves as a temporary storage place for hydrogens from $NADH + H^+$. The conversion of pyruvate to lactic acid restores some NAD^+, but a lactic acid buildup adds still further to the body's acid burden.

Liver metabolism clears most of the ethanol from the blood. However, about 10 percent is excreted through the breath and in the urine. This is the basis for the breath-analyzing test for drunkenness administered by the police. The amount of alcohol in the breath is in proportion to that in the bloodstream. In most states, legal drunkenness is set at 0.10 percent or lower. Table FP6–1 shows the blood-alcohol levels that correspond with progressively greater intoxication.

Figure FP6–3 illustrates alcohol's effects on the brain. Brain cells are particularly sensitive to excessive exposure to alcohol. Like liver cells, they die; however, unlike liver cells, brain cells cannot regenerate. This is one reason for the permanent brain damage observed in some heavy drinkers.

It is lucky that the brain centers respond to ethanol in the order described in Figure FP6–3 because an individual passes out before drinking enough to reach a lethal dose. It is possible, though, to drink fast enough that the effects continue to accelerate after one has gone to sleep. The occasional death that takes place during a drinking contest is attributed to this effect. The drinker drinks fast enough, before passing out, to receive a lethal dose.

Ethanol interferes with a multitude of chemical and hormonal reactions in the body. It depresses production of antidiuretic hormone (ADH) by the pituitary gland in the brain. Loss of body water leads to thirst, and thirst leads to more drinking. The only fluid that will relieve dehydration is water, but the thirsty drinker may choose another alcoholic beverage instead. A person who

fatty liver: an early stage of liver deterioration seen in several diseases, including kwashiorkor and alcoholic liver disease. Fatty liver is characterized by accumulation of fat in the liver cells.

fibrosis: an intermediate stage of liver deterioration seen in several diseases, including viral hepatitis and alcoholic liver disease. In fibrosis, the liver cells lose their function and assume the characteristics of connective tissue cells (fibers).

cirrhosis (seer-OH-sis): advanced liver disease, in which liver cells have died, hardened, and turned orange; often associated with alcoholism.
cirrhos = an orange

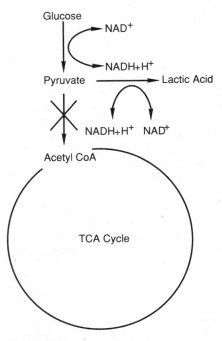

Figure FP6–2 Blocked Metabolism of Pyruvate to Acetyl CoA
Pyruvate is converted to lactic acid if the pathway to acetyl CoA is blocked.

Table FP6–1 Alcohol Doses and Brain Responses

Number of Drinks	Blood Alcohol (%)	Effect on Brain
2	0.05	Judgment impaired
4	0.10	Control impaired
6	0.15	Muscle coordination and reflexes impaired
8	0.20	Vision impaired
12	0.30	Drunk, out of control
14 or more	0.50 to 0.60	Amnesia, finally death

antidiuretic hormone (ADH): a hormone produced by the pituitary gland in response to dehydration (or a high sodium concentration in the blood); stimulates the kidneys to reabsorb more water and so excrete less. This ADH should not be confused with the enzyme alcohol dehydrogenase, which is also abbreviated ADH.

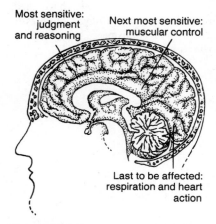

Most sensitive: judgment and reasoning

Next most sensitive: muscular control

Last to be affected: respiration and heart action

Figure FP6—3 Alcohol's Effects on the Brain
When ethanol flows to the brain, it first sedates the frontal lobe, the reasoning part. As the ethanol molecules diffuse into the cells of this lobe, they interfere with reasoning and judgment. If the drinker drinks faster than the rate at which the liver can oxidize the ethanol, then the speech and vision centers of the brain become sedated, and the area that governs reasoning becomes more incapacitated. Later, the cells of the brain responsible for large-muscle control are affected; at this point, people "under the influence" stagger or weave when they try to walk. Finally, the conscious brain is completely subdued, and the person "passes out." Now, luckily, the person can drink no more; this is fortunate because a higher dose's anesthetic effect could reach the deepest brain centers that control breathing and heartbeat, and the person could die.

tries to use alcoholic beverages to quench thirst, however, only worsens the problem. The smart drinker, then, either drinks beer (which contains plenty of water), or drinks mixers or chasers with wine or hard liquor. Better still, the drinker alternates alcoholic beverages with glasses of water and limits the total amount consumed.

The water loss caused by ADH depression involves loss of more than just water. The water takes with it magnesium, potassium, calcium, and zinc, depleting the body's reserves.

Ethanol also depresses appetite by the euphoria it produces, as well as by its attack on the mucosa of the stomach, so that heavy drinkers usually eat poorly, if at all. With a large portion of their energy fuel coming from the empty kcalories of alcohol, they find it difficult to obtain the essential nutrients. Thus, some of their malnutrition is due to lack of food—but even if they eat well, the direct effects of alcohol will take their toll because ethanol affects every tissue's metabolism of nutrients. Stomach cells oversecrete histamine and acid, becoming vulnerable to ulcer formation. Intestinal cells fail to absorb thiamin, folacin, and vitamin B_{12}. Liver cells lose efficiency in activating vitamin D, and alter their production and excretion of bile. Rod cells in the retina, which normally process retinol (the vitamin A alcohol) to retinal (its aldehyde form) needed in vision, process ethanol to acetaldehyde instead. The kidneys excrete increased quantities of magnesium, calcium, potassium, and zinc.

Acetaldehyde interferes with nutrient metabolism, too. For example, it dislodges vitamin B_6 from its protective binding protein so that it is destroyed, creating a secondary vitamin B_6 deficiency and, thereby, lowered production of red blood cells.

In summary, ethanol hinders the absorption, alters the metabolism, and increases the excretion of many nutrients, so that malnutrition can occur even in the well-fed drinker. It disturbs many normal body processes—many more than have been enumerated here. Since the liver is a crossroads for all nutrients in the body, its domination by ethanol or injury results in many side effects. Table FP6—2 lists some long-term effects of alcohol abuse.

Tobacco

Young people searching for role models may be taken in by the highly persuasive advertisements distributed by the tobacco industry. In their efforts to achieve sophistication, young people imitate these attractive advertising models, adopting the habit of smoking tobacco. A person whose mind is open to using tobacco begins by trying it once. That one time is followed by another, and in a short while, because nicotine is a powerfully addictive drug, the person becomes a user for life.[23]

Statistics on smoking are impressive. Each day, 5000 children light up for the first time—some of them only seven or eight years old, in a hurry to grow up. In 1968, 3 million teenagers were smoking; by 1978, that number had more than doubled.[24] Cigarette smoking among high school seniors peaked in the mid-1970s, declined until 1980, and seems to have leveled out. Surveys of high school seniors report that seven of ten have tried cigarettes, and one in five

Table FP6–2   Long-Term Effects of Alcohol Abuse

Hepatitis and cirrhosis.
Vitamin and trace mineral deficiencies.
Brain damage.
Psychological depression.
Loss of testicular function and damage to the adrenal glands, leading
to feminization and sexual impotence in men.
Failure of the ovaries and early menopause in women.
Hypertension and an increased risk of stroke.
Increased risk of cancer of the tongue, mouth, esophagus, and liver.
Intestinal inflammation; ulcers.
Deterioration of muscles, including the heart muscle.
Sedation of the bone marrow, with consequent blood abnormalities.
Reduced capacity for exercise; heart pain sooner with exercise.
Suppression of the immune system; reduced resistance to disease.
Kidney damage; bladder damage; prostate gland damage.
Failure to maintain the skin's health; rashes and sores.
Increased susceptibility to lung infections.
Adverse drug reactions.

Adapted from M. J. Eckardt and coauthors, Health hazards associated with alcohol consumption, *Journal of the American Medical Association* 246 (1981): 648–666.

smoke cigarettes regularly.[25] This shift in smoking behavior reflects society's reassessment of a previously accepted normative behavior. A folder written by young people for young people describes how smokers rationalize their choice to smoke:

▶ I'm young now. Why not smoke? I can quit later.
▶ I don't inhale. Smoking can't hurt me.
▶ Smoking makes me look grown-up and mature.
▶ I smoke filter cigarettes; that will protect me.
▶ My parents smoke. Why shouldn't I?
▶ If I don't spend the money on cigarettes, I'll spend it on something else.
▶ All my friends smoke. Why shouldn't I?[26]
▶ It keeps me from biting my nails.
▶ It keeps me from eating. Smoking is better than putting on weight.
▶ It gives me something to do when I'm mad or bored or hurt or unhappy or restless.

Each of these reasons may be invalid, but the new smoker believes them.

Cigarette smoking is a pervasive health problem causing thousands of people to suffer from cancer and diseases of the cardiovascular, digestive, and respiratory systems. These effects are beyond the scope of this text, but there are a few nutrition connections to be explored. Smoking cigarettes does influence hunger, body weight, and nutrient status. There are also links between nutrients and lung cancer.

Smoking a cigarette eases feelings of hunger. Nicotine inhibits the hunger contractions of the stomach and causes a temporary, but rapid, rise in blood-glucose concentrations.[27] So when smokers receive a hunger signal, they can quiet it with a cigarette instead of food. Such behavior ignores body signals and deters energy and nutrient intake.

Indeed, smokers tend to weigh less than nonsmokers and to gain weight upon cessation of smoking.[28] This phenomenon is not easily explained. Common belief held that smokers weighed less because they ate less; that cigarette smoking affected their eating behaviors. When they quit smoking, they began to eat more, and therefore gained weight. However, studies have indicated that smokers actually consume at least as many kcalories per day as nonsmokers.[29] Some smokers show only a slight increase in their energy intakes after cessation, while others increase their energy intakes by more than 200 kcalories per day.[30] However, increased energy intake does not fully account for the weight gains seen upon cessation.[31]

The lower body weight and subsequent weight gain upon cessation of smoking appear to be due to effects of cigarette smoking beyond those on food intake. One study suggests that smoking and nicotine lower the efficiency of energy storage or increase the metabolic rate.[32] Researchers have found that smoking increases daily energy expenditure by approximately 10 percent, even though changes in physical activity or basal metabolic rate were not noted.[33] Any increase noted in metabolic rate does not appear to be dose related. If it were, heavy smokers would be the lightest in weight of all smokers. Such is not the case; moderate smokers (15 to 24 cigarettes per day) are the lightest.[34] The effects of cigarette smoking on metabolic rate are not clear, nor are they always evident.[35]

Another possible metabolic explanation for the body weight effects of smoking involves the enzyme lipoprotein lipase. Lipoprotein lipase is the enzyme on the fat cells that is responsible for hydrolyzing triglycerides from blood-borne lipoproteins, making fatty acids available for fat storage. Smokers have higher lipoprotein lipase activity than nonsmokers. When researchers measured the activity of this enzyme in smokers before and after they quit smoking, they found a striking correlation.[36] The higher the enzyme activity when smoking, the greater the weight gain upon cessation.

Weight gain is often a concern for people contemplating giving up cigarettes. The decision to quit weighs unhealthy smoking against unattractive (and potentially unhealthy) weight gain. The message to smokers wanting to quit is to adjust diet and exercise habits in order to maintain weight during and after cessation.

Smokeless or chewing tobacco is gaining popularity in this country, especially among young people. In addition to the cancer problems such a practice presents, these tobacco products contain large quantities of sodium. Sodium is added to the tobacco for flavor and may be found at levels comparable to that found in dill pickles or cured bacon.

Nutrient intakes of smokers and nonsmokers differ. Smokers have been found to have lower intakes of dietary fiber, vitamins, and minerals, even when their energy intakes are quite similar.[37] The association between smoking and low vitamin intake may be noteworthy, considering the altered metabolism of vitamin C in smokers and the protective effect of beta-carotene against lung cancer.

Results of one research study indicate that the vitamin C requirement of smokers may exceed that of nonsmokers. The plasma concentration of vitamin C in smokers is commonly low, and the metabolic turnover of vitamin C in smokers is higher than in nonsmokers; that is, smokers break down vitamin C faster, thus requiring more vitamin C to achieve steady body pools comparable to those of nonsmokers.[38] This study concludes that smokers require a daily intake of at least 140 milligrams of vitamin C and that nonsmokers require about 100 milligrams, both higher values than current recommendations.

Recent research findings suggest that beta-carotene, a precursor to vitamin A found in vegetables, has anticancer activity.[39] Specifically noted is an inverse correlation between dietary carotene and the incidence of lung cancer. That is, the risk of lung cancer is greatest for smokers who have the lowest intake of carotene. Of course conclusions from such evidence cannot be made in haste. Teenagers cannot be led to believe that as long as they eat their carrots they can safely smoke their cigarettes. However, it is important to encourage teenagers to eat foods rich in carotene, a nutrient many of them lack in their diets.

The teen years are similar to an obstacle course, both requiring careful consideration of the pathways and the consequences that follow each decision. To make the best choice, adolescents need to learn of the associated risks and benefits of various behaviors. Perhaps the most effective way to educate teens is by example. The teen years are a time of identity formation, a time of seeking and emulating models. Adults who enthusiastically maintain their own health can have a positive impact on teenagers. Teenagers who realize that a life of health and happiness begins today are on their way. The rapid changes of the teen years offer a flexibility and opportunity to make positive choices that will improve the rest of life's journey.

Focal Point 6 Notes

1. Data presented in this discussion are from the national surveys of roughly 17,000 high school seniors entitled Monitoring the Future: A Continuing Study of the Lifestyles and Values of Youth, funded by the National Institute on Drug Abuse, conducted every spring since 1975, as cited in L. D. Johnston, P. M. O'Malley, and J. G. Bachman, Psychotherapeutic, licit, and illicit use of drugs among adolescents, *Journal of Adolescent Health Care* 8 (1987): 36–51.
2. Johnston, O'Malley, and Bachman, 1987.
3. L. J. King, J. D. Teale, and V. Marks, Biochemical aspects of cannabis, in *Cannabis and Health*, ed. J. D. Graham (New York: Academic Press, 1976).
4. L. E. Hollister, Marihuana in man: Three years later, *Science* 172 (1971): 21–29.
5. King, Teale, and Marks, 1976; Hollister, Marihuana in man, 1971.
6. N. C. Doyle, Marihuana and the lungs, a bulletin distributed by the American Lung Association, November 1979.
7. E. L. Abel, Effects of marihuana on the solution of anagrams, memory and appetite, *Nature* 231 (1971): 260–261; C. T. Tart, Marihuana intoxication: Common experiences, *Nature* 226 (1970): 701–704.
8. L. E. Hollister, Hunger and appetite after single doses of marihuana, alcohol, and dextroamphetamine, *Clinical Pharmacology and Therapeutics* 12 (1971): 44–49; J. D. P. Graham and D. M. F. Li, The pharmacology of cannabis and cannabinoids, in *Cannabis and Health*, ed. J. D. Graham (New York: Academic Press, 1976).
9. Hollister, Hunger and appetite, 1971.
10. L. E. Hollister, Health aspects of cannabis, *Pharmacological Reviews* 38 (1986): 1–20.
11. Marihuana: Truth on health problems, *Science News* 22 (1975): 117.
12. Johnston, O'Malley, and Bachman, 1987.
13. Johnston, O'Malley, and Bachman, 1987.
14. Johnston, O'Malley, and Bachman, 1987.
15. J. M. Jonas and M. S. Gold, Cocaine abuse and eating disorders, *Lancet* 1 (1986): 390–391.
16. Alcohol and the Adolescent, a pamphlet available from National Council on Alcoholism, 733 Third Avenue, New York, NY 10017; B. Bower, Teen drug use: Ups and downs, *Science News* 128 (1985): 310; Johnston, O'Malley, and Bachman, 1987.
17. Johnston, O'Malley, and Bachman, 1987.
18. Parts of this discussion are adapted from E. N. Whitney and E. M. N. Hamilton, *Understanding Nutrition*, 4th ed. (St. Paul, Minn.: West, 1987).
19. A. B. Eisenstein, Nutritional and metabolic effects of alcohol, *Journal of the American Dietetic Association* 81 (1982): 247–251.
20. F. Iber, In alcoholism, the liver sets the pace, *Nutrition Today*, January/February 1971, pp. 2–9.
21. C. S. Lieber, Liver adaptation and injury in alcoholism, *New England Journal of Medicine* 228 (1973): 356–361.
22. H. L. Bleich and E. S. Boro, Metabolic and hepatic effects of alcohol, *New England Journal of Medicine* 296 (1977): 612–616.
23. Parts of this discussion are adapted from F. S. Sizer and E. N. Whitney, *Life Choices: Health Concepts and Strategies* (St. Paul, Minn.: West, 1988).

24. R. Keeshan, Children and smoking, in *Smoking and Health,* proceedings of a conference commemorating the 20th anniversary of the first Surgeon General's Report on Smoking and Health, 11 January 1984, available from the American Council on Science and Health, 47 Maple Street, Summit, NJ 07901.

25. Johnston, O'Malley, and Bachman, 1987.

26. The first several bullet items are adapted from *8 Reasons Young People Smoke,* HHS brochure no. 200-75-0516, available from the Superintendent of Documents, Government Printing Office, Washington, DC 20402.

27. L. Willian-Olsson, Smoking and platelet stickiness (letter), *Lancet* 2 (1965): 908–909.

28. R. M. Carney and A. P. Goldberg, Weight gain after cessation of cigarette smoking: A possible role for adipose-tissue lipoprotein lipase, *New England Journal of Medicine* 310 (1984): 614–616.

29. D. R. Jacobs and S. Gottenborg, Smoking and weight: The Minnesota lipid research clinic, *American Journal of Public Health* 71 (1981): 391–396.

30. A. M. Fehily, K. M. Phillips, and J. W. G. Yarnell, Diet, smoking, social class, and body mass index in the Caerphilly Heart Disease Study, *American Journal of Clinical Nutrition* 40 (1984): 827–833; B. A. Stamford and coauthors, Effects of smoking cessation on weight gain, metabolic rate, caloric consumption, and blood lipids, *American Journal of Clinical Nutrition* 43 (1986): 486–494.

31. Stamford and coauthors, 1986.

32. J. T. Wack and J. Rodin, Smoking and its effect on body weight and the systems of caloric regulation, *American Journal of Clinical Nutrition* 35 (1982): 366–380.

33. A. Hofstetter and coauthors, Increased 24-hour energy expenditure in cigarette smokers, *New England Journal of Medicine* 314 (1986): 79–82.

34. Fehily, Phillips, and Yarnell, 1984.

35. Stamford and coauthors, 1986.

36. Carney and Goldberg, 1984.

37. Fehily, Phillips, and Yarnell, 1984.

38. A. B. Kallner, D. Hartmann, and D. H. Hornig, On the requirements of ascorbic acid in man: Steady-state turnover and body pool in smokers, *American Journal of Clinical Nutrition* 34 (1981): 1347–1355.

39. Dietary carotene and the risk of lung cancer, *Nutrition Reviews* 40 (1982): 265–268.

Appendix A

Nutrition Assessment

Nutrition assessment evaluates a person's health from a nutrition perspective. Many factors influence or reflect nutrition status. Consequently, a skilled dietitian or other qualified health care professional must gather information from many sources, using several nutrition assessment techniques. These techniques include:

▸ History taking.

▸ Anthropometric measurements.

▸ Physical examinations.

▸ Biochemical analyses (laboratory tests).

These methods involve collecting data in a variety of ways and interpreting each finding in relation to the others in order to create a total picture.

The accurate gathering of this information and its careful interpretation are the basis for a meaningful evaluation. The more information gathered about a person, the more accurate the assessment will be. Gathering information is a time-consuming process, and time is often a rare commodity in the health care setting. Nutrition care is only one part of total care. It may not be practical or essential to collect detailed information on each person.

A strategic compromise is to screen clients by collecting preliminary data. Data such as height-weight and hematocrit are easy to obtain and can alert health care workers to potential problems. Nutrition screening identifies clients who will require additional nutrition assessment (see Figure A–1).

This appendix provides a sample of the procedures, standards, charts, and forms commonly used in nutrition assessment.* The section entitled Nutrition Assessment during Pregnancy demonstrates the usefulness and importance of nutrition assessment procedures and tools during pregnancy.

nutrition screening: the use of preliminary nutrition assessment techniques to identify people who are malnourished or who are at risk for malnutrition.

Historical Data

Clues about present nutrition status become evident with a careful review of a person's historical data (see Table A–1). Even when the data are subjective, they reveal important facts about a person. A thorough history provides a sense of the whole person. An adept history taker uses the interview not only to gather facts, but to establish a rapport, exploring a person's history from

*Parts of this discussion have been adapted with permission from E. N. Whitney, C. B. Cataldo, and S. R. Rolfes, *Understanding Normal and Clinical Nutrition* 2nd ed. (St. Paul, Minn.: West, 1987).

Figure A–1   Nutrition Screening
A preliminary evaluation screens for possible nutrition disorders. If results of initial tests are abnormal, follow up tests are conducted to further evaluate the disorder. If results of these tests indicate no nutrition disorder, a reevaluation is conducted at a later time. If results indicate abnormalities, steps are taken to correct them.

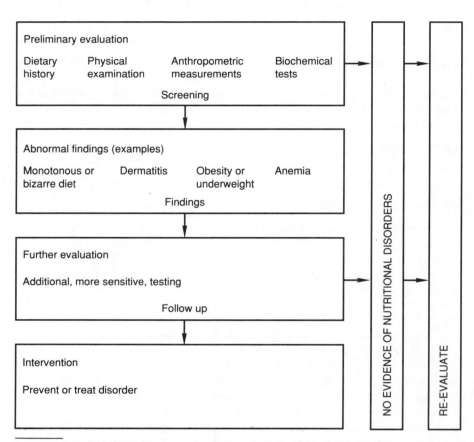

Source: Adapted from S. J. Fomon and coauthors, *Nutritional Disorders of Children: Prevention, Screening, and Followup,* DHEW Publication no. (HSA) 76-5612 (Washington, D.C.: Government Printing Office, 1976), inside front cover.

several angles: medical, socioeconomic, drug, and diet. A history identifies risk factors associated with poor nutrition status (see Table A–2). Form A–1 shows the kinds of questions asked to collect such information. As you can see, many aspects of a person's life have an impact on nutrition status and provide clues to possible problems.

Medical and social histories can often be obtained from records completed by the attending physician, nurse, or other health care workers. Additional information can be gathered through an interview.

The drug history requires special attention. Hundreds of drugs interact with nutrients, creating the possibility of imbalances or deficiencies. They must not be overlooked in assessing a person's nutrition status. Form A–2 elicits the

Table A–1   Historical Data Used in Standard Nutrition Assessments

Histories	Identifies
Medical	Diseases that affect nutrition status

Diet
    24-hour recall
    food diary
    food frequency record
	Nutrient intake excesses or deficiencies

Socioeconomic	Personal, financial, and environmental interferences with food intake
Drug	Medications that affect nutrition status

necessary information regarding drugs and Table A–3 identifies commonly used drugs and their effects on nutrition.

Medical History

The assessor can obtain medical histories from records completed by the attending physician, nurse, or other health care provider. In addition, conversations with the client can uncover valuable medical information previously overlooked because "no one asked" or because the client was too upset on admission to think clearly.

An accurate, complete medical history can reveal any conditions that place a client at risk for malnutrition. Diseases can have either long- or short-term effects on nutrition status by interfering with ingestion, digestion, absorption, metabolism, or excretion of nutrients.

Socioeconomic History

Socioeconomic factors profoundly affect nutrition status. The wealth of a social class influences the diet of the people. In general, the adequacy of the diet diminishes as income decreases. At some point, the ability to purchase the foods required to meet nutrient needs is lost; an inadequate income contributes to an inadequate diet. Agencies use poverty indexes to identify people at risk for poor nutrition and to qualify people for government food assistance programs.

Decreased income affects not only the power to purchase foods, but also food storage and preparation facilities. A skilled assessor will note whether a person has access to a refrigerator and stove. Inadequate transportation to grocery stores can also be an obstacle to meal preparation for low-income people.

Drug History

The important interactions of foods and drugs require that special attention be paid to the drug history. Hundreds of drugs interact with nutrients, increasing

Table A–2   Risk Factors for Poor Nutrition Status

Medical History	Diet History	Social/Economic History of Family	Drug History
Alcoholism	Anorexia nervosa	Eating alone	Antibiotics
Anorexia	Bulimia	Inadequate food budget	Anticancer agents
Cancer	Frequently eating out	Inadequate food preparation facilities	Anticonvulsants
Chewing or swallowing difficulties (including poorly fitted dentures, dental caries, and missing teeth)	Inadequate food intake	Inadequate food storage facilities	Antihypertensive agents
Circulatory problems	Intravenous fluids (other than total parenteral nutrition) for 10 or more days	Poor education	Catabolic steroids
Constipation	No intake for 10 or more days	Poor self-concept	Oral contraceptives
Diabetes	Poor appetite	Transportation unavailable	Vitamin and other nutrient preparations
Diarrhea	Restricted or fad diets		
Diseases of the GI tract			
Drug addiction			
Fever			
Heart disease			
Hormonal imbalance			
Hyperlipidemia			
Hypertension			
Infection			
Kidney disease			
Liver disease			
Lung disease			
Mental retardation or deterioration			
Multiple pregnancies[a]			
Nausea			
Neurologic disorders			
Overweight			
Pancreatic insufficiency			
Paralysis			
Physical disability			
Pregnancy[a]			
Radiation therapy			
Recent major illness			
Recent major surgery			
Recent weight loss or gain			
Smokes cigarettes			
Surgery of the GI tract			
Trauma			
Ulcers			
Underweight			
Vomiting			

[a]See also Chapter 2.

Form A–1   History

Name _____   Today's date _____
Address _____   Age _____
        _____   Sex _____
        _____   Phone _____
Date of last medical checkup _____   Height _____
Reason for coming in _____   Weight _____
        _____   Usual Weight _____

PERSONAL DATA

1. Last grade of school completed _____ Still in school? _____
2. Are you employed? _____ Occupation _____
3. Does someone else live at your home? _____ Who? _____
4. Do you smoke in any way? _____ How much? _____
5. Have your recently lost or gained more than 10 lbs? _____ If yes, please
   explain how _____
6. Are you pregnant? _____ How many months? _____
7. How may pregnancies have you carried to term? _____
8. Are your menstrual periods normal? _____ If not, please explain _____
   _____
9. Have you been told that you have (check any that apply):
   Diabetes _____ High blood pressure _____ Hardening of the arteries _____
   Lung disease _____ Kidney disease _____ Liver disease _____ Ulcers _____
   Cancer _____ Other _____
10. Do you eat at regular times each day? _____ How many times per day? _____
11. Do you usually eat snacks? _____ When? _____
12. Where do you usually eat your meal?
    Morning _____ Noon _____ Night _____
    With whom?
    Morning _____ Noon _____ Night _____
13. Would you say your appetite is good? _____ Fair? _____ Poor? _____
    If poor, please explain _____
14. What foods do you particularly dislike? _____
15. Are there foods you don't eat for other reasons? _____
16. Do you have any difficulty eating? _____
17. How would you describe your feelings about food? _____
    _____
    _____
18. Who prepares your meals? _____
19. Are you, or is any member of your family, on a special diet? _____
    If yes, who and what kind? _____
20. Do you drink alcohol? _____ How many drinks per day? _____
    Do you ever drink alcohol excessively? _____ How often? _____
21. Do you take any kind of medication, either prescribed by a doctor or over the
    counter, for any condition? _____
22. How would you describe your exercise habits?
    Kind of exercise _____ How intense? _____
    How long at a time? _____ How often? _____
23. Are there any other facts about your lifestyle that you think might be related to
    your nutritional health? _____ Explain _____
    _____

Form A–2   Drug History

1a. Do you have any health problems for which you are taking prescription medications at the present time? Yes ___ No ___
If yes:

Health problem	Proprietary name of drug	Generic name of drug	Dose Frequency	Duration of intake

1b. Are you taking any other medication a doctor has prescribed (name of drug unknown, reason for taking unknown)?
Yes ___ No ___
If yes:

Description of drug	Dose	Frequency	Duration of intake

2a. Have you taken prescription medication for any of the health problems listed below within the past three months?
Yes ___ No ___
If yes:

Health problem	Drug name	Duration of intake	When discontinued	Reason for stopping	Still taking*
Asthma.					
Arthritis					
High blood pressure					
Fluid retention					
Infection (specify)					
Tuberculosis					
Malaria					
Psoriasis					
Colitis					
High cholesterol					
Parkinson's disease					
Liver disease					
Kidney disease					
Blood disease					
Bone disease					
Gout					
Blood clots					
Diabetes					
Other (specify)					

*Check (√) if still taking.

2b. Have you taken any other medication within the past three months that a doctor has prescribed (name of drug unknown, reason for taking unknown)? Yes ___ No ___

Description	Dose	Frequency	Duration of intake

3a. Do you take medications, self-prescribed, for any reason? Yes ___ No ___
If yes:

Complaint	Constantly	Frequently	Occasionally
Constipation			
Indigestion			
Headache			
Nervousness			
Insomnia			
Pain			
Menstrual cramps			
Colds and sinus trouble			
Other (state)			

Form A–2   (continued)

3b. If response to 3a is positive in one or more categories, what medication do you take ro relieve these complaints, and how much do you need to gain relief?

Complaint	*Drug*	*Dose*	*Frequency*	*Duration*
Constipation				
Indigestion				
Headache				
Nervousness				
Insomnia				
Pain				
Menstrual cramps				
Colds and sinus trouble				
Other (state)				

4. Are you taking birth control pills now ? Yes ___[a] No ___
If yes:
Name:
Duration of intake:
Have you taken birth control pills within the past six months? Yes ___ No ___
If yes:
Name:
Duration of intake:
Date discontinued:
Reason for stopping:

Source: Adapted from D. Roe, *Drug-Induced Nutritional Deficiencies* (Westport, Conn.: AVI Publishing Company, 1976), Table 4.2, pp. 106–108.

[a]A yes answer to this question would indicate reduced menstrual blood loss, possible consequent iron conservation, and reduced risk of pregnancy. Chapter 1's discussion on oral contraceptives shows that their overall effect on nutrition status is minimal.

Table A–3   Selected Drug-Nutrient Interactions[a]

Drug	Nutrient	Effect on Nutrition
Alcohol	Energy	➡ intake
	Protein	➡ intake
	Fat	➡ buildup in liver
		➡ absorption
	Thiamin	➡ absorption
		➡ storage
	Vitamin B_6	➡ activation
	Folacin	➡ absorption
		➡ utilization
	Vitamin B_{12}	➡ absorption
	Magnesium	➡ urinary excretion
	Zinc	➡ urinary excretion
Amphetamines	Many nutrients affected	➡ intake Anorexia, dry mouth, metallic taste, nausea, vomiting

Table A–3   (continued)

Drug	Nutrient	Effect on Nutrition
Analgesics		
Aspirin	Folacin	↓ serum levels
		Altered transport
	Vitamin C	↑ urinary excretion
	Thiamin	↑ urinary excretion
	Vitamin K	↑ urinary excretion
	Iron	May cause blood loss
Antacids		
Aluminum hydroxide	Phosphorus	↓ absorption
Other types	Thiamin	↑ destruction
Anticoagulants	Vitamin K	↓ conversion to active form
Anticonvulsants	Folacin	↓ serum levels
	Vitamin B$_6$	↓ serum levels
	Vitamin B$_{12}$	↓ serum levels
	Vitamin D	↓ conversion to active forms
	Vitamin K	↑ requirement
Antimicrobials (antibiotics)		
Chloramphenicol	Riboflavin	↑ requirement (?)
	Vitamin B$_6$	↑ requirement (?)
	Vitamin B$_{12}$	↑ requirement (?)
Neomycin	Fats	↓ absorption
	Nitrogen	↓ absorption
	Carbohydrates	↓ absorption
	Folacin	↓ absorption
	Vitamin B$_{12}$	↓ absorption
	Fat-soluble vitamins	↓ absorption
	Calcium	↓ absorption
	Iron	↓ absorption
	Potassium	↓ absorption
	Vitamin K	↓ intestinal synthesis
Penicillin	Potassium	↑ urinary excretion
Tetracycline	Fat	↓ absorption
	Amino acids	↓ absorption
	Calcium	↓ absorption
	Iron	↓ absorption
	Magnesium	↓ absorption
	Zinc	↓ absorption
	Niacin	↑ urinary excretion
	Riboflavin	↑ urinary excretion
	Folacin	↑ urinary excretion
	Vitamin C	↑ urinary excretion
Antineoplastic agents		
5-Fluorouracil	Protein	↓ absorption
		↓ synthesis

Table A–3   (continued)

Drug	Nutrient	Effect on Nutrition
Methotrexate and pyrimethamine	Folacin	Folacin antagonist
	Vitamin B_{12}	← absorption
	Fat	← absorption
	Many nutrients affected	← intake
		Anorexia, nausea, vomiting, mouth sores
Antitubercular drugs		
Cycloserine	Vitamin B_6	Vitamin B_6 antagonist
	Protein	← synthesis
	Calcium	← absorption (?)
	Magnesium	← absorption (?)
	Vitamin B_6	← serum levels (?)
	Folacin	← serum levels (?)
	Vitamin B_{12}	← serum levels (?)
Isonicotinic acid hydrazide (INH)	Vitamin B_6	Vitamin B_6 antagonist
		↑ urinary excretion
		Causes deficiency
	Niacin	Causes deficiency
	Vitamin B_{12}	← absorption
		← serum levels
Para-aminosalicylic acid	Folacin	← absorption
	Vitamin B_{12}	← absorption
	Fat	← absorption
	Iron	← absorption
Chelating agents		
Penicillamine	Vitamin B_6	↑ requirement
		↑ urinary excretion
	Zinc	↑ urinary excretion
	Iron	↑ urinary excretion
	Copper	↑ urinary excretion
	Many nutrients affected	← intake
		Alterations in taste: anorexia, nausea, vomiting
Cholesterol-lowering agents		
Cholestyramine	Fat and cholesterol	← absorption
	Fat-soluble vitamins	← absorption
	Folacin	← absorption
	Iron	← absorption
	Vitamin B_{12}	← absorption
		← blood levels
	Calcium	↑ urinary excretion
		← blood levels
Clofibrate	Vitamin B_{12}	← absorption
	Iron	← absorption
	Many nutrients affected	← intake
		Alterations in taste; nausea and GI irritation

Table A–3   (continued)

Drug	Nutrient	Effect on Nutrition
Colchicine	Fat	↓ absorption
	Vitamin A	↓ absorption
	Folacin	↓ absorption
	Vitamin B$_{12}$	↓ absorption
	Sodium	↓ absorption
	Potassium	↓ absorption
Corticosteroids	Vitamin D	↑ metabolism
		↑ requirement
	Vitamin B$_6$	↑ requirement
	Vitamin C	↑ requirement
		↑ urinary excretion
	Calcium	↓ absorption
		↑ urinary excretion
	Phosphorus	↓ absorption
	Zinc	↑ urinary excretion
		↓ serum levels
	Glucose	↑ serum levels
	Triglycerides	↑ serum levels
	Cholesterol	↑ serum levels
	Potassium	↑ urinary excretion
	Nitrogen	↑ urinary excretion
Diuretics		
Furosemide	Calcium	↑ urinary excretion
	Sodium	↑ urinary excretion
	Potassium	↓ serum levels
	Chloride	↓ serum levels
	Magnesium	↓ serum levels
	Zinc	↑ serum levels
		↓ storage in liver
Mercurials	Thiamin	↑ urinary excretion
	Calcium	↑ urinary excretion
	Sodium	↑ urinary excretion
	Potassium	↑ urinary excretion
	Chloride	↑ urinary excretion
	Magnesium	↑ urinary excretion
Thiazides	Sodium	↑ urinary excretion
	Potassium	↓ blood levels
	Chloride	↓ blood levels
	Calcium	↑ urinary excretion
		↑ blood levels
	Magnesium	↑ urinary excretion
	Phosphorus	↓ blood levels
	Glucose	↑ blood levels (?)
Triamterene	Sodium	↑ urinary excretion
	Folacin	↓ serum levels
	Vitamin B$_{12}$	↓ serum levels
Glutethimide	Vitamin D	↑ metabolism
Hydralazine hydro-chloride	Vitamin B$_6$	↑ urinary excretion

Table A–3   (continued)

Drug	Nutrient	Effect on Nutrition
Hypoglycemics		
Phenformin hydrochloride and Metformin	Vitamin B_{12}	⬇ absorption
Laxatives		
Cathartics	Fat	⬇ absorption
	Glucose	⬇ absorption
	Vitamin D	⬇ absorption
	Calcium	⬇ absorption
	Potassium	⬇ absorption
Mineral oil	Fat-soluble vitamins	⬇ absorption
	Carotene	⬇ absorption
Levodopa	Amino acids	⬆ requirement
	Vitamin B_6	⬆ requirement
	Vitamin C	⬆ requirement
	Sodium	⬇ urinary excretion
	Potassium	⬇ urinary excretion
Oral contraceptives	Vitamin B_6	⬆ requirement
		⬇ blood levels
	Riboflavin	⬆ requirement
		⬇ blood levels
	Folacin	⬇ absorption
		⬇ blood levels
	Vitamin B_{12}	⬇ blood levels
	Vitamin C	⬇ blood levels
	Vitamin A	⬆ blood levels
	Calcium	⬆ absorption
	Iron	⬆ serum levels
	Copper	⬆ serum levels
	Magnesium	⬇ blood levels (?)
	Zinc	⬇ blood levels (?)
Potassium salts	Vitamin B_{12}	⬇ absorption
Sulfonamides		
Salicylazosulfapyridine	Folacin	⬇ absorption
		⬇ blood levels
	Iron	⬇ blood levels
Others	Folacin	⬇ intestinal synthesis
	Vitamin K	⬇ intestinal synthesis
	B vitamins	⬇ intestinal synthesis

[a] ⬆ = increases: ⬇ = decreases; (?) = possible effect.

Adapted from: R. E. Hodges, *Nutrition in Medical Practice* (Philadelphia: Saunders, 1980), pp 323–331; R. C. Theuer and J. J. Vitale, Drug and nutrient interactions, in *Nutritional Support of Medical Practice*. eds. H. A. Schneider. C. F. Anderson, and D. B. Coursin (Hagerstown, Md.: Harper and Row, 1977), pp. 297–305; D. A. Roe. *Drug Induced Nutritional Deficiencies* (Westport, Conn. AVI, 1985).

the possibility of imbalances or deficiencies. Table A–3 identifies commonly used drugs and their effects on nutrition.

Drugs demand consideration in assessing a person's nutrition status. If a person is taking any drug, the assessor records on the drug history form the name of the drug; the dose, the frequency, and duration of intake; the reason for taking the drug; and signs of any adverse effects. Form A–2 is used to elicit the necessary information regarding drugs.

Diet History

A diet history provides a record of a person's food intake. The accurate recording of such data requires skill. Trained dietitians often use food models or photos and measuring devices to help clients identify serving sizes of food consumed. Besides the type of food and quantity consumed, the assessor will want to know how the food was prepared. Food choices are an important part of lifestyle and often represent an expression of personal philosophy. The assessor who asks nonjudgmental questions about food intake encourages trust and the likelihood of accurate information.

There are several methods of obtaining food intake data, including the 24-hour recall, the usual intake record, the food frequency checklist, and the food diary. The assessor compares food intakes with standards; in this case, the standards are recommended nutrient intakes. The question to answer is how closely the person's diet meets the recommendations. Are any nutrients excessive or deficient? Besides identifying possible nutrient imbalances, diet histories provide valuable clues about how a person will accept diet changes should they be necessary. Information about what and how a person eats provides the background for realistic and attainable nutrition goals.

Food intake data are often obtained by using the 24-hour recall. The assessor asks the client to recount everything eaten or drunk in the past 24 hours or for the previous day. (Form A–3 shows a typical 24-hour recall form.) This method is commonly used in nutrition surveys to obtain estimates of the typical food intakes of large numbers of people in given populations. Its limit is in providing enough accurate information to allow generalizations about an individual's usual food intake.

An advantage of the 24-hour recall is that it is easy to obtain. It is also less frustrating to elicit information about the past 24 hours than to require a person to estimate intake over a longer period of time. However, the previous day's intake may not be the usual intake; the person may be unable to accurately estimate the amounts of food eaten; or the person may conceal facts about food consumption. As a result, sometimes the information gathered in a 24-hour recall does not truly reflect a person's usual intake.

To obtain data about a person's usual intake pattern, an inquiry might begin with "What is the first thing you usually eat or drink during the day?" Similar questions follow until a typical daily intake pattern emerges. This method is similar to the 24-hour recall and uses the same form (Form A–3). A skilled and patient interviewer can derive much useful information from a person's usual intake pattern. For a person whose intake varies widely from day to day, however, it may be difficult to answer the questions, and in such a case, the data may be useless in estimating nutrient intake. However, the usual

Form A–3   Food Intake for a 24-Hour Recall or Usual Intake Pattern

Name and address _____   Date _____

_____

_____

Did you take a vitamin/mineral supplement? _____

If yes, what kind? _____   Dose _____

Please record the amount and type of foods and beverages consumed today. [Or: Please record the amount and type of foods and beverages you typically consume each day.]

Food	Amount (c, tbsp, or piece)	Description (how cooked, how served)

intake method is useful in verifying food intake when the past 24 hours have been atypical.

Another approach is to use a food frequency checklist. The purpose of this record is to ascertain how often an individual eats a specific type of food per day, week, or month. The assessor uses a long list of foods, asking clients to state how often they eat a certain food or type of food. This information helps pinpoint food groups, and therefore nutrients, that may be excessive or deficient in the diet. If used with the usual intake or 24-hour recall, the food frequency record permits double-checking the accuracy of the information obtained. Form A–4 is a food frequency checklist.

Still another alternative is the food diary. (Form A–5 provides an example.) Completion of a diary often helps to determine factors associated with food intake (time of day, place eaten, others present, mood). The assessor instructs the person keeping the diary to write down the required information immediately after eating. A food diary works well with cooperative people, but requires considerable time and effort on their part.

A prime advantage of the food diary is that the diary keeper assumes an active role and may for the first time begin to see and understand personal food habits. It also provides the assessor with an accurate picture of the diary keeper's lifestyle and factors that affect food intake. For these reasons, food diaries are particularly useful in outpatient counseling for such nutrition problems as overweight, underweight, or food allergy. The major disadvantages stem from poor compliance in recording the data and conscious or unconscious changes in eating habits that may occur while the diary is being kept.

Form A–4   Food Frequency Checklist

The following information will help us to understand your regular eating habits so that we may offer you the best service possible. If you have any doubt about some items, be sure to underestimate the "goodness" of your habits rather than to overestimate.

1. How many times *per week* do you eat the following foods? Circle the appropriate number:

                                                          PER WEEK
Poultry... 0 <1 1 2 3 4 5 6 7 8 9 >9 ____
Fish .... 0 <1 1 2 3 4 5 6 7 8 9 >9 ____
Hot dogs .... 0 <1 1 2 3 4 5 6 7 8 9 >9 ____
Bacon .... 0 <1 1 2 3 4 5 6 7 8 9 >9 ____
Lunch meat...................................... 0 <1 1 2 3 4 5 6 7 8 9 >9 ____
Sausage... 0 <1 1 2 3 4 5 6 7 8 9 >9 ____
Pork or ham .... 0 <1 1 2 3 4 5 6 7 8 9 >9 ____
Salt pork.. 0 <1 1 2 3 4 5 6 7 8 9 >9 ____
Liver... 0 <1 1 2 3 4 5 6 7 8 9 >9 ____
Beef or veal .... 0 <1 1 2 3 4 5 6 7 8 9 >9 ____
Other meats (which?) _____ .... 0 <1 1 2 3 4 5 6 7 8 9 >9 ____
Eggs .... 0 <1 1 2 3 4 5 6 7 8 9 >9 ____
Fast foods?...................................... 0 <1 1 2 3 4 5 6 7 8 9 >9 ____

2. How many times *per day* do you eat the following foods? Circle the appropriate number:

                                                          PER DAY
Bread, toast, rolls, muffins .... 0 <1 1 2 3 4 5 6 7 8 9 >9 ____
Milk (including on cereal) .... 0 <1 1 2 3 4 5 6 7 8 9 >9 ____
Yogurt or tofu................................... 0 <1 1 2 3 4 5 6 7 8 9 >9 ____
Cheese or cheese dishes........................ 0 <1 1 2 3 4 5 6 7 8 9 >9 ____
Sugar, jam, jelly, syrup, honey .... 0 <1 1 2 3 4 5 6 7 8 9 >9 ____
Butter or margarine............................. 0 <1 1 2 3 4 5 6 7 8 9 >9 ____

3. How many times *per week* do you eat the following foods? Circle the appropriate number:

                                                          PER WEEK
Fruit or fruit juice .... 0 <1 1 2 3 4 5 6 7 8 9 >9 ____
Vegetables other than potato................... 0 <1 1 2 3 4 5 6 7 8 9 >9 ____
Potatoes and other starchy vegetables.......... 0 <1 1 2 3 4 5 6 7 8 9 >9 ____
Salads or raw vegetables....................... 0 <1 1 2 3 4 5 6 7 8 9 >9 ____
Cereal (which kind?) _____ .... 0 <1 1 2 3 4 5 6 7 8 9 >9 ____
Pancakes or waffles .... 0 <1 1 2 3 4 5 6 7 8 9 >9 ____
Rice or other cooked grains..................... 0 <1 1 2 3 4 5 6 7 8 9 >9 ____
Noodles (macaroni, spaghetti) .... 0 <1 1 2 3 4 5 6 7 8 9 >9 ____
Crackers or pretzels .... 0 <1 1 2 3 4 5 6 7 8 9 >9 ____
Sweet rolls or doughnuts .... 0 <1 1 2 3 4 5 6 7 8 9 >9 ____
Cooked dry beans or peas....................... 0 <1 1 2 3 4 5 6 7 8 9 >9 ____
Peanut butter or nuts .... 0 <1 1 2 3 4 5 6 7 8 9 >9 ____
Milk or milk products............................ 0 <1 1 2 3 4 5 6 7 8 9 >9 ____
TV dinners, pot pies, other prepared meals .... 0 <1 1 2 3 4 5 6 7 8 9 >9 ____
Sweet bakery goods (cake, cookies)............... 0 <1 1 2 3 4 5 6 7 8 9 >9 ____
Snack foods (potato or corn chips)................ 0 <1 1 2 3 4 5 6 7 8 9 >9 ____
Candy .... 0 <1 1 2 3 4 5 6 7 8 9 >9 ____
Soft drinks (which?) _____ .... 0 <1 1 2 3 4 5 6 7 8 9 >9 ____

Form A—4 (continued)

Coffee or tea . . . . 0 <1 1 2 3 4 5 6 7 8 9 >9 ____
Frozen sweets (which?) _____ . . . . 0 <1 1 2 3 4 5 6 7 8 9 >9 ____
Instant meals such as breakfast bars or diet meal
beverages (which?) _____ . . . . 0 <1 1 2 3 4 5 6 7 8 9 >9 ____
Wine . . . . 0 <1 1 2 3 4 5 6 7 8 9 >9 ____
Beer. . . . . 0 <1 1 2 3 4 5 6 7 8 9 >9 ____
Whiskey, vodka, rum, etc. . . . . 0 <1 1 2 3 4 5 6 7 8 9 >9 ____

4. What specific kinds of the following foods do you eat most often? Include the name of the food; whether it is fresh, canned, or frozen; and how it is prepared.

   Fruits and fruit juices _____
   Vegetables _____
   Milk and milk products _____
   Meats _____
   Breads and cereals _____
   Desserts _____
   Snack foods _____

5. Please list the names of any liquid, powder, or pill form of vitamin or mineral product you take, and state how often you take it. Please list also any diet supplement you use (such as protein milk shakes or brewer's yeast), how much you use, and how often you use it. _____

6. Is there anything else we should know about your food/nutrient intake? _____
_____

Form A—5 Food Diary

Name _____
Date _____

Time	Place	With Whom	Emotional State	Hungry or Not Hungry	Food Eaten (Amount)

(etc.)

After collecting food intake data, the assessor determines nutrient intake, if appropriate. Food composition tables provide nutrient values for comparison with standards such as the RDA (see Appendix B). The comparison is made by a skilled dietitian, who estimates or manually calculates the amount of each nutrient obtained from each food or uses a diet analysis computer program.

A computer diet analysis tends to imply an accuracy greater than is possible from data as uncertain as those that provide the starting information. Nutrient contents of foods listed in tables of food composition are averages, and for some nutrients, complete data are not available. Foods vary.

In addition, the nutrient content of foods as reported in food composition tables does not reflect the amount of the nutrient absorbed. Iron is a case in point. Iron is classified as having high, medium, or low availability based on a method of estimating absorbable iron in a meal.[1] This method sums the amount of total iron, heme iron, nonheme iron, ascorbic acid, meat, poultry, and fish. Figure A–2 explains how to calculate iron absorption from a meal.

Furthermore, the person who reports eating "a serving" of greens may not know the difference between 1/4 cup and 2 whole cups; only trained individuals can accurately estimate serving sizes. Children tend to remember the serving sizes of foods they like as being larger than serving sizes of foods they dislike.[2]

Thus, there are many opportunities for error when comparing nutrient intakes with nutrient needs in this way. Most history takers learn to use shortcut systems to obtain rough estimates of nutrient intakes and then use the calculation method to pinpoint any suspected nutrient deficiencies or imbalances.

An estimate of nutrient intakes from a diet history, combined with other sources of information, allows the assessor to confirm or eliminate the possibility of suspected nutrition problems. The assessor must constantly remember that a sufficient intake of a nutrient does not guarantee adequate nutrient status for an individual. Likewise, insufficient intake does not always indicate deficiency, but does alert the assessor to a possible problem. Each person digests, absorbs, metabolizes, and excretes nutrients in a unique way; individual needs vary.

Anthropometric Data

anthropometric: relating to measurement of the physical characteristics of the body, such as height and weight.
anthropos = human
metric = measuring

Anthropometrics are physical measurements that provide an indirect assessment of body composition and development (see Table A–4). Health care providers compare measurements taken on an individual with standards specific for gender and age or with previous measures of the individual. These standards derive from measurements taken on a population of people. Measurements taken periodically and compared with previous measurements reveal patterns and indicate changes in an individual's status.

Anthropometric measurements are easy to take and require minimal equipment. However, the skills of the measurer limit their accuracy and value. Mastering the correct techniques requires proper instruction and practice to ensure reliability. Furthermore, significant changes in measurements are slow

Figure A–2   Calculation of Iron Absorbed from Meals

Three factors go into the calculation of the amount of iron absorbed from a meal: first, how much of the iron in the meal was heme and how much was nonheme iron; second, how much vitamin C was in the meal; and third, how much total meat, fish, and poultry (MFP) was consumed. (It is assumed your iron stores are moderate; otherwise, you'd have to take this into consideration, too.) Answer these six questions:

1. How much iron was from animal tissues (MFP)? _____ mg
2. Forty percent of this, on the average, is heme iron. _____ mg heme iron
3. How much iron was from other sources? _____ mg
4. This, plus 60 percent of (1), is nonheme iron. _____ mg + .60 × mg
   = mg nonheme iron
5. How much vitamin C was in the meal? Less than 25 milligrams is low; 25 to 75 milligrams is medium; more than 75 milligrams is high.
6. How much MFP was in the meal? Less than 1 ounce lean MFP is low; 1 to 3 ounces is medium; more than 3 ounces is high.*

Now calculate:

You absorbed 23 percent of the heme iron (2), or _____ mg.

Now, take your best score from (5) and (6). If either vitamin C or MFP was high or if both were medium, the availability of your nonheme iron was high. If neither was high but one was medium, the availability of your nonheme iron was medium. If both were low, your nonheme iron had poor availability. You absorbed:

High availability: 8 percent of the nonheme iron.
Medium availability: 5 percent.
Poor availability: 3 percent.
   Your total: _____ mg nonheme iron absorbed

Add the two together:

   _____ mg heme iron absorbed
   _____ mg nonheme iron absorbed
Total = _____ mg iron absorbed

The RDA assumes you will absorb 10 percent of the iron you ingest. Thus, if you are a man of any age or a woman over 50 years old (RDA 10 milligrams), you need to absorb 1 milligram per day; if you are a woman 11 to 50 years old (RDA 18 milligrams), you need to absorb 1.8 milligrams. If you have higher menstrual losses than the average woman, you may still need more.

---

*Note on #6: We have adapted the calculation of Monsen and coauthors, stating it in ounces. Her actual numbers are less than 23 grams cooked meat, low; 23 to 46 grams, medium; and 69 grams or more, high.

Table A–4   Anthropometric Measures Used in Standard Nutrition Assessments

Measurement	Reflects
Height-weight	Overnutrition and undernutrition
	Growth in children
%IBW, %UBW, Recent weight change	Overnutrition and undernutrition
Midarm circumference	Muscle mass and subcutaneous fat
Fatfold	Subcutaneous fat and total body fat
Midarm muscle circumference	Muscle mass (i.e., protein status)
Head circumference	Brain growth and development in children

to occur in adults. When changes do occur, they represent prolonged changes in nutrient intake.

Height-Weight

Height and weight are the most commonly used anthropometric measurements. Length measurements for infants and height measurements for children are particularly valuable in assessing growth, and therefore nutrition status (as described in Chapter 4). For adults, height measurement helps to estimate desirable weight and to interpret other assessment data.

For infants and children younger than three, special equipment is available to measure length. The barefoot infant lies on a measuring board that has a fixed headboard and movable footboard attached at right angles to the surface (see Figure A–3). Care is taken to ensure that the infant's head is against the headboard and legs are held securely at the knees. Since this is difficult to accomplish, two people are needed to obtain an accurate measurement. Many health care providers, however, use a less accurate method: with the infant lying on a flat surface, a nonstretchable measuring tape is run along the side of the infant from the top of the head to the heel of the foot.

The procedure for measuring a child who can stand erect and cooperate is the same as for an adult. The best way to measure standing height is to have

1 in = 2.54 cm.

Figure A–3   Length Measurement of an Infant
An infant is measured lying down by use of a length measuring device with a fixed headboard and movable footboard. Note that two people are needed to measure the infant's length.

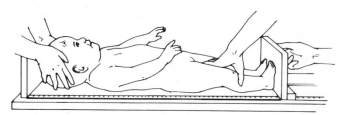

Reprinted with permission of Ross Laboratories, Columbus, Ohio 43216.

the person stand against a flat wall alongside an affixed, nonstretchable measuring tape or stick (see Figure A–4). The person stands erect, without shoes, with heels together. The person's line of sight should be horizontal, with the heels, buttocks, shoulders, and head touching the wall. The assessor carefully checks the height measurement and immediately records the result in either inches or centimeters. Such a practice prevents misplacing or forgetting the measurement.

The measuring rod of a scale is an acceptable but, because of its movability, less accurate means to measure height. The assessor follows the same general procedure, asking the person to face away from the scale and to take extra care to stand erect.

Unfortunately, it is a common practice in many health care institutions to ask clients how tall they are, rather than measuring their height. Self-reported height is often inaccurate and should be used only as a last resort when measurement is impractical (in the case of an uncooperative client, an emergency admission, or the like).

Special beam balance and electronic scales are available to measure infants' weights (see Figure A–5). Their design allows for infants to lie or sit on the scales. Weighing infants naked, without diapers, is standard procedure. To weigh children who can stand, health care providers use the same procedure as for an adult. Beam balance scales provide accurate weight measurements (see Figure A–6). Standardized conditions increase the usability of repeated weight measurements. Weighing a person at the same time of day (preferably before breakfast), in the same amount of clothing (without shoes), after having voided, and on the same scale increases reliability. Bathroom scales are inaccurate and inappropriate in a professional setting. As with all measurements, the assessor records observed weight immediately, in either pounds or kilograms.

To measure head circumference, the assessor places a nonstretchable tape around the largest part of the infant's or child's head. The tape surrounds the head, passing just over the eyebrow ridges, just over the point where the ears attach, and around the occipital prominence at the back of the head. Measurements are recorded immediately in either inches or centimeters.

Growth retardation (indicated by height, weight, and head circumference measures) in infants and young children is an important sign of poor nutrition status. Health professionals generally evaluate physical development by monitoring the growth rate of a child and comparing this rate to standard charts. Standard charts compare weight to height; ideally, height and weight are in roughly the same percentile. Although individual growth measurements vary, in general, the growth curve follows along the same percentile throughout childhood. In growth-retarded children, height and weight ideally increase to reach higher percentiles. In overweight children, the goal is for weight to remain stable as height increases, until weight becomes appropriate for height.

To evaluate growth in infants and children, an assessor uses charts such as Figures A–7 (A and B), A–8 (A and B), A–9 (A and B), and A–10 (A and B). The assessor follows these steps to plot a weight measurement on a percentile graph:

▶ Selects the appropriate chart based on age and gender. (When length is measured, the birth to 36 months chart is used; when height is measured, the 2 to 18 years chart is used.)

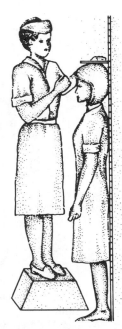

Figure A–4   Height Measurement of an Older Child or Adult
Height is measured most accurately when the person stands against a flat wall to which a measuring tape has been affixed. When the person is taller than the measurer, the measurer can stand on a stool to help ensure that the proper height measurement is obtained.

1 kg = 2.2 lb.
1 lb = 454 g.

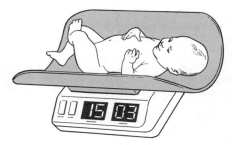

Figure A–5   Weight Measurement of an Infant
Infants sit or lie down on scales that are designed to hold them while they are being weighed.

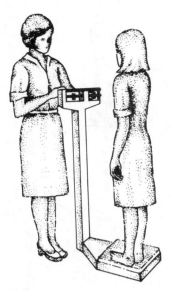

Figure A–6 Weight Measurement of an Older Child or Adult
Whenever possible, children and adults are measured on beam balance scales to ensure accuracy.

Figure A–7A Girls: Birth to 36 Months Physical Growth NCHS Percentiles—Length and Weight for Age

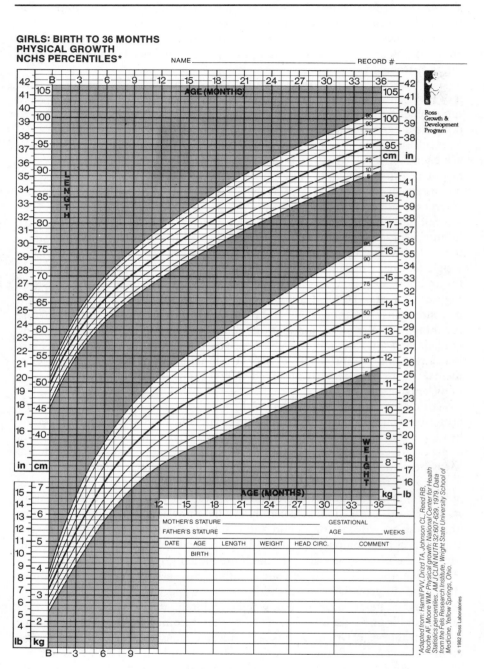

Figure A–7B   Boys: Birth to 36 Months Physical Growth NCHS Percentiles—Length and Weight for Age

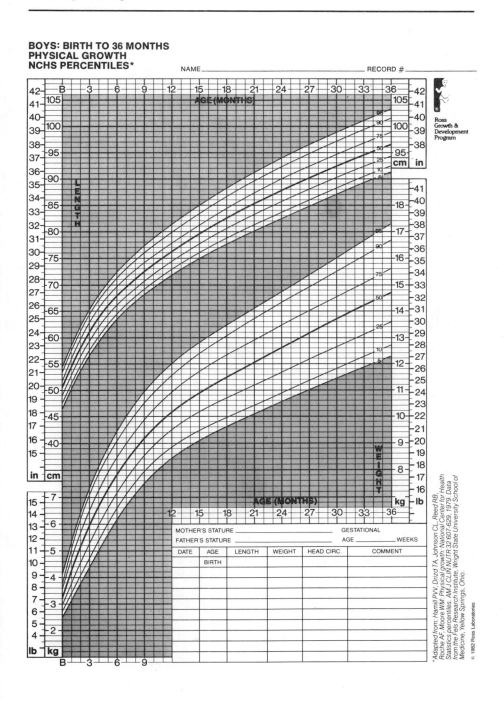

Figure A–8A   Girls: Birth to 36 Months Physical Growth NCHS Percentiles—Head Circumference for Age and Weight for Length

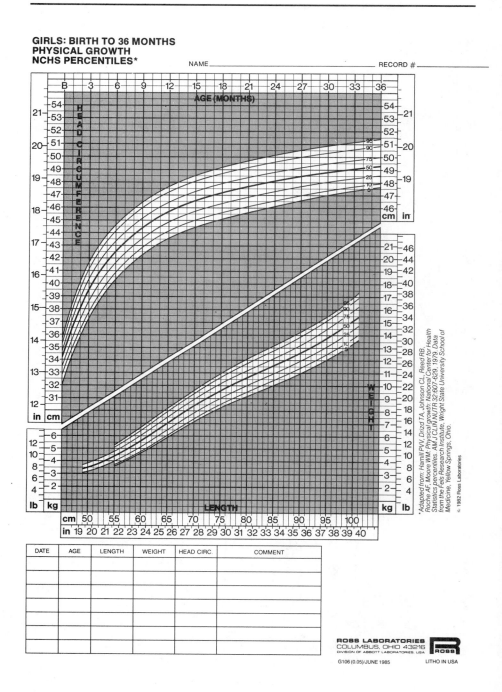

Figure A–8B   Boys: Birth to 36 Months Physical Growth NCHS Percentiles—Head Circumference for Age and Weight for Length

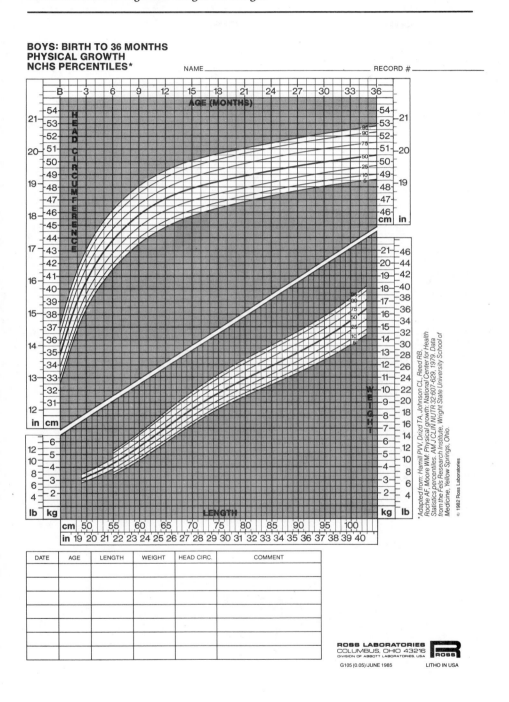

Figure A–9A   Girls: 2 to 18 Years Physical Growth NCHS Percentiles—Height and Weight for Age

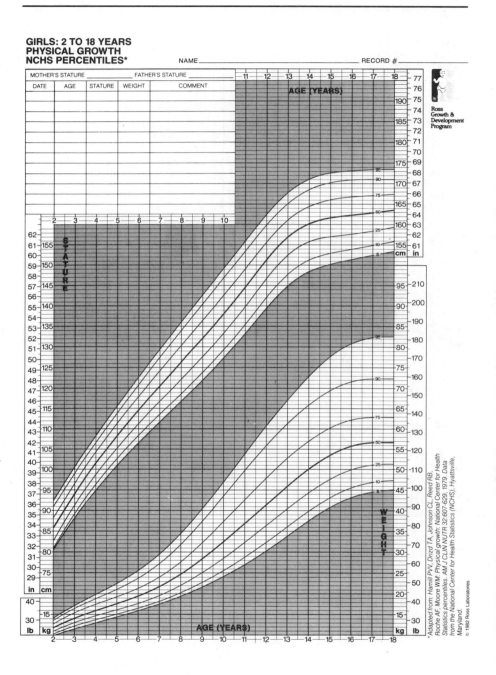

Figure A–9B Boys: 2 to 18 Years Physical Growth NCHS Percentiles—Height and Weight for Age

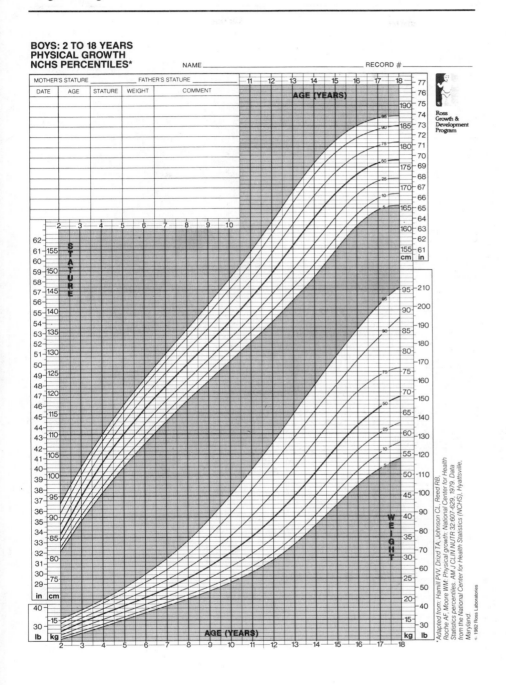

Figure A–10A   Girls: Prepubescent Physical Growth NCHS Percentiles—Weight for Height

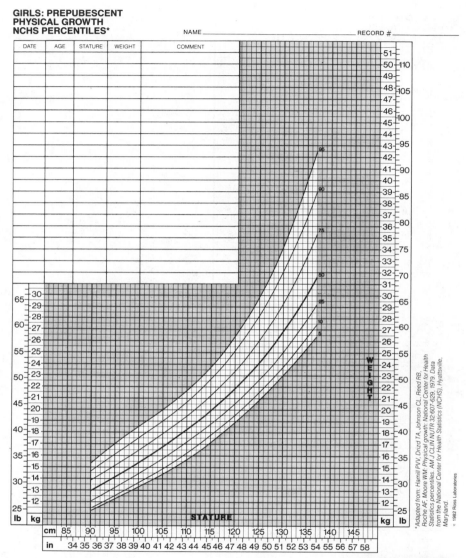

Figure A–10B   Boys: Prepubescent Physical Growth NCHS Percentiles—Weight for Height

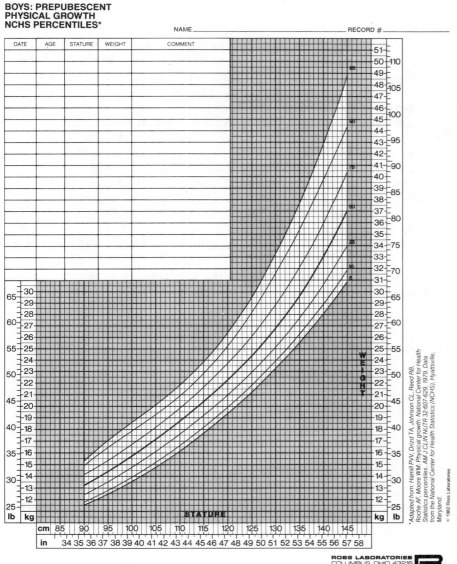

BOYS: PREPUBESCENT PHYSICAL GROWTH NCHS PERCENTILES*

ROSS LABORATORIES
COLUMBUS, OHIO 43216
DIVISION OF ABBOTT LABORATORIES, USA

G107 (0.05)/JUNE 1985   LITHO IN USA

► Locates the child's age on the bottom or top of the chart.

► Locates the child's weight in pounds or kilograms on the lower left or right side of the chart.

► Marks the chart where the age and weight lines intersect.

To assess length, height, or head circumference, the assessor follows the same procedure, using the appropriate figure.

With height, weight, and head circumference measures plotted on growth percentile charts, a skilled clinician can begin to interpret the data. Percentile charts divide the measures of a population into 100 equal parts. Thus, half of the population falls above the 50th percentile, and half falls below. This design allows for comparisons among people of similar characteristics, such as age and gender. For example, a six-month-old, female infant whose weight is at the 75th percentile weighs more than 75 percent of the female infants her age.

Head circumference is generally measured in children under three years of age. Since the brain is rapidly growing during early infancy, researchers believe that malnourished children will have fewer brain cells and a smaller head circumference.[3] The assessor plots head circumference measurements on a percentile growth chart; head circumference percentile should be similar to the child's weight and height percentiles.

Health care providers compare weight measurements for adults with standard weight-for-height tables (see Table A–5), which are specific for height, gender, and frame size. To use the height-weight table, the assessor refers to a table of frame sizes such as the one based on elbow breadth (Table

Table A–5 1983 Metropolitan Height and Weight Tables

Weights at ages 25-29 based on lowest mortality. Weights in pounds according to frame (in indoor clothing weighing 5 pounds for men or 3 pounds for women, shoes with 1-inch heels. For frame size standards, see Table A–7.

Men					Women				
Height		Small Frame	Medium Frame	Large Frame	Height		Small Frame	Medium Frame	Large Frame
Feet	Inches				Feet	Inches			
5	2	128–134	131–141	138–150	4	10	102–111	109–121	118–131
5	3	130–136	133–143	140–153	4	11	103–113	111–123	120–134
5	4	132–138	135–145	142–156	5	0	104–115	113–126	122–137
5	5	134–140	137–148	144–160	5	1	106–118	115–129	125–140
5	6	136–142	139–151	146–164	5	2	108–121	118–132	128–143
5	7	138–145	142–154	149–168	5	3	111–124	121–135	131–147
5	8	140–148	145–157	152–172	5	4	114–127	124–138	134–151
5	9	142–151	148–160	155–176	5	5	117–130	127–141	137–155
5	10	144–154	151–163	158–180	5	6	120–133	130–144	140–159
5	11	146–157	154–166	161–184	5	7	123–136	133–147	143–163
6	0	149–160	157–170	164–188	5	8	126–139	136–150	146–167
6	1	152–164	160–174	168–192	5	9	129–142	139–153	149–170
6	2	155–168	164–178	172–197	5	10	132–145	142–156	152–173
6	3	158–172	167–182	176–202	5	11	135–148	145–159	155–176
6	4	162–176	171–187	181–207	6	0	138–151	148–162	158–179

Source: Reproduced with permission of Metropolitan Life Insurance Company. Source of basic data: *1979 Build Study,* Society of Actuaries and Association of Life Insurance Medical Directors of America, 1980.

A–6) or the one that compares wrist circumference to height (see Figure A–11 and Table A–7). The height and weight tables use a weight range, rather than pinpointing one weight. This is a good reminder that there is no one "perfect" weight for anyone.

The height-weight tables are useful for identifying both undernutrition and overnutrition. A standard derived from height and weight, which is especially useful for estimating the risk to health associated with overnutrition, is the body mass index (BMI). Figure A–12 presents a nomogram for determining the BMI.

The table of average weights for height is less useful in cases where a person has weighed much more or much less than the average throughout life. To assess such a person's weight, it may be more informative to compare the present weight not with an "ideal" body weight, but with the person's usual body weight. The percentages of a person's actual weight compared with an ideal or usual body weight are useful indicators of malnutrition (Table A–8).

To calculate the percent ideal body weight (% IBW), a comparison is made between a person's actual weight and the ideal weight. This provides a rough estimate of the degree of overnutrition or undernutrition. A %IBW greater

body mass index (BMI): an index of a person's weight in relation to height, determined by dividing the weight in kilograms by the square of the height in meters:

$$BMI = \frac{Weight\ (kg)}{Height^2\ (m)}.$$

$$\%\ IBW = \frac{Actual\ weight}{Ideal\ weight^*} \times 100.$$

*Use the midpoint of the ideal weight range; some assessors use the upper end of the range for people who are overweight and the lower end of the range for people who are underweight.

Table A–6   How to Determine Your Body Frame by Elbow Breadth

To make a simple approximation of your frame size, do the following. Extend your arm, and bend the forearm upward at a 90-degree angle. Keep the fingers straight, and turn the inside of your wrist away from the body. Place the thumb and index finger of your other hand on the two prominent bones on *either side* of your elbow. Measure the space between your fingers against a ruler or a tape measure[a] Compare the measurements with the following standards.

These standards represent the elbow measurements for medium-framed men and women of various heights. Measurements smaller than those listed indicate you have a small frame, and larger measurements indicate a large frame.

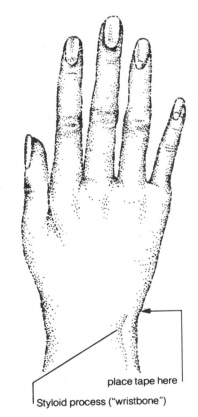

Figure A–11   Wrist circumference
The wrist circumference is measured as shown above.

place tape here

Styloid process ("wristbone")

Men

Height in 1-Inch Heels	Elbow Breadth
5 ft 2 inches to 5 ft 3 inches	2½ to 2⅞ inches
5 ft 4 inches to 5 ft 7 inches	2⅝ to 2⅞ inches
5 ft 8 inches to 5 ft 11 inches	2¾ to 3 inches
6 ft 0 inches to 6 ft 3 inches	2¾ to 3⅛ inches
6 ft 4 inches and over	2⅞ to 3¼ inches

Women

Height in 1-Inch Heels	Elbow Breadth
4 ft 10 inches to 4 ft 11 inches	2¼ to 2½ inches
5 ft 0 inches to 5 ft 3 inches	2¼ to 2½ inches
5 ft 4 inches to 5 ft 7 inches	2⅜ to 2⅝ inches
5 ft 8 inches to 5 ft 11 inches	2⅜ to 2⅝ inches
6 ft 0 inches and over	2½ to 2¾ inches

---

[a]For the most accurate measurement, have your physician measure your elbow breadth with a caliper.

Source: Metropolitan Life Insurance Company.

Table A–7　Frame Size from Height-Wrist Circumference Ratios (r)

	Male r Values[a]	Female r Values[a]
Small	>10.4	>11.0
Medium	9.6–10.4	10.1–11.0
Large	<9.6	<10.1

$$^a r = \frac{\text{Height (cm)}}{\text{Wrist circumference (cm)}_b}$$

[b]The wrist is measured where it bends (distal to the styloid process), on the right arm.

Source: Adapted for J. P. Grant, Patient selection, *Handbook of Total Parenteral Nutrition* (Philadelphia: Saunders, 1980), p. 15.

Figure A–12　Nomogram for Body Mass Index

Weights and heights are without clothing. With clothes, add 5 pounds for men or 3 pounds for women, and 1 inch in height for shoes. Draw a straight line or place a ruler from your height (left) to your weight (right). At the point where it crosses the BMI line, read your body mass index. A body mass index greater than 27.2 for men or 26.9 for women indicates obesity.

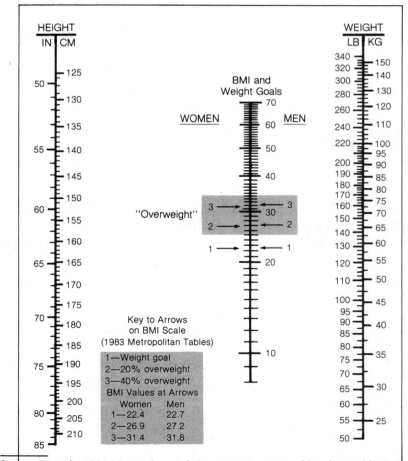

Source: From the 1983 Metropolitan Life Insurance Company tables, designed by B. T. Burton and W. R. Foster, Health implications of obesity, an NIH Consensus Development Conference, *Journal of the American Dietetic Association* 85 (1985): 1117–1121.

Table A–8   **Weight as an Indicator of Malnutrition**

%IBW[a]	%UBW[b]	Degree of Undernutrition
80–90%	85–95%	Mildly depleted
70–79%	75–84%	Moderately depleted
<70%	<75%	Severely depleted

[a]Percent ideal body weight.
[b]Percent usual body weight.

Source: Adapted from J. P. Grant, Patient selection, *Handbook of Total Parenteral Nutrition* (Philadelphia: Saunders, 1980), p. 11.

than 115 to 120 is indicative of obesity; less than 90 is indicative of undernutrition.

A more valuable parameter for assessing weight measurements is the percent usual body weight (%UBW), which considers what is normal for a particular individual. The client, family, friends, and older medical records are sources of such information. A health care provider may inadvertently overlook malnutrition in an obese person when using %IBW rather than %UBW.

$$\%UBW = \frac{\text{Actual weight}}{\text{Usual weight}} \times 100.$$

To determine any recent weight change, the assessor compares the %UBW to the time period over which a change, if any, has occurred. A 5 percent weight loss might be significant if it occurred within a month, yet might be insignificant if it occurred over five months.

In children, estimations of body fat can be obtained from several indexes. Two such indexes are the growth charts and body mass index mentioned earlier; they are most useful in assessing a child according to that individual child's own growth and development.

Another index used to evaluate childhood obesity is the Eid index. The Eid (named for the person who developed it) index is a percentage weight at the age when the child's height is on the 50th percentile. To determine this index, find the child's actual height on the height-for-age chart and note the age when his or her height is at the 50th percentile. Then find the 50th percentile weight for that age on the weight-for-age chart. The child's actual weight is then compared to this weight and calculated as a percentage. This index assumes the child is at the age appropriate for his height and then asks if the weight is appropriate for that age. The formula is:

$$\frac{\text{Actual weight}}{\substack{\text{50th percentile weight} \\ \text{for the age at which the child's height} \\ \text{is on the 50th percentile}}} \times 100.$$

Another index, the developmental index, recognizes that growth does not occur consistently over time or from child to child. It also recognizes that normal growth involves weight gain. A child who gains weight may actually decrease in percentage overweight if height increases and weight gain is less than expected. Similarly, two children who lose the same amount of weight may differ in their percent overweight if one has grown developmentally and the other has not. This index calculates an adjusted weight change as a ratio of expected to actual changes in height. The adjusted weight is:

$$\text{Actual weight change} - \frac{\text{Actual height change}}{\text{Expected height change}} \times \text{Expected weight change} \;.$$

A careful visual assessment of a child can determine whether these measures are even required. Often the best clinical assessment of obesity is the trained eye.[4] It is quite likely that those who are visually identified as obese are also obese by other criteria. When a child does not appear obese or if the assessment is questionable, both weight-for-height and triceps fatfold measurements should be used to confirm the diagnosis.

Height and weight are well-recognized anthropometrics. Others include the midarm circumference and fatfold measurements.

Midarm Circumference and Fatfold Measurements

An assessor measures midarm circumference with a nonstretchable tape around the arm midway between the shoulder and the elbow (see Figure A–13 and Table A–9). The midarm circumference measures muscle mass and subcutaneous fat. This measurement decreases with both acute and chronic undernutrition and increases with obesity.

Approximately half the fat in the body is located directly beneath the skin. In some parts of the body, this fat is more loosely attached; a person can pull it up between the thumb and forefinger. These sites provide an opportunity to measure fatfold thickness. By estimating subcutaneous fat, the assessor can approximate total body fat. Fatfold thickness has a high correlation with other, more sophisticated methods of measuring total body fat, such as underwater weighing, radioactive potassium counting, and total body water. However, careful training in the use of fatfold calipers is critical to obtaining accurate measurements.

Since fat stores decrease slowly with inadequate energy intake, short-term depletion of subcutaneous fat is undetectable. Detectable depletion reflects either long-term undernutrition or intentional weight loss.

The most commonly used site for measuring fatfold thickness is the triceps area, because the upper midarm is easily accessible. To measure fatfold, a trained technician follows a standard procedure using reliable calipers as illustrated in Figure A–14. Fatfold measurements from a specific area of the body are then used to estimate total body fat. Triceps fatfold percentiles are given in Table A–10. Together with the midarm circumference, triceps fatfold enables an assessor to calculate the derived midarm muscle circumference.

The midarm muscle circumference derives from a mathematical equation; it is not directly measurable. The equation assumes the arm to be circular, subtracting the fatfold measure from the midarm circumference (see Figures A–15 and A–16 and Table A–11). The derived midarm muscle circumference permits an estimate of muscle mass and, thus, represents protein nutriture.

Midarm circumference, fatfold measurements, and the derived midarm muscle circumference are reproducible measurements if an assessor follows standard procedures. Accurately following standard procedure requires prac-

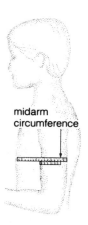

midarm circumference

Figure A–13 How to Measure the Midarm Circumference
Ask the subject to let his or her arm hang loosely to the side. Place the measuring tape horizontally around the arm at the midpoint mark. This measurement is the midarm circumference.

Table A–9   Midarm Circumference (MAC) (centimeters)

Age	Male 5th	25th	50th	75th	95th	Female 5th	25th	50th	75th	95th
<1	reliable data unavailable					reliable data unavailable				
1–1.9	14.2	15.0	15.9	17.0	18.3	13.8	14.8	15.6	16.4	17.7
2–2.9	14.1	15.3	16.2	17.0	18.5	14.2	15.2	16.0	16.7	18.4
3–3.9	15.0	16.0	16.7	17.5	19.0	14.3	15.8	16.7	17.5	18.9
4–4.9	14.9	16.2	17.1	18.0	19.2	14.9	16.0	16.9	17.7	19.1
5–5.9	15.3	16.7	17.5	18.5	20.4	15.3	16.5	17.5	18.5	21.1
6–6.9	15.5	16.7	17.9	18.8	22.8	15.6	17.0	17.6	18.7	21.1
7–7.9	16.2	17.7	18.7	20.1	23.0	16.4	17.4	18.3	19.9	23.1
8–8.9	16.2	17.7	19.0	20.2	24.5	16.8	18.3	19.5	21.4	26.1
9–9.9	17.5	18.7	20.0	21.7	25.7	17.8	19.4	21.1	22.4	26.0
10–10.9	18.1	19.6	21.0	23.1	27.4	17.4	19.3	21.0	22.8	26.5
11–11.9	18.6	20.2	22.3	24.4	28.0	18.5	20.8	22.4	24.8	30.3
12–12.9	19.3	21.4	23.2	25.4	30.3	19.4	21.6	23.7	25.6	29.4
13–13.9	19.4	22.8	24.7	26.3	30.1	20.2	22.3	24.3	27.1	33.8
14–14.9	22.0	23.7	25.3	28.3	32.3	21.4	23.7	25.2	27.2	32.2
15–15.9	22.2	24.4	26.4	28.4	32.0	20.8	23.9	25.4	27.9	32.2
16–16.9	24.4	26.2	27.8	30.3	34.3	21.8	24.1	25.8	28.3	33.4
17–17.9	24.6	26.7	28.5	30.8	34.7	22.0	24.1	26.4	29.5	35.0
18–18.9	24.5	27.6	29.7	32.1	37.9	22.2	24.1	25.8	28.1	32.5
19–24.9	26.2	28.8	30.8	33.1	37.2	21.1	24.7	26.5	29.0	34.5
25–34.9	27.1	30.0	31.9	34.2	37.5	23.3	25.6	27.7	30.4	36.8
35–44.9	27.8	30.5	32.6	34.5	37.4	24.1	26.7	29.0	31.7	37.8
45–54.9	26.7	30.1	32.2	34.2	37.6	24.2	27.4	29.9	32.8	38.4
55–64.9	25.8	29.6	31.7	33.6	36.9	24.3	28.0	30.3	33.5	38.5
65–74.9	24.8	28.5	30.7	32.5	35.5	24.0	27.4	29.9	32.6	37.3

Source: Adapted from A. R. Frisancho, New norms of upper limb fat and muscle areas for assessment of nutritional status, *American Journal of Clinical Nutrition* 34 (1981): 2540–2545.

tice, however. For best results, the same person would measure the same client routinely.

To assess protein-energy malnutrition (PEM), health care providers employ several lab tests with these anthropometric measures. Table A–12 shows the depletion of different compartments depending on whether the person has kwashiorkor (from protein deficiency as reflected in skeletal muscle and visceral protein), marasmus (from energy deficiency as reflected in body fat), or a mixture of the two. A form, such as Form A–6, summarizes the anthropometric and biochemical data used to classify PEM.

Physical Data

The assessor searches for clues to a person's nutrition status by examining the person for physical signs of malnutrition. Such an examination requires knowledge and skill to identify the signs and their associated nutrient deficiency or toxicity. Many physical signs are nonspecific; they can reflect

Figure A–14 How to Measure the Triceps Fatfold

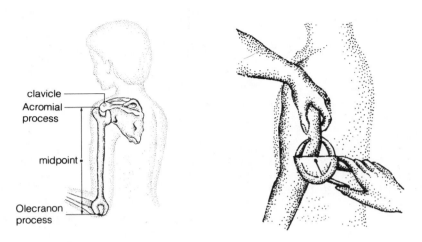

A. Find the midpoint of the arm:
1. Ask the subject to bend his or her arm at the elbow and lay the hand across the stomach. (If he or she is right-handed, measure the left arm, and vice versa.)
2. Feel the shoulder to locate the acromial process. It helps to slide your fingers along the clavicle to find the acromial process. The olecranon process is the tip of the elbow.
3. Place a measuring tape from the acromial process to the tip of the elbow. Divide this measurement by 2 and mark the midpoint of the arm with a pen.
B. Measure the fatfold:
1. Ask the subject to let his or her arm hang loosely to the side.
2. Grasp a fold of skin and subcutaneous fat between the thumb and forefinger slightly above the midpoint mark. Gently pull the skin away from the underlying muscle. (This step takes a lot of practice. If you want to be sure you don't have muscle as well as fat, ask the subject to contract and relax his muscle. You should be able to feel if you are pinching muscle.)
3. Place the calipers over the fatfold at the midpoint mark and read the measurement to the nearest 1.0 mm in two to three seconds. (If using plastic calipers, align pressure lines and read measurement to the nearest 1.0 mm in two to three seconds.)
4. Repeat steps 2 to 4 twice more. Add the three readings and then divide by 3 to find the average.

more than one nutrient deficiency or nonnutrition conditions. For this reason, physical findings alone cannot diagnose a nutrition problem. Instead, their value is in revealing possible problems for other assessment techniques to confirm, or to confirm other assessment measures.

Many tissues and organs can reflect signs of malnutrition. Physical signs of malnutrition appear most rapidly in parts of the body where cell replacement occurs at a high rate, such as in the hair, skin, and digestive tract. Table A–13 lists the signs of vitamin malnutrition.

Table A–10   Triceps Fatfold Percentiles (millimeters) for Males and Female.

Age	Male 5th	25th	50th	75th	95th	Female 5th	25th	50th	75th	95th
1–1.9	6	8	10	12	16	6	8	10	12	16
2–2.9	6	8	10	12	15	6	9	10	12	16
3–3.9	6	8	10	11	15	7	9	11	12	15
4–4.9	6	8	9	11	14	7	8	10	12	16
5–5.9	6	8	9	11	15	6	8	10	12	18
6–6.9	5	7	8	10	16	6	8	10	12	16
7–7.9	5	7	9	12	17	6	9	11	13	18
8–8.9	5	7	8	10	16	6	9	12	15	24
9–9.9	6	7	10	13	18	8	10	13	16	22
10–10.9	6	8	10	14	21	7	10	12	17	27
11–11.9	6	8	11	16	24	7	10	13	18	28
12–12.9	6	8	11	14	28	8	11	14	18	27
13–13.9	5	7	10	14	26	8	12	15	21	30
14–14.9	4	7	9	14	24	9	13	16	21	28
15–15.9	4	6	8	11	24	8	12	17	21	32
16–16.9	4	6	8	12	22	10	15	18	22	31
17–17.9	5	6	8	12	19	10	13	19	24	37
18–18.9	4	6	9	13	24	10	15	18	22	30
19–24.9	4	7	10	15	22	10	14	18	24	34
25–34.9	5	8	12	16	24	10	16	21	27	37
35–44.9	5	8	12	16	23	12	18	23	29	38
45–54.9	6	8	12	15	25	12	20	25	30	40
55–64.9	5	8	11	14	22	12	20	25	31	38
65–74.9	4	8	11	15	22	12	18	24	29	36

Source: Adapted from A. R. Frisancho, New norms of upper limb fat and muscle areas for assessment of nutritional status, *American Journal of Clinical Nutrition* 34 (1981): 2540–2545.

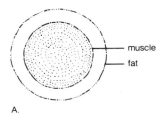

A.

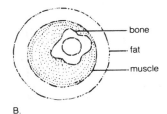

B.

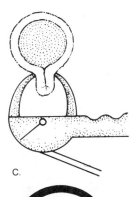

C.

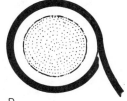

D.

Figure A–15   How to Derive Midarm Muscle Circumference

A. The arm is visualized as an inner circle of muscle surrounded by an outer circle of fat.
B. In reality, the arm is not circular, and there is some bone, but the simplified picture is approximately correct.
C. This measurement (the fatfold) gives you two times the thickness of the fat.
D. This measurement (the tape-measured outer circumference of the arm) gives you the outer circumference (muscle plus fat).
E. An equation then derives the *circumference of the muscle,* an index of the body's total skeletal muscle mass. The equation is:

midarm muscle circumference (cm) =
midarm circumference (cm) − [0.314* × triceps fatfold (mm)]

*This factor converts the fatfold measurement to a circumference measurement and millimeters to centimeters.

Figure A–16 Nomograms for Determination of Midarm Muscle Circumference (MAMC)

To obtain muscle circumference using either nomogram, lay ruler between values of arm circumference and fatfold and read off muscle circumference.

Arm Circumference (cm)

Arm Muscle Circumference (cm)

Triceps Fatfold (mm)

Arm Circumference (cm)

Arm Muscle Circumference (cm)

Triceps Fatfold (mm)

Source: Reproduced with permission from J. Gurney and D. Jelliffe, Arm anthropometry in nutritional assessment; nomogram for rapid calculation of muscle circumference and cross-sectional muscle and fat areas, *American Journal of Clinical Nutrition* 26 (1973): 912, as adapted by A. Grant, *Nutritional Assessment Guidelines,* 2nd ed., 1979 (available from P.O. Box 25057, Northgate Station, Seattle, WA 98125).

Table A–11   Midarm Muscle Circumference (MAMC)(centimeters)

	Male					Female				
Age	5th	25th	50th	75th	95th	5th	25th	50th	75th	95th
1–1.9	11.0	11.9	12.7	13.5	14.7	10.5	11.7	12.4	13.9	14.3
2–2.9	11.1	12.2	13.0	14.0	15.0	11.1	11.9	12.6	13.3	14.7
3–3.9	11.7	13.1	13.7	14.3	15.3	11.3	12.4	13.2	14.0	15.2
4–4.9	12.3	13.3	14.1	14.8	15.9	11.5	12.8	13.6	14.4	15.7
5–5.9	12.8	14.0	14.7	15.4	16.9	12.5	13.4	14.2	15.1	16.5
6–6.9	13.1	14.2	15.1	16.1	17.7	13.0	13.8	14.5	15.4	17.1
7–7.9	13.7	15.1	16.0	16.8	19.0	12.9	14.2	15.1	16.0	17.6
8–8.9	14.0	15.4	16.2	17.0	18.7	13.8	15.1	16.0	17.1	19.4
9–9.9	15.1	16.1	17.0	18.3	20.2	14.7	15.8	16.7	18.0	19.8
10–10.9	15.6	16.6	18.0	19.1	22.1	14.8	15.9	17.0	18.0	19.7
11–11.9	15.9	17.3	18.3	19.5	23.0	15.0	17.1	18.1	19.6	22.3
12–12.9	16.7	18.2	19.5	21.0	24.1	16.2	18.0	19.1	20.1	22.0
13–13.9	17.2	19.6	21.1	22.6	24.5	16.9	18.3	19.8	21.1	24.0
14–14.9	18.9	21.2	22.3	24.0	26.4	17.4	19.0	20.1	21.6	24.7
15–15.9	19.9	21.8	23.7	25.4	27.2	17.5	18.9	20.2	21.5	24.4
16–16.9	21.3	23.4	24.9	26.9	29.6	17.0	19.0	20.2	21.6	24.9
17–17.9	22.4	24.5	25.8	27.3	31.2	17.5	19.4	20.5	22.1	25.7
18–18.9	22.6	25.2	26.4	28.3	32.4	17.4	19.1	20.2	21.5	24.5
19–24.9	23.8	25.7	27.3	28.9	32.1	17.9	19.5	20.7	22.1	24.9
25–34.9	24.3	26.4	27.9	29.8	32.6	18.3	19.9	21.2	22.8	26.4
35–44.9	24.7	26.9	28.6	30.2	32.7	18.6	20.5	21.8	23.6	27.2
45–54.9	23.9	26.5	28.1	30.0	32.6	18.7	20.6	22.0	23.8	27.4
55–64.9	23.6	26.0	27.8	29.5	32.0	18.7	20.9	22.5	24.4	28.0
65–74.9	22.3	25.1	26.8	28.4	30.6	18.5	20.8	22.5	24.4	27.9

Source: Adapted from A. R. Frisancho, New norms of upper limb fat and muscle areas for assessment of nutritional status, *American Journal of Clinical Nutrition* 34 (1981): 2540–2545.

Table A–12   Anthropometric and Biochemical Measures Used to Assess Protein-Energy Malnutrition (PEM)

	Body Compartment Measured		
Measure	Body Fat	Skeletal Muscle	Visceral Protein
Anthropometrics			
Weight[a]	x	x	
Triceps skinfold	x		
Midarm circumference	x	x	
Midarm muscle circumference		x	
Lab tests			
Serum albumin			x
Serum transferrin			x
Total lymphocyte count			x
Creatinine–height index[b]		x	

[a]A standard table of weight for height appears in Table A–5.
[b]The amount of creatinine excreted is thought to reflect total skeletal mass. It therefore should be proportional to height. If creatinine excreted (for a person of a given height) is low, this reflects depleted skeletal muscle. Table A–15 and A–16 present standards.

Form A–6   Nutrition Assessment Summary

Date _____   Admitting date _____
Client _____   Room _____
Height _____   Admitting weight _____
Current weight _____   Usual body weight _____
Admitting diagnosis _____

Somatic protein and fat	Client value	Degree of depletion			
		None	Mild	Moderate	Severe
Weight as % IBW					
Weight as % UBW					
Midarm circumference					
Triceps fatfold					
Midarm muscle circumference					
Urinary creatinine					
Creatinine-height index					
Visceral protein					
Serum albumin					
Total iron binding capacity					
Transferrin (serum or calculated)					
Total lymphocyte count					
Cell mediated immunity					

Nitrogen balance: _____

Protein–energy nutrition status

☐ Adequate
☐ Marasmus
   Somatic protein and fat depleted;
   visceral protein adequate

☐ Kwashiorkor
   Somatic protein and fat adequate;
   visceral protein depleted
☐ Kwashiorkor-marasmus mix
   Somatic and visceral protein depleted

Other findings and comments
(Include pertinent food intake data, other laboratory tests, and physical findings.)

_____

_____
Signature of Assessor

Table A–13 Physical Findings Associated with Vitamin Deficiencies

Vitamin	Disease	Area Affected	Main Effects	Technical Names
Thiamin	Beriberi	Nervous system	Mental confusion Peripheral paralysis Loss of ankle and knee jerk reflexes	
		Muscles	Weakness Wasting Painful calf muscles	
		Cardiovascular system	Edema Enlarged heart Death from cardiac failure	
Riboflavin	Ariboflavinosis	Facial skin	Dermatitis around nose and lips Cracking of corners of mouth	Cheilosis (kee-LOH-sis)
		Eyes	Hypersensitivity to light Reddening of cornea	Photophobia
		GI tract	Magenta tongue	
Niacin	Pellagra	Skin	Bilateral symmetrical dermatitis, especially on body parts exposed to sun	
		Tongue	Loss of surface features, swelling, edema	Glossitis (gloss-EYE-tis)
		GI tract	Diarrhea	
		Nervous system	Irritability Mental confusion, progressing to psychosis or delirium	
Vitamin B$_6$	(No name)	Skin	Dermatitis	
			Cracking of corners of mouth	Cheilosis
			Irritation of sweat glands	
		Tongue	Smoothness (atrophy of surface structures)	Glossitis
		Nervous system	Abnormal brainwave pattern Convulsions	
Folacin	(No name)	Tongue	Smoothness, swelling, cracks	Glossitis
		GI tract	Diarrhea (loss of villi and their enzymes)	
		Nervous system	Fatigue, depression, confusion	
		Blood	Anemia (characterized by large cells)	Macrocytic anemia
		Immune system	Suppression; infections likely	
Vitamin B$_{12}$	(No name)[a]	Tongue	Smoothness, swelling, cracks	Glossitis
		Blood	Anemia (characterized by large cells)	Macrocytic anemia
		Skin	Hypersensitivity	
		Nervous system	Degeneration of peripheral nerves	

Table A–13 (continued)

Vitamin	Disease	Area Affected	Main Effects	Technical Names
Pantothenic acid	(No name)	GI tract	Vomiting, GI distress	
		Nervous system	Insomnia, fatigue	
Biotin	(No name)	Skin	Scaly dermatitis, drying, loss of hair	
		Nervous system	Depression, lassitude, muscle pains	
		GI tract	Anorexia, nausea	
		Cardiovascular system	Abnormal heart action	
Vitamin C	Scurvy	Gums	Bleeding, spongy, receding	
		Skin	Small red or purple skin hemorrhages	Petechiae Ecchymoses
Vitamin A		Eye		
		Retina	Night blindness	
		Membranes	Failure to secrete mucopolysaccharide causes changes in epithelial tissue	Hyperkeratinization
		General	Drying (mildest form)	Xerosis
			Triangular grey spots on eye	Bitot's spots
			Irreversible drying and degeneration of the cornea causes blindness (most severe)	Keratomalacia
			The eye's symptoms of vitamin A deficiency are collectively know as:	Xerophthalmia
		Skin	Hair follicles plug with keratin, forming white lumps	Hyperkeratosis
		GI tract	Changes in lining; diarrhea	
		Respiratory tract	Changes in lining; infections	
		Urogenital tract	Changes in lining favor calcium deposition, resulting in kidney stones, bladder disorders	
			Infections of bladder and kidney	
			Infections of vagina	
		Bones	Bone growth ceases; shapes of bones change; joints are painful	
		Teeth	Enamel-forming cells malfunction; teeth develop cracks and tend to decay; dentin-forming cells atrophy	
		Nervous system	Brain and spinal cord grow too fast for stunted skull and spine; injury to brain and nerves causes paralysis	
		Immune system	Depression of immune reactions	
		Blood	Anemia, often masked by dehydration	

Table A–13 (continued)

Vitamin	Disease	Area Affected	Main Effects	Technical Names
Vitamin D	Rickets	Bones	Faulty calcification, resulting in misshapen bones (bowing of legs) and retarded growth	
			Enlargement of ends of long bones (knees, wrists)	
			Deformities of ribs (bowed, with beads or knobs)	
			Delayed closing of fontanel, resulting in rapid enlargement of head	
		Blood	Decreased calcium and/or phosphorus	
		Teeth	Slow eruption; teeth not well-formed; tendency to decay	
		Muscles	Lax muscles resulting in protrusion of abdomen; muscle spasms	
		Excretory system	Increased calcium in stools; decreased calcium in urine	
		Glandular system	Abnormally high secretion of parathyroid hormone	
	Osteomalacia	Bones	Softening effect: deformities of limbs, spine, thorax, and pelvis; demineralization; pain in pelvis, lower back, and legs; bone fractures	,
		Blood	Decreased calcium and/or phosphorus; increased alkaline phosphatase	
		Muscles	Involuntary twitching; muscle spasms	
Vitamin E		Blood	Red blood cells break open	Erythrocyte hemolysis
Vitamin K	Hemorrhagic disease	Blood	Blood cannot clot	

[a]The name *pernicious anemia* refers to the vitamin B_{12} deficiency caused by lack of intrinsic factor, but not to that caused by inadequate dietary intake.

Biochemical (Lab) Data

Biochemical or clinical lab tests help to determine what is happening inside the body (see Table A–14). Blood and urine samples measure nutrients or metabolites (end products or enzymes) that reflect nutrient status.

Detecting subclinical deficiencies is a difficult and complicated task primarily because multiple deficiencies often occur simultaneously. One of the goals of nutrition assessment is to uncover early signs of malnutrition long before a classical deficiency disease develops. Biochemical measurements are useful in detecting subclinical malnutrition.

subclinical deficiency: a nutrient deficiency in the early stages, before the outward signs have appeared.

Table A–14   Laboratory Tests Used in Standard Nutrition Assessments

Lab Test	Reflects
Urinary creatinine excretion	Skeletal muscle mass (i.e., malnutrition) and a standard for other measures
Albumin	Protein status
Transferrin	Protein and iron status
Total lymphocyte count	Protein status
Nitrogen balance	Protein status
Vitamin and mineral tests	Vitamin and mineral status

Protein-Energy Malnutrition

serum: the watery portion of the blood that remains after removal of the cells and clot-forming material.

plasma: unclotted blood. In most cases, serum and plasma concentrations are similar. Lab technicians usually prefer serum samples because plasma samples occasionally clog mechanical blood analyzers.

The most common lab tests used in hospitals today for nutrition assessment help to uncover protein-energy malnutrition. These tests include urinary creatinine excretion, serum albumin, serum transferrin, total lymphocyte count, and nitrogen balance.

Urinary creatinine excretion   Creatinine is a breakdown product of an energy source that is present specifically in skeletal muscle. Its excretion occurs at a constant rate determined by the amount of skeletal muscle and therefore reflects skeletal muscle mass. As skeletal muscle atrophies during malnutrition, creatinine excretion decreases.

Standards for creatinine excretion, based on sex and height, are given in Tables A–15 and A–16. Assessors use these standards and measured urinary creatinine to derive the creatinine-height index (CHI):

$$\frac{\text{Measured urinary creatinine (24-hr sample)}}{\text{Standard creatinine for height and sex}} \times 100.$$

The CHI is a percentage of the standard; generally, acceptable values are 90 to 100 percent. The CHI measurement is one way to evaluate protein nutrition status in children.[5] Children suffering from protein-energy malnutrition have a low CHI. Standards for children are based on expected creatinine excretion of healthy children of normal height.

Creatinine excretion is also used to determine whether other urinary lab test results are appropriate to the size of the individual's skeletal muscle mass. The measurement of urinary creatinine requires a 24-hour urine collection, which may be difficult to obtain. The test is invalid if the subject shows signs of kidney disease since the disease might reduce the body's ability to excrete creatinine.

Albumin   Albumin accounts for over 50 percent of the total serum proteins. It helps to maintain fluid and electrolyte balance and to transport many nutrients, hormones, drugs, and other compounds. Albumin synthesis depends

Table A–15 Creatinine-Height Index Standards for Men

Height		Small Frame			Medium Frame			Large Frame		
in	cm	Ideal weight (kg)	Creatinine (g/24 h)	(mmol/d)[a]	Ideal weight (kg)	Creatinine (g/24 h)	(mmol/d)[a]	Ideal weight (kg)	Creatinine (g/24 h)	(mmol/d)[a]
61	154.9	52.7	1.21	10.7	56.1	1.29	11.4	60.7	1.40	12.4
62	157.5	54.1	1.24	11.0	57.7	1.33	11.8	62.0	1.43	12.6
63	160.0	55.4	1.27	11.2	59.1	1.36	12.0	63.6	1.46	12.9
64	162.5	56.8	1.31	11.6	60.4	1.39	12.3	65.2	1.50	13.3
65	165.1	58.4	1.34	11.8	62.0	1.43	12.6	66.8	1.54	13.6
66	167.6	60.2	1.39	12.3	63.9	1.47	13.0	68.9	1.59	14.1
67	170.2	62.0	1.43	12.6	65.9	1.52	13.4	71.1	1.64	14.5
68	172.7	63.9	1.47	13.0	67.7	1.56	13.8	72.9	1.68	14.9
69	175.3	65.9	1.52	13.4	69.5	1.60	14.1	74.8	1.72	15.2
70	177.8	67.7	1.56	13.8	71.6	1.65	14.6	76.8	1.77	15.6
71	180.3	69.5	1.60	14.1	73.6	1.69	14.9	79.1	1.82	16.1
72	182.9	71.4	1.64	14.5	75.7	1.74	15.4	81.1	1.87	16.5
73	185.4	73.4	1.69	14.9	77.7	1.79	15.8	83.4	1.92	17.0
74	187.9	75.2	1.73	15.3	80.0	1.85	16.4	85.7	1.97	17.4
75	190.5	77.0	1.77	15.6	82.3	1.89	16.7	87.7	2.02	17.9

[a]To convert urinary creatinine measures (g/24 h) to standard international units (mmol/d) multiply by 8.840.

Source: *A. Grant and S. DeHoog Nutritional Assessment and Support*, 3rd ed., 1985 (available from P.O. Box 25057, Northgate Station, Seattle, WA 98125).

Table A–16 Creatinine-Height Index Standards for Women

Height		Small Frame			Medium Frame			Large Frame		
in	cm	Ideal weight (kg)	Creatinine (g/24 h)	(mmol/d)[a]	Ideal weight (kg)	Creatinine (g/24 h)	(mmol/d)[a]	Ideal weight (kg)	Creatinine (g/24 h)	(mmol/d)[a]
56	142.2	43.2	0.79	7.0	46.1	0.83	7.3	50.7	0.91	8.0
57	144.8	44.3	0.80	7.1	47.3	0.85	7.5	51.8	0.93	8.2
58	147.3	45.4	0.82	7.2	48.6	0.88	7.8	53.2	0.96	8.5
59	149.8	46.8	0.84	7.4	50.0	0.90	8.0	54.5	0.98	8.7
60	152.4	48.2	0.87	7.7	51.4	0.93	8.2	55.9	1.01	8.9
61	154.9	49.5	0.89	7.9	52.7	0.95	8.4	57.3	1.03	9.1
62	157.5	50.9	0.92	8.1	54.3	0.98	8.7	58.9	1.06	9.4
63	160.0	52.3	0.94	8.3	55.9	1.01	8.9	60.6	1.09	9.6
64	162.5	53.9	0.97	8.6	57.9	1.04	9.2	62.5	1.13	10.0
65	165.1	55.7	1.00	8.8	59.8	1.08	9.5	64.3	1.16	10.3
66	167.6	57.5	1.04	9.2	61.6	1.11	9.8	66.1	1.19	10.5
67	170.2	59.3	1.07	9.5	63.4	1.14	10.1	67.9	1.22	10.8
68	172.7	61.4	1.11	9.8	65.2	1.17	10.3	70.0	1.26	11.1
69	175.2	63.2	1.14	10.1	67.0	1.21	10.7	72.0	1.30	11.5
70	177.8	65.0	1.17	10.3	68.9	1.24	11.0	74.1	1.33	11.8

[a]To convert urinary creatinine measures (g/24 h) to standard international units (mmol/d) multiply by 8.840.

Source: *A. Grant and S. DeHoog Nutritional Assessment and Support*, 3rd ed., 1985 (available from P.O. Box 25057, Northgate Station, Seattle, WA 98125).

on the existence of functioning liver cells and on an appropriate supply of amino acids. Because there is so much albumin in the body and because it is not broken down quickly, albumin concentrations change slowly. Therefore, albumin is a useful indicator of prolonged protein depletion. Unlike creatinine, albumin levels can reflect the protein status of the blood and internal organs. Standards for determining the severity of serum albumin depletion are given in Table A–17.

Many other conditions besides malnutrition can depress albumin concentration, including eclampsia, liver disease, advanced kidney disease (nephrotic syndrome), infection, cancer, and burns. Therefore, as is true for all nutrition assessment measurements, albumin alone cannot determine protein status, but rather serves as one indicator among many.

Transferrin   Transferrin is a protein that transports iron between the intestine and sites of hemoglobin synthesis and degradation. Researchers consider it a more sensitive indicator of protein malnutrition than albumin because it responds more promptly to changes in protein intake and has a smaller body pool.

Transferrin concentration is inversely related to iron stores; concentration is high in iron deficiency and low when iron storage is excessive. Therefore, the presence of abnormal iron nutriture makes interpretation of the transferrin level as an indicator of protein status difficult. Liver disease, nephrotic syndrome, and burns cause decreases in transferrin levels; iron deficiency, pregnancy, and blood loss elevate values. Standards for determining the severity of transferrin depletion are given in Table A–17.

Lymphocyte count   Various forms of protein-energy malnutrition and individual nutrient deficiencies depress the immune system. The total number of lymphocytes appears to decrease as protein depletion occurs, so the total lymphocyte count is one useful index in nutrition assessment.

Total lymphocyte count (mm³) = WBC (mm³) × %lymphocytes.

Nitrogen balance   Nitrogen balance studies are useful in estimating the degree of protein depletion and repletion in the body. Normally, adults are in nitrogen

Table A–17   Relationship between Degree of Undernutrition and Serum Proteins

Degree of Depletion	Albumin (g/100 ml)	(nmol/L)[a]	Transferrin (mg/100 ml)	(g/L)[b]
Mild	2.8-3.4	104–126	150-200	1.50–2.00
Moderate	2.1-2.7	79–100	100-149	1.00–1.49
Severe	<2.1	79	<100	<1.00

[a]To convert albumin (g/100 ml) to standard units (nmol/L) multiply by 37.06.
[b]To convert transferrin (mg/100 ml) to standard units (g/L) multiply by 0.01.

balance. Nitrogen balance is usually positive during pregnancy, growth, and recovery from disease. Nitrogen balance is usually negative during malnutrition and following trauma.

A simple approach to measuring nitrogen is to measure urine urea nitrogen (UUN) in a 24-hour urine collection. During the same 24-hour period, an accurate record of the subject's protein (nitrogen) intake must be kept to complete the balance study.

To calculate nitrogen intake, divide protein intake (in grams) by 6.25 (grams of nitrogen per gram of protein). Nitrogen output per day equals the UUN plus a factor of 4 grams to account for nitrogen lost through the lungs, hair, skin, nails, and nonurea nitrogen losses in the urine. The equation for nitrogen balance is:

$$\text{N balance} = \frac{\text{Protein (g)}}{6.25} - (\text{UUN g} + 4 \text{ g}).$$

As with creatinine excretion, the kidneys must be functioning properly for UUN measurement to be accurate. Additionally, clinicians must consider abnormally high nitrogen losses (as seen in clients with severe burns) if this test is to be valid.

Nitrogen balance studies provide a prime example of the need for communication and cooperation between various health care providers and departments. A nitrogen balance study is invalid if anyone fails to measure even one urine specimen or record even one meal's food intake. To repeat the entire procedure is most inconvenient to the client and the staff.

Laboratory tests add a valuable dimension to nutrition assessment. However, as emphasized earlier, many factors influence lab tests; therefore, a single test cannot assess nutrition status. The combination of many laboratory tests with histories, anthropometric measures, and physical findings provides for a total picture that becomes clearer with careful interpretation. Laboratory tests are particularly useful in assessing vitamin and mineral status when combined with physical findings. Vitamin and mineral levels present in the blood and urine sometimes represent recent intake rather than long-term intake. This makes detecting a subclinical deficiency difficult. Furthermore, many nutrients interact; the amounts of other nutrients in the body can affect a lab value for a particular nutrient. Table A–18 summarizes the biochemical tests used to assess vitamin-mineral status.

Iron Deficiency

Because iron deficiency is the most common deficiency disease, it is important to understand its assessment. For practical reasons, clinicians define iron status in terms of hemoglobin concentration. (Hemoglobin is the iron-containing pigment of the red blood cells. Its function is to carry oxygen.) An assumption is made that if insufficient iron limits hemoglobin production, then iron must be insufficient for other iron-requiring molecules as well. In addition, hemoglobin is relatively easy to measure. Unfortunately, limited hemoglobin production is the final stage of iron deficiency development (see Table A–19). Thus, a clear picture of iron status, especially early deficiency, requires several

Nitrogen (N) balance:
 N intake = N output.
Positive N balance:
 N intake > N output.
Negative N balance:
 N intake < N output.

Table A–18   Laboratory Tests Useful for Assessing Some Vitamin and Mineral Deficiencies

Vitamins	Tests
Vitamin A	Serum vitamin A, serum carotene, retinol binding protein
Thiamin	Erythrocyte transketolase, urinary thiamin
Riboflavin	Erythrocyte glutathione reductase, urinary riboflavin
Niacin	Urinary N-methylnicotinamide, urinary 2-pyridone
Vitamin B_6	Tryptophan load test, serum vitamin B_6, urinary vitamin B_6, blood transaminase
Folacin	Erythrocyte folate, vitamin B_{12} status, serum free folate, urinary formiminoglutamic acid
Vitamin B_{12}	Deoxyuridine suppression test, serum vitamin B_{12}, erythrocyte vitamin B_{12}, methymalonic acid excretion
Vitamin C	Leukocyte vitamin C, serum vitamin C
Vitmain D	Serum alkaline phosphatase
Vitamin E	Erythrocyte hemolysis test, plasma or serum tocopherol
Vitamin K	Prothrombin time

Minerals	Tests
Calcium	Serum calcium; bone tests under development
Potassium	Serum potassium
Magnesium	Serum magnesium, urinary magnesium
Iron	Hemoglobin, hematocrit, total iron-binding capacity (TIBC) % transferrin saturation, erythrocyte protoporphyrin, leukocyte ferritin, serum iron, mean corpuscular volume (MCV)
Iodine	Serum protein-bound iodine, radioiodine uptake
Zinc	Serum or plasma zinc, hair zinc

Table A–19   Stages of Iron Deficiency Development

Stage	Detected by	Reflects
Stores depleted	↓ Serum ferritin	Liver and bone marrow stores
Transport iron diminished	↓ Transferrin saturation	Iron binding capacity Serum iron
Hemoglobin production limited	↑ Erythrocyte protoporphyrin	Detectable anemia Microcytosis

Source: Adapted from P. R. Dallman, Diagnostic criteria for iron deficiency, in *Iron Nutrition Revisited—Infancy, Childhood, Adolescence,* Report of the 82nd Ross Laboratories Conference on Pediatric Research, (Columbus, Ohio.: Ross, 1981).

biochemical measures. Biochemical tests used to detect iron deficiency include hematocrit, mean corpuscular volume, hemoglobin, mean corpuscular hemoglobin concentration, erythrocyte protoporphyrin, serum iron, total iron-binding capacity, transferrin saturation, and serum ferritin. Recommended screening ages to detect iron deficiency in children are one, between two and three, five, and adolescence.[6]

It is important to remember that nonnutrient conditions influence both physical signs and biochemical measures. This appendix does not list all the conditions that can affect a particular lab test, but mentions the values associated with nutrient deficiencies and excesses. Of particular importance in assessing iron status during any stage of the life cycle is the changing chemistry of the blood. For this reason, assessment values for various age groups and for pregnancy differ.

Hematocrit Hematocrit is commonly used to diagnose iron deficiency, even though it is an inconclusive measure of iron status. To measure the hematocrit, a clinician spins a volume of blood in a centrifuge to separate the red blood cells from the plasma. The packed red cell volume is the hematocrit and represents a percentage of the total blood volume. Table A–20 provides values used to assess hematocrit status. Low values indicate incomplete hemoglobin formation, which is evident in microcytic, hypochromic red blood cells.

Microcytic = abnormally small cell.
Normocytic = normal-sized cell.
Macrocytic = abnormally large cell.
Hypochromic = under color.

Mean corpuscular volume A direct or calculated measure of the mean copuscular volume (MCV) determines the average size of a red blood cell (RBC). Such a measure helps to classify the type of nutrient anemia. The equation to calculate mean corpuscular volume is:

$$MCV = \frac{hematocrit}{RBC\ count} \times 10.$$

High MCV values indicate macrocytosis, which accompanies folacin and vitamin B_{12} deficiencies. Low MCV values indicate microcytosis and reflect poor iron status. (Other, nonnutrient factors can also affect MCV.)

Table A–20 Hematocrit Values[a]

Age	Sex	Deficient	Acceptable
< 2 yr	(M-F)	< 0.28	0.31 or >
2–5 yr	(M-F)	< 0.30	0.34 or >
6–12 yr	(M-F)	< 0.30	0.36 or >
13–16 yr	(M)	< 0.37	0.40 or >
	(F)	< 0.31	0.36 or >
> 16 yr	(M)	< 0.37	0.44 or >
	(F)	< 0.31	0.38 or >
trimester 2		< 0.30	0.35 or >
trimester 3		< 0.30	0.33 or >

[a]To convert hematocrit values (%) to standard units, multiply by 0.01.

Hemoglobin   Hemoglobin is a more direct measure of iron deficiency than hematocrit. Its shortcoming is that is falls with other nutrient anemias as well. Table A–21 provides hemoglobin values used in nutrition assessment.

Mean corpuscular hemoglobin concentration   Mean corpuscular hemoglobin concentration (MCHC) reflects the average amount of hemoglobin in a red blood cell. Like mean corpuscular volume, its measurement is either direct or calculated. To calculate mean corpuscular hemoglobin concentration:

$$MCHC = \frac{hemoglobin \times 100}{hematocrit}.$$

Low values indicate hypochromia, which accompanies iron deficiency.

Erythrocyte protoporphyrin   The iron-containing portion of the hemoglobin molecule is heme, which is a combination of iron and protoporphyrin. Protoporphyrin accumulates in the blood when iron supplies are inadequate for the formation of heme. Lab technicians can measure erythrocyte protoporphyrin directly; high values indicate iron deficiency.

Serum iron   Lab technicians can also measure serum iron directly. Elevated values indicate iron overload; reduced values indicate iron deficiency.

Total iron-binding capacity   Iron travels through the blood bound to the protein transferrin. Total iron-binding capacity is a measure of the total amount of iron that transferrin can carry. Lab technicians measure iron-binding capacity directly. Elevated values are seen in iron deficiency and pregnancy; reduced values are indicative of iron overload and malnutrition.

Transferrin saturation   The percentage of transferrin saturation is an indirect measure; the mathematical equation uses serum iron and total iron-binding capacity measures as follows:

Table A–21   Hemoglobin Values (gm/100ml)

Age	Sex	Deficient	Acceptable
< 2 yr	(M-F)	< 9.0	10.0 or >
2–5 yr	(M-F)	< 10.0	11.0 or >
6–12 yr	(M-F)	< 10.0	11.5 or >
13–16 yr	(M)	< 12.0	13.0 or >
	(F)	< 10.0	11.5 or >
> 16 yr	(M)	< 12.0	14.0 or >
	(F)	< 10.0	12.0 or >
trimester 2		< 9.5	11.0 or >
trimester 3		< 9.0	10.5 or >

$$\text{Percent transferrin} = \frac{\text{serum iron} \times 100}{\text{total iron-binding capacity}}.$$

Low values accompany iron deficiency anemia.

Serum ferritin   Serum ferritin measures provide a noninvasive estimate of iron stores. Such information is most valuable to iron assessment. The procedure is rarely used, however, because it requires special equipment and a skilled technician.

Nutrition Assessment During Pregnancy

Perhaps at no other time in life is the motivation to take care of oneself so great as it is during the unique time of pregnancy. The health and well-being of two individuals are inseparable at this time. Many women willingly abstain from smoking and drinking, and pay more attention to their eating habits than ever before. The wise health professional will offer guidance to support this motivation and enhance the chances of an optimal pregnancy and birth.

Maternal nutrition assessment may begin by observing the physical appearance of the woman, but it certainly does not end there. If a woman is not eating well, questions about the extent of her nutrition knowledge, family income, and availability of food will help determine why. A medical, social, drug, and diet history can provide such information. Of special concern in assessing maternal nutrition status are:[7]

▸ *Age*. Adolescents (17 years of age and under) and women over 30 are at higher risk for complications of pregnancy.

▸ *Age at onset of menstruation*. The average age of menarche today is 13 years. Delayed menarche has been associated with poor childhood nutrition, which in turn predicts a possible problem pregnancy.

▸ *Prepregnancy weight*. Normal weight for height presents the best prognosis. Women who are 10 percent below or 20 percent above the standard weight for height and age present a greater risk for a poor pregnancy outcome.

▸ *Pattern and amount of weight gained in prior pregnancies*. This will help determine potentially high-risk individuals.

▸ *Length of time between pregnancies*. Intervals of less than one year deplete nutrient stores.

▸ *Birthweights of previous infants*. Low birthweights and high birthweights indicate nutrition problems.

▸ *Smoking, drug, or alcohol use*. Ideally, there will have been none before or during pregnancy. In any case, the less, the better.

▸ *Alternative dietary practices and food patterns*. These include adherence to diets that severely restrict kcalories or exclude one or more food groups and the use of vitamin-mineral supplements in amounts above the RDA, unless prescribed by a health care provider for a specific reason.

symphysis-fundus measure: the distance from the junction of the pubic bones on midline in front to the uppermost part of the uterus.

preeclampsia: an abnormal condition of pregnancy characterized by edema, increasing hypertension, and protein in the urine.

Two of the most important anthropometric measures predictive of the birthweight of a child are the mother's prepregnancy weight and the amount and pattern of her weight gain or loss during previous pregnancies. Normal weight gains related to duration of the pregnancy in weeks are shown in Figure A–17. Patterns of weight gain that deviate from these require further investigation. Figure A–18 presents a new chart to monitor maternal weight gain based on the adequacy of prepregnant weight for height.

During pregnancy, growth is measured by a variety of indirect methods. Most commonly, uterine growth is judged by maternal weight gain and the symphysis-fundus measure. Placental weight can be estimated by measuring the human placental lactogen hormone, which generally correlates with fetal weight. The best estimator of fetal size during pregnancy is ultrasound measurement.

The "physiological anemia of pregnancy" results from the great increase in the mother's blood volume. The volume occupied by red blood cells does not increase as much as that occupied by the plasma, so the number of cells per milliliter is lower than in the nonpregnant state. Serum protein concentration decreases, while values for iron, folacin, and vitamin D are variable, depending on supplementation. Values for vitamin A, vitamin E, and serum copper rise.[8]

During pregnancy, serum zinc concentrations decline. As with iron, however, the decline represents a physiological adaptation to pregnancy due in part to maternal-fetal transfer of zinc and maternal plasma volume expansion.[9] Gestational stage must be considered when evaluating maternal zinc status since values change as pregnancy progresses.

No single biochemical test accurately reflects an individual's zinc status. A minimal assessment of zinc status should therefore include an estimate of dietary zinc and a measure of serum zinc.[10] A 24-hour urinary zinc excretion measure would provide additional useful information.

The edema of pregnancy is also "physiological" (that is, expected and normal)—provided it is not accompanied by indicators of preeclampsia such as high blood pressure or protein in the urine. This normal edema results from high estrogen, which promotes water retention, and low serum albumin, which lowers osmotic pressure.

The altered carbohydrate metabolism resembles that of diabetes, but is normal for pregnancy. Glucose is the primary fuel for the developing fetus. As a result of the large fetal energy demand, glucose transfers rapidly from mother to fetus, causing a fall in maternal fasting blood glucose levels. At the same time, maternal tissues place a greater reliance on fat to meet energy needs. Hormonal responses during pregnancy also alter maternal carbohydrate metabolism. Due to a rise in glucocorticoids, estrogen, progesterone, and human placental lactogen, maternal tissues become insulin-resistant. Consequently, with food intake, pregnant women have larger outputs of insulin than do nonpregnant women.[11]

Unfortunately, pregnancy norms have not been established for all biochemical tests. Chapter 2 discusses the treatment of truly abnormal conditions.

In recent years, new techniques and methodologies have greatly enhanced early detection and treatment of disease and nutrition disorders. Women with chronic conditions, such as diabetes or heart disease, today can deliver normal, healthy infants, while only a few years ago pregnancy was not even an option for many of them.

Figure A–17 Prenatal Weight Gain Grid
The standard prenatal weight gain grid plots the ideal rate of weight gain during pregnancy for most women.

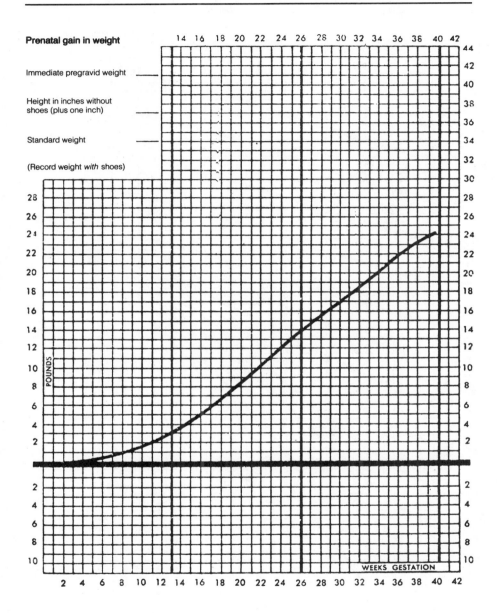

How extensively should maternal assessment be pursued? The amount appropriate for an individual varies, depending on factors such as prior pregnancies, age, and weight. Table A–22 offers a hierarchy of priorities. All pregnancies require a minimal nutrition assessment. If such an evaluation reveals inadequacies, then additional tests should be conducted.

Figure A–18   New Prenatal Weight Gain Grid
Chart to monitor weight gain during pregnancy considering prepregnancy weight and height.

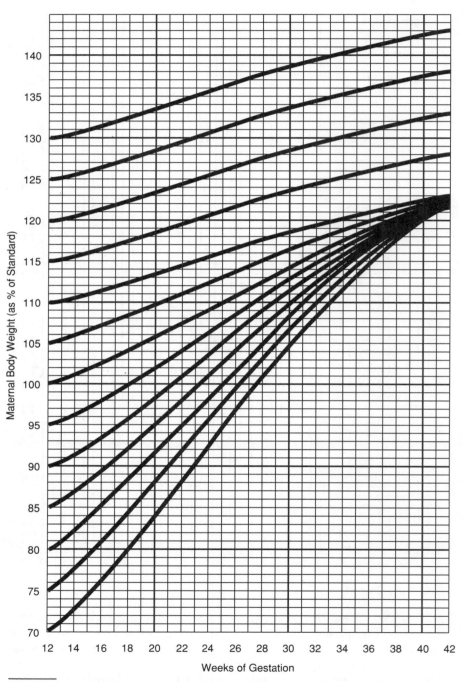

Source: Adapted from P. Rosso, A new chart to monitor weight gain during pregnancy, *American Journal of Clinical Nutrition* 41 (1985): 644–652.

Table A–22   Levels of Maternal Nutrition Assessment

Level of Approach	Dietary	History: Medical and Socioeconomic	Clinical Evaluation	Laboratory Evaluation
Minimal	Present basic diet: meal patterns; fad or abnormal diets; supplements	Obstetrical: Age: parity; interval between pregnancies; previous obstetrical history Medical: Intercurrent diseases and illnesses; drug use; smoking history Family and social: Size of family; "wanted" pregnancy; socioeconomic status	Prepregnancy weight; weight gain pattern during pregnancy; signs and symptoms of gross nutritional deficiencies	Hemoglobin; hematocrit
Mid-level	The above, plus semi-quantitative determination of food intake	The above, plus occupational patterns; utilization of maternity care and family planning services	The above, plus screening for intercurrent disease	The above, plus blood smear; RBC indices; serum iron; sickle preparation
In-depth level	The above, plus household survey data; dietary history; quantitative 24-hour recall		The above, plus special anthropometric measurements of skinfold, arm circumference, etc.	The above, plus folate and other vitamin levels

Source: American Public Health Association, Inc., *Nutritional Assessment in Health Programs*, ed. G. Christakis, (Washington, D.C.: American Public Health, Assoc. Inc., 1974) p. 62.

Cautions About Nutrition Assessment

To give all the details of nutrition assessment procedures would entail writing another textbook. Whole graduate courses are taught in the subject, requiring hundreds of pages of reading. However, any student of nutrition should know the basics of a proper nutrition assessment procedure, for two reasons.

First, competent medical care includes attention to nutrition. Physicians should either employ a person skilled in nutrition assessment techniques or refer all patients to such a person to ensure the sound nutrition health of their clients. Health care facilities should make nutrition assessment a routine part of the initial workup on every client so that nutrition handicaps will not hinder the response to medical treatment and the recovery from illness.

Second, because nutrition is such a popular subject today, fraudulent practices are even more abundant than they have been in the past (and they have always been rampant). The knowledgeable consumer needs to know what procedures to expect in a nutrition assessment and what kinds of information they yield. This appendix has presented the basics of nutrition assessment for these reasons.

This caution is added: the tests outlined here yield information that becomes meaningful only when integrated into a whole picture by a skilled, experienced, and educated interpreter. Sources of error are many, from the taking of the initial data to their reporting and analysis. Each assessment method and measure stands only as a part of the whole, to confirm or eliminate the possibility of suspected nutrition problems. For example, the assessor must constantly remember that a sufficient intake of a nutrient does not guarantee adequate nutrient status for an individual. Conversely, the apparent inadequate intake of a nutrient does not, by itself, establish that a deficiency exists.

Similarly, many uncertainties, such as the calibration of the equipment, the skills of the measurer, and the perspective of the interpreter, limit the accuracy and value of anthropometric measures. This is also true of the results of the physical examination. Physical signs suggestive of malnutrition are nonspecific: they can reflect nutrient deficiencies or may be totally unrelated to nutrition. Assessors must interpret physical findings in light of other assessment findings. Finally, the usefulness of biochemical tests is also limited; the assessor must use caution in interpreting results. Vitamin and mineral blood concentrations may reflect disease processes, abnormal hormone levels, or other aberrations rather than dietary intake. Even if concentrations do reflect dietary intake, they may reflect what the person has been eating recently and not give a true picture of the person's nutrient status. Such complications sometimes make it difficult to detect a subclinical deficiency. Furthermore, many nutrients interact. The assessor has to keep in mind that an abnormal lab value for one nutrient may reflect abnormal status of other nutrients. The final diagnosis is therefore appropriately tentative, and its confirmation comes only after careful remedial steps to successfully alleviate the observed problems.

The responsible use of nutrition assessment procedures is far from the kind of experience people may encounter when they walk into a "nutrition clinic" and receive a "nutrition assessment" by a "nutritionist." People today are easily led to believe that computers or hair analysis will accurately determine their nutrition status. They do not understand all the processes involved in doing such tests, but they see that the "experts" seem to know a lot and that the systems in operation are very complicated, and so they think there must be some validity to the "results."

A single example of a fraudulent nutrition assessment technique is hair analysis—except in strictly limited applications. Hair analyses are still in the experimental stage. Researchers are studying hair analyses to determine what their validity and usefulness may be. One way in which nutrition researchers can use hairs for nutrition assessment is to pull them out and measure the size or protein content of the roots. This provides a clue to protein nutrition status because hair roots diminish in size and protein content early in a developing protein deficiency. However, the minerals in the shaft of the hair do not accurately reflect the body's total content of minerals—except for some toxic metal contaminants and possibly zinc—and then only for populations, not individuals. Hair analysis is a valuable method in research and shows promise as an assessment tool if researchers can solve the problems. At present, however, it is not suitable for use in individual nutrition assessments. In several instances, hair contents of minerals do *not* reflect body content in any consistent way.[12] Too many confounding variables interfere: air and water pollution, shampoos and dyes, water hardness, and many others.

Hair analysis is only one example of the many ways unscrupulous practitioners elicit belief and extract money from unsuspecting, uninformed people. The guiding rule for the cautious consumer is to be skeptical. If the consumer does not understand, or has not heard of, the method a "nutritionist" is using to test nutrition status, it may not reflect limited knowledge. The test may simply be a fraud.

Appendix A Notes

1. E. R. Monsen and coauthors, Estimation of available dietary iron, *American Journal of Clinical Nutrition* 31 (1978): 134–141.
2. J. T. Dwyer, E. A. Krall, 2nd K. A. Coleman, The problem of memory in nutritional epidemiology research, *Journal of the American Dietetic Association* 87 (1987): 1509–1512.
3. M. B. Stoch and P. M. Smythe, 15-year developmental study on effects of severe undernutrition during infancy on subsequent physical growth and intellectual functioning, *Archives of Disease in Childhood* 51 (1976): 327–336.
4. W. H. Dietz, Jr., Childhood obesity: Susceptibility, cause, and management, *Journal of Pediatrics* 103 (1983): 676–686.
5. H. E. Sauberlich, R. P. Dowdy, and J. H. Skala, *Laboratory Tests for the Assessment of Nutritional Status*, (Boca Raton, Fla.: CRC Press, Inc., 1974), pp. 95–96.
6. P. R. Dallman, M. A. Siimes, and A. Stekel, Iron deficiency in infancy and childhood, *American Journal of Clinical Nutrition* 33 (1980): 86–118.
7. G. Christakis, *Nutritional Assessment in Health Programs* (Washington, D.C.: American Public Health Association, 1977), pp. 58–59.
8. J. C. King, Dietary risk patterns during pregnancy, *Nutrition Update* 1 (1983): 205–226.
9. C. A. Swanson and J. C. King, Zinc and pregnancy outcome, *American Journal of Clinical Nutrition* 46 (1987): 763–771.
10. Swanson and King, 1987.
11. King, 1983.
12. R. S. Gibson, B. M. Anderson, and C. A. Scythes, Regional differences in hair zinc concentrations: A possible effect of water hardness, *American Journal of Clinical Nutrition* 37 (1983): 37–42; K. M. Hambidge, Hair analyses: Worthless for vitamins, limited for minerals, *American Journal of Clinical Nutrition* 36 (1982): 943–949.

Appendix B

Recommended Nutrient Intakes (RDA, RNI, RDI)

Many countries have developed nutrient standards. Those of the United States (the Recommended Dietary Allowances, or RDA) and Canada (the Recommended Nutrient Intakes, or RNI) are examples. The main RDA table is presented on the inside front cover of this book. The energy RDA are presented here in Table B–1. The remaining RDA appear in Table B–2 and are expressed as ranges of recommended intakes because there is less information on which to base allowances.

Table B–3 presents the U.S. RDA for adults and children over four years of age. The Food and Drug Administration derived the U.S. RDA from the RDA for use on food labels. The U.S. RDA are about equal to the highest numbers for each nutrient in the RDA table. For most nutrients, the U.S. RDA are the same as the RDA for an adult man. For iron, however, the woman's RDA is higher so the woman's RDA is used.

The Canadian recommendations are in Tables B–4 and B–5. The Canadian recommendations differ from the RDA in some respects, partly because of differences in interpretation of the data they were derived from and partly because conditions in Canada differ somewhat from those in the United States.

As you can see from the inside front cover, the latest edition of the RDA was published in 1980. In 1985 a new RDA committee re-examined the 1980 RDA in order to issue the 1985 RDA. The committee completed its work and incorporated many changes in its report, including creating more specific age categories, lowering the quantity of milk used as a standard for breastfeeding infants, lowering the quantity of fat reserve required during pregnancy, and using new height and weight standards. The committee was guided by an awareness that applications of the RDA were expanding, and by a need to keep recommendations at a level that could be met, with careful planning, from available foods.

The committee's report was withheld from publication due to scientific differences of opinion between the committee and its reviewers.[1] Such disagreement among scientists is not uncommon; scientists using different, equally sound assumptions and measures can arrive at divergent conclusions and recommendations.

Another reason for postponing publication of the 1985 edition involves changing the overall approach for assessing nutrient intake to satisfy "the known nutritional needs of practically all healthy persons." Past RDA com-

---

1. F. Press, Postponement of the 10th edition of the RDAs, *Journal of the American Dietetic Association* 85 (1985): 1644–1645.

Table B–1   Mean Heights and Weights and Recommended Energy Intakes (United States)

Age	Weight		Height		Energy Needs[a]	
(years)	(kg)	(lb)	(cm)	(in)	(kcal)	(MJ)[b]
Infants						
0.0-0.5	6	13	60	24	kg × 115 (95–145)	kg × 0.48
0.5–1.0	9	20	71	28	kg × 105 (80–135)	kg × 0.44
Children						
1–3	13	29	90	34	1,300 (900–1,800)	5.5
4–6	20	44	112	44	1,700 (1,300–2,300)	7.1
7–10	28	62	132	52	2,400 (1,650–3,300)	10.1
Males						
11–14	45	99	157	62	2,700 (2,000–3,700)	11.3
15–18	66	145	176	69	2,800 (2,100–3,900)	11.8
19–22	70	154	177	70	2,900 (2,500–3,300)	12.2
23–50	70	154	178	70	2,700 (2,300–3,100)	11.3
51–75	70	154	178	70	2,400 (2,000–2,800)	10.1
76+	70	154	178	70	2,050 (1,650–2,450)	8.6
Females						
11–14	46	101	157	62	2,200 (1,500–3,000)	9.2
15–18	55	120	163	64	2,100 (1,200–3,000)	8.8
19–22	55	120	163	64	2,100 (1,700–2,500)	8.8
23–50	55	120	163	64	2,000 (1,600–2,400)	8.4
51–75	55	120	163	64	1,800 (1,400–2,200)	7.6
76+	55	120	163	64	1,600 (1,200–2,000)	6.7
Pregnant					+300	
Lactating					+500	

[a]The energy allowances for the young adults are for men and women doing light work. The allowances for the two older age groups represent mean energy needs over these age spans, allowing for a 2 percent decrease in basal (resting) metabolic rate per decade and a reduction in activity of 200 kcal per day for men and women between 51 and 75 years, 500 kcal for men over 75 years, and 400 kcal for women over 75. The customary range of daily energy output, shown in parentheses, is based on a variation in energy needs of ± 400 kcal at any one age, emphasizing the wide range of energy intakes appropriate for any group of people. Energy allowances for children through age 18 are based on median energy intakes of children these ages followed in longitudinal growth studies. The values in parentheses are tenth and ninetieth percentiles of energy intake, to indicate the range of energy consumption among children of these ages.

[b]MJ stands for megajoules (1 MJ = 1,00 kJ).

mittees were given the responsibility of defining recommendations at minimal levels that would avoid deficiencies. With recent developments in the relationships between nutrition and health, especially as nutrition influences the aging process and chronic diseases, a more comprehensive approach is warranted.[2] A group of scientists, including members of this RDA committee, have developed what they are calling the recommended dietary intakes (RDI). You will see reference to the RDI in this text and in others; they are provided in Table B–6 through B–12.

2. Press, 1985.

Table B–2   Estimated Safe and Adequate Daily Dietary Intakes of Additional Selected Nutrients (United States)[a]

Age (years)	Vitamins			Electrolytes		
	Vitamin K (μg)	Biotin (μg)	Pantothenic acid (mg)	Sodium (mg)	Potassium (mg)	Chloride (mg)
0–0.5	12	35	2	115–350	350–925	275–700
0.5–1	10–20	50	3	250–750	425–1,275	400–1,200
1–3	15–30	65	3	325–975	550–1,650	500–1,500
4–6	20–40	85	3–4	450–1,350	775–2,325	700–2,100
7–10	30–60	120	4–5	600–1,800	1,000–3,000	925–2,775
11+	50–100	100–200	4–7	900–2,700	1,525–4,575	1,400–4,200
Adults	70–140	100–200	4–7	1,100–3,300	1,875–5,625	1,700–5,100

Age (years)	Trace Elements[b]					
	Chromium (mg)	Selenium (mg)	Molybdenum (mg)	Copper (mg)	Manganese (mg)	Fluoride (mg)
0–0.5	0.01–0.04	0.01–0.04	0.03–0.06	0.5–0.7	0.5–0.7	0.1–0.5
0.5–1	0.02–0.06	0.02–0.06	0.04–0.08	0.7–1.0	0.7–1.0	0.2–1.0
1–3	0.02–0.08	0.02–0.08	0.05–0.1	1.0–1.5	1.0–1.5	0.5–1.5
4–6	0.03–0.12	0.03–0.12	0.06–0.15	1.5–2.0	1.5–2.0	1.0–2.5
7–10	0.05–0.2	0.05–0.2	0.1–0.3	2.0–2.5	2.0–3.0	1.5–2.5
11+	0.05–0.2	0.05–0.2	0.15–0.5	2.0–3.0	2.5–5.0	1.5–2.5
Adults	0.05–0.2	0.05–0.2	0.15–0.5	2.0–3.0	2.5–5.0	1.5–4.0

[a]Because there is less information on which to base allowances, these figures are not given in the main table of the RDA and are provided here in the form of ranges of recommended intakes.
[b]Since the toxic levels for many trace elements may be only several times usual intakes, the upper levels for the trace elements given in this table should not habitually be exceeded.

Table B–3   The U.S. RDA

Nutrient	The U.S. RDA
Nutrients that *must* appear on the label[a]	
protein (g), PER ≥ casein[b]	45
protein (g), PER < casein	65
vitamin A (RE)	1,000
vitamin C (ascorbic acid) (mg)	60
thiamin (vitamin B$_1$) (mg)	1.5
riboflavin (vitamin B$_2$) (mg)	1.7
niacin (mg)	20
calcium (g)	1.0
iron (mg)	18
Nutrients that *may* appear on the label	
vitamin D (IU)	400
vitamin E (IU)	30
vitamin B$_6$ (mg)	2.0
folic acid (folacin) (mg)	0.4
vitamin B$_{12}$ (μg)	6
phosphorus (g)	1.0
iodine (μg)	150
magnesium (mg)	400
zinc (mg)	15
copper (mg)	2
biotin (mg)	0.3
pantothenic acid (mg)	10

[a]whenever nutrition labeling is required.
[b]PER is an index of protein quality

Source: Adapted from *Food Technology* 28 (7): 5, 1974.

Table B–4   Recommended Nutrient Intakes for Canadians, 1983 (formerly Canadian *Dietary Standard, 1975*)

| Age | Sex | Weight (kg) | Protein (g/day)[a] | Fat-Soluble Vitamins | | |
				Vitamin A (RE/day)[b]	Vitamin D (µg/day)[c]	Vitamin E (mg/day)[d]
Months						
0-2	Both	4.5	11[f]	400	10	3
3-5	Both	7.0	14[f]	400	10	3
6-8	Both	8.5	17[f]	400	10	3
9-11	Both	9.5	18	400	10	3
Years						
1	Both	11	19	400	10	3
2-3	Both	14	22	400	5	4
4-6	Both	18	26	500	5	5
7-9	M	25	30	700	2.5	7
	F	25	30	700	2.5	6
10-12	M	34	38	800	2.5	8
	F	36	40	800	2.5	7
13-15	M	50	50	900	2.5	9
	F	48	42	800	2.5	7
16-18	M	62	55	1,000	2.5	10
	F	53	43	800	2.5	7
19-24	M	71	58	1,000	2.5	10
	F	58	43	800	2.5	7
25-49	M	74	61	1,000	2.5	9
	F	59	44	800	2.5	6
50-74	M	73	60	1,000	2.5	7
	F	63	47	800	2.5	6
75 +	M	69	57	1,000	2.5	6
	F	64	47	800	2.5	5
Pregnancy (additional)						
1st Trimester			15	100	2.5	2
2nd Trimester			20	100	2.5	2
3rd Trimester			25	100	2.5	2
Lactation (additional)			20	400	2.5	3

Recommended intakes of certain nutrients are not listed in this table because of the nature of the variables upon which they are based. For nutrients not shown, the following amounts are recommended: thiamin, 0.4 mg/1,000 kcal (0.48/5,000 kJ); riboflavin, 0.5 mg/1,000 kcal (0.6 mg/5,000 kJ); niacin, 7.2 NE/1,000 kcal (8.6 NE/5,000 kJ); vitamin B_6, 15 µg, as pyridoxine, per gram of protein; phosphorus, same as calcium. Recommended intakes during periods of growth are taken as appropriate for individuals representative of the mid-point in each age group. All recommended intakes are designed to cover individual variations in essentially all of a healthy population subsisting upon a variety of common foods available in Canada.

[a]The primary units are expressed per kilogram of body weight. The figures shown here are examples.
[b]One retinol equivalent (RE) corresponds to the biological activity of 1 µg of retinol, 6 µg of B-carotene or 12 µg of other carotenes.
[c]Expressed as cholecalciferol or ergocalciferol.
[d]Expressed as d-α-tocopherol equivalents, relative to which B- and γ-tocopherol and α-tocotrienol have activities of 0.5, 0.1 and 0.3 respectively.

Source: *Recommended Nutrient Intakes for Canadians,* Health and Welfare Canada (Ottawa: Canadian Government Publishing Centre, 1984), Table X.1, pp. 179–180.

Table B-4 (continued)

Age	Water-Soluble Vitamins			Minerals				
	Vitamin C (mg/day)	Folacin (μg/day)[e]	Vitamin B_{12} (μg/day)	Calcium (mg/day)	Magnesium (mg/day)	Iron (mg/day)	Iodine (μg/day)	Zinc (mg/day)
Months								
0-2	20	50	0.3	350	30	0.4[g]	25	2[h]
3-5	20	50	0.3	350	40	5	35	3
6-8	20	50	0.3	400	50	7	40	3
9-11	20	55	0.3	400	50	7	45	3
Years								
1	20	65	0.3	500	55	6	55	4
2-3	20	80	0.4	500	70	6	65	4
4-6	25	90	0.5	600	90	6	85	5
7-9	35	125	0.8	700	110	7	110	6
	30	125	0.8	700	110	7	95	6
10-12	40	170	1.0	900	150	10	125	7
	40	180	1.0	1,000	160	10	110	7
13-15	50	150	1.5	1,100	210	12	160	9
	45	145	1.5	800	200	13	160	8
16-18	55	185	1.9	900	250	10	160	9
	45	160	1.9	700	215	14	160	8
19-24	60	210	2.0	800	240	8	160	9
	45	175	2.0	700	200	14	160	8
25-49	60	220	2.0	800	250	8	160	9
	45	175	2.0	700	200	14[i]	160	8
50-74	60	220	2.0	800	250	8	160	9
	45	190	2.0	800	210	7	160	8
75+	60	205	2.0	800	230	8	160	9
	45	190	2.0	800	220	7	160	8
Pregnancy (additional)								
1st Trimester	0	305	1.0	500	15	6	25	0
2nd Trimester	20	305	1.0	500	20	6	25	1
3rd Trimester	20	305	1.0	500	25	6	25	2
Lactation (additional)	30	120	0.5	500	80	0	50	6

[e]Expressed as total folate.
[f]Assumption that the protein is from breast milk or is of the same biological value as that of breast milk and that between 3 and 9 months adjustment for the quality of the protein is made.
[g]It is assumed that breast milk is the source of iron up to 2 months of age.
[h]Based on the assumption that breast milk is the source of zinc for the first 2 months.
[i]After the menopause the recommended intake is 7 mg/day.

Table B–5 Average Energy Requirements (Canada)

Age	Sex	Average Height (cm)	Average Weight (kg)	kcal/kg[b]	MJ/kg[b]	Requirements[a] kcal/day	MJ/day	kcal/cm	MJ/cm
Months									
0–2	Both	55	4.5	120–100	0.50–0.42	500	2.0	9	0.04
3–5	Both	63	7.0	100–95	0.42–0.40	700	2.8	11	0.05
6–8	Both	69	8.5	95–97	0.40–0.41	800	3.4	11.5	0.05
9–11	Both	73	9.5	97–99	0.41	950	3.8	12.5	0.05
Years									
1	Both	82	11	101	0.42	1100	4.8	13.5	0.06
2–3	Both	95	14	94	0.39	1300	5.6	13.5	0.06
4–6	Both	107	18	100	0.42	1800	7.6	17	0.07
7–9	M	126	25	88	0.37	2200	9.2	17.5	0.07
	F	125	25	76	0.32	1900	8.0	15	0.06
10–12	M	141	34	73	0.30	2500	10.4	17.5	0.07
	F	143	36	61	0.25	2200	9.2	15.5	0.06
13–15	M	159	50	57	0.24	2800	12.0	17.5	0.07
	F	157	48	46	0.19	2200	9.2	14	0.06
16–18	M	172	62	51	0.21	3200	13.2	18.5	0.08
	F	160	53	40	0.17	2100	8.8	13	0.05
19–24	M	175	71	42	0.18	3000	12.4		
	F	160	58	36	0.15	2100	8.8		
25–49	M	172	74	36	0.15	2700	11.2		
	F	160	59	32	0.13	1900	8.0		
50–74	M	170	73	31	0.13	2300	9.6		
	F	158	63	29	0.12	1800	7.6		
75 +	M	168	69	29	0.12	2000	8.4		
	F	155	64	23	0.10	1500	6.0		

[a]Requirements can be expected to vary within a range of ±30 percent; based on expected patterns of activity.
[b]First and last figures are averages at the beginning and at the end of the 3–month period.

Source: *Recommended Nutrient Intakes for Canadians*, 1984, Table II.1, pp. 22–23.

Table B–6   Comparison of the RDI and RDA for Adults

	62–kg woman		76–kg man	
	RDI	*RDA*	*RDI*	*RDA*
Vitamin A				
(retinol, μg*)	600	800	700	1000
Folate (mcg)	190	400	240	400
Vitamin B$_{12}$ (μg)	2	3	2	3
Vitamin C (mg)	30	60	40	60
Vitamin K (μg)	35	70–140	45	70–140
Iron (mg)	15	18	10	10

*1 μg retinol or 1 retinol equivalent (RE) = 3.33 IU

Source: Adapted from V. Herbert, Recommended dietary intakes (RDI) of folate in humans, *American Journal of Clinical Nutrition* 45 (1987): 661–670; V. Herbert, Recommended dietary intakes (RDI) of vitamin B$_{12}$ in humans, *American Journal of Clinical Nutrition* 45 (1987): 671–678; V. Herbert, Recommended dietary intakes (RDI) of iron in humans, *American Journal of Clinical Nutrition* 45 (1987): 679–686; J. A. Olson, Recommended dietary intakes (RDI) of vitamin K in humans, *American Journal of Clinical Nutrition* 45 (1987): 687–692; J. A. Olson and R. E. Hodges, Recommended dietary intakes (RDI) of vitamin C in humans, *American Journal of Clinical Nutrition* 45 (1987): 693–703; J. A. Olson, Recommended dietary intakes (RDI) of vitamin A in humans, *American Journal of Clinical Nutrition* 45 (1987): 704–716; Food and Nutrition Board, Committee on Dietary Allowance, *Recommended Dietary Allowances,* 9th ed. (Washington D.C.: National Academy of Sciences, 1980).

Table B–7   Vitamin A RDI and RDA Compared

Age/Condition	RDI (μg)	RDA (μg)
Infants, 0–24 mo.	375	400–420
Children, 2–6 yr.	400	400
Children, 6–9 yr.	500	500–700
Males, 10–11 yr.	600	700–1000
Males, 12–70+ yr.	700	1000
Females, 10–70+ yr.	600	700–800
Pregnancy, 6–9 mo.	+200	+200
Lactation, 0–5 mo.	+400	+400
Lactation, 6+ mo.	+320	+400

Source: Adapted from J. Olson, Recommended dietary intakes (RDI) of vitamin A, *American Journal of Clinical Nutrition* 45 (1987): 704–716; Food and Nutrition Board, Committee on Dietary Allowance, *Recommended Dietary Allowances,* 9th ed. (Washington D.C.: National Academy of Sciences, 1980).

Table B–8   Folacin RDI and RDA Compared

Age/Condition	RDI	RDA
Infants, 0–6mo.	3.6 μg/kg	30 μg/day
Infants, 6 mo.–1 yr.	3.6 μg/kg	45 μg/day
Children, 1–3 yr.	3.3 μg/kg	100 μg/day
Children, 4–6 yr.	3.3 μg/kg	200 μg/day
Children, 7–10 yr.	3.3 μg/kg	300 μg/day
Males, 11–51+ yr.	3.0 μg/kg	400 μg/day
Females, 11–51+ yr.	3.0 μg/kg	400 μg/day
Pregnancy	500 μg/kg	800 μg/day
Lactation	3 μg/kg +100 μg/day	500 μg/day

Source: Adapted from V. Herbert, Recommended dietary intakes (RDI) of folate in humans, *American Journal of Clinical Nutrition* 45 (1987): 661–670; Food and Nutrition Board, Committee on Dietary Allowance, *Recommended Dietary Allowances,* 9th ed. (Washington D.C.: National Academy of Sciences, 1980).

Table B–9   Vitamin B_{12} and RDI and RDA Compared

Age/Condition	RDI	RDA
Infants, 0–6 mo.	0.06 μg/kg	0.5 μg/day
Infants, 6 mo.–1 yr.	0.06 μg/kg	1.5 μg/day
Children, 1–3 yr.	0.06 μg/kg	2.0 μg/day
Children, 4–6 yr.	0.06 μg/kg	2.5 μg/day
Children, 7–10 yr.	0.06 μg/kg	3.0 μg/day
Males, 11–51+ yr.	2 μg/kg	3.0 μg/day
Females, 11–51+ yr.	2 μg/kg	3.0 μg/day
Pregnancy, 0–2.9 mo.	2 μg/kg	4.0 μg/day
Pregnancy, 3–9 mo.	2.5 μg/kg	4.0 μg/day
Lactation	2.5 μg/kg	4.0 μg/day

Source: Adapted from V. Herbert, Recommended dietary intakes of vitamin B_{12}, *American Journal of Clinical Nutrition* 45 (1987): 671–678; Food and Nutrition Board, Committee on Dietary Allowance, *Recommended Dietary Allowances,* 9th ed. (Washington D.C.: National Academy of Sciences, 1980).

Table B–10   Vitamin C RDI and RDA Compared

Age/Condition	RDI	RDA
Infants, 1–12 mo.	25 mg	35 mg
Children, 1–9 yr.	25 mg	45 mg
Males, 10–11 yr.	30 mg	45–50 mg
Males, 12–17 yr.	40 mg	50–60 mg
Females, 10–17 yr.	30 mg	45–60 mg
Males, 18–70+ yr.	40 mg	60 mg
Females, 18–70+ yr.	30 mg	60 mg
Pregnancy, 3–6 mo.	+ 5 mg	+20 mg
Pregnancy, 6–9 mo.	+10 mg	+20 mg
Lactation, 0–6 mo.	+25 mg	+40 mg
Lactation, 6+ mo.	+20 mg	+40 mg

Source: Adapted from J. A. Olson and R. E. Hodges, Recommended dietary intakes (RDI) of Vitamin C in humans, *American Journal of Clinical Nutrition* 45 (1987): 693–703; Food and Nutrition Board, Committee on Dietary Allowance, *Recommended Dietary Allowances,* 9th ed. (Washington D.C.: National Academy of Sciences, 1980).

Table B–11   Vitamin K RDI and RDA Compared

Age/Condition	RDI	RDA
Infants, 0–12 mo.	10 μg	10–20 μg
Children, 1–3 yr.	15 μg	15–30 μg
Children, 4–6 yr.	20 μg	20–40 μg
Children, 7–10 yr.	25 μg	30–60 μg
Adolescents, 11–14 yr.	30 μg	50–100 μg
Adolescents, 15–18 yr.	35 μg	50–100 μg
Males, 19–70+ yr.	45 μg	70–140 μg
Females, 19–70+ yr.	35 μg	70–140 μg
Pregnancy	+10 μg	—
Lactation	+20 μg	—

Source: Adapted from J. A. Olson, Recommended dietary intakes (RDI) of vitamin K in humans, *American Journal of Clinical Nutrition* 45 (1987): 687–692; Food and Nutrition Board, Committee on Dietary Allowance, *Recommended Dietary Allowances,* 9th ed. (Washington D.C.: National Academy of Sciences, 1980).

Table B–12   Iron RDI and RDA Compared

Age/Condition	RDI (mg)	RDA (mg)
Infants, 0–3 mo.	—	10
Infants, 3–6 mo.	6.6	10
Infants, 6–12 mo.	8.8	15
Children, 1–9 yr.	10.0	10–15
Males, 10–17 yr.	12.0	10–18
Males, 18–70+ yr.	10.0	10
Females, 10–50 yr.	15.0	18
Females, 51–70+ yr.	10.0	10
Pregnancy	45.0	30–60
Lactation	15.0	30–60

Source: Adapted from: V. Herbert, Recommended dietary intakes (RDI) of iron in humans, *American Journal of Clinical Nutrition* 45 (1987): 679–686; Food and Nutrition Board, Committee on Dietary Allowance, *Recommended Dietary Allowances,* 9th ed. (Washington D.C.: National Academy of Sciences, 1980).

Appendix C

Food Group Plans

Nutrient recommendations such as those presented in Appendix B are one of the tools used in planning diets, but other tools are needed to translate nutrients into food. Food group plans tell people what kinds of foods to eat and how much to eat. They help to make the diet adequate and balanced. The most familiar food group plan fits all foods into four groups and a miscellaneous category as shown in Table C–1. Each food group contains foods that are similar in origin and that supply a characteristic array of nutrients. These foods are whole foods that form the foundation of a healthy diet: milk and milk products, fruits and vegetables, starches and grains, and meats and meat alternates. The plan suggests for adults a two, four, four, two pattern of servings from each group, although other patterns are possible and desirable for individuals.

The miscellaneous category contains foods that do not fit into the four food groups. Among them are butter, margarine, cream, salad dressing, ketchup, jam and jelly, coffee, tea, herbs, soft drinks, alcoholic beverages, and others. These items may contain a few nutrients, but they are so greatly diluted with fat, sugar, or water, or used in such small quantities, that they make little contribution to nutrition.

Other food group plans are available. Canada has one of its own—Canada's Food Guide, shown in Table C–2. Table C–3 shows a food group plan specifically for vegetarians. The modified food group plan shown in Table C–4 may be appropriate for those who spend many kcalories in vigorous physical activity.

Table C–1 The Four Food Group Plan

Food Group	Servings/ Day (Adult)	Sample Foods	Main Nutrients
Milk and milk products	2[a]	(A) Nonfat milk, buttermilk, lowfat milk, plain yogurt (B) whole milk, cheese, fruit-flavored yogurt, cottage cheese (C) custard, milkshake, pudding, ice cream	Protein, riboflavin, vitamin B_{12},[b] calcium, magnesium
Fruits and vegetables	4[c]	(A) Apricot, bean sprouts, broccoli, Brussels sprouts, cabbage, cantaloupe, carrots, cauliflower, cucumber, grapefruit, green beans, green peas, leafy greens (spinach, mustard, and collard greens), lettuce, mushrooms, orange, orange juice, peach, strawberries, tomato, winter squash (B) apple, banana, canned fruit, corn, pear, potato (C) avocado, dried fruit, sweet potato	Vitamins A and C,[d] folacin, fiber
Grains (whole-grain and enriched bread and cereal products)	4[c]	(A) Whole grain and enriched breads, rolls, tortillas (B) rice, cereals, pastas (macaroni, spaghetti), bagel (C) pancake, muffin, cornbread, biscuit, presweetened cereals	Thiamin,[f] niacin, iron, zinc, fiber
Meat and meat alternates	2	(A) Poultry, fish, lean meat (beef, lamb, pork), dried peas and beans, eggs (B) beef, lamb, pork, luncheon meats, refried beans (C) hot dogs, peanut butter, nuts	Protein, thiamin, riboflavin, niacin, vitamins B_6 and B_{12},[b] folacin, magnesium, zinc

Note: Foods labeled (A) are lowest in kcalories, (C) highest, (B) in between. A miscellaneous category includes foods that tend to be high in fat, salt, sugar, alcohol, and, in most cases, kcalories. Foods high in fat include margarine, salad dressing, oils, mayonnaise, cream, cream cheese, butter, gravy, and sauces. Foods high in salt include potato chips, corn chips, pretzels, pickles, olives, bouillon, prepared mustard, soy sauce, steak sauce, salt, and seasoned salt. Foods high in sugar include cake, pie, cookies, doughnuts, sweet rolls, candy, soft drinks, fruit drinks, jelly, syrup, gelatin desserts, sugar, and honey. Alcoholic beverages include wine, beer, and liquor. Other miscellaneous foods, not high in kcalories, include spices, herbs, coffee, tea, and diet soft drinks.

[a] For children up to 9, 2 to 3 c; for children 9–12, 3 to 4 c; for teenagers and pregnant women, 3 to 4 c; for nursing mothers, 4 c or more; for women past 50, 3 to 5 c.

[b] Vitamin B_{12} is contributed only by foods that come from animals.

[c] One should be rich in vitamin C; at least one every other day should be rich in vitamin A.

[d] Dark green and deep orange vegetables are especially reliable vitamin A sources; other fruits and vegetables are not. For vitamin C, citrus fruits, green leafy vegetables, and selected other fruits and vegetables are superior sources.

[e] Enriched or, preferably, whole-grain products only. Whole grains include wheat, oats, rice, barley, millet, rye, and bulgur.

[f] If the recommended four or more servings are eaten, these foods contribute significant nutrients to the diet. They also contribute most of the complex carbohydrate of the diet. Whole-grain products are preferred over refined enriched products.

Sources: Adapted from *Building a Better Diet,* Food and Nutrition Service, USDA Program Aid No. 1241, 1979; and Food Group Chart, © Dairy Council of California (0020N, 1983, distributed by National Dairy Council).

Table C–2 Canada's Food Guide

Food Group	Servings/Day (Adult)
Milk and milk products	2[a]
Meat, fish, poultry, and alternates	2
Fruits and vegetables	4–5[b]
Breads and cereals	3–5

[a]A serving is 250 ml, or about 1 c. Milk group servings differ; for children up to age 11, 2 to 3 servings; adolescents, 3 to 4 servings; pregnant and nursing women, 3 to 4 servings.
[b]Include at least two vegetables.

Source: *Canada's Food Guide Handbook,* revised (Health and Welfare Canada, 1985).

Table C–3 Four Food Group Plan for the Vegetarian

Food Group	Servings/Day (Adult)
Milk and milk products	2[a]
Protein-rich foods	2[b]
Legumes	2[c]
Fruits/vegetables	4[d]
Breads/cereals (whole-grain only)	4

[a]If not using milk or milk products, use soy milk fortified with calcium and vitamin B_{12}.
[b]Examples of protein-rich foods: cheeses and tofu.
[c]Legumes (2 c daily) should be eaten in addition to protein-rich foods, to help women meet iron requirements.
[d]Include 1 c dark greens daily to help women meet iron requirements.

Source: Adapted from *Vegetarian Food Choices* (Gainesville: Shands Teaching Hospital and Clinics, Food and Nutrition Service, University of Florida, 1976).

Table C–4 Modified Four Food Group Plan

Food Group	Servings/Day (Adult)
Milk and milk products	2
Meat, fish, or poultry	2[a]
Legumes	2[b]
Fruits/vegetables	4
Grains	4[c]

[a]Servings size is 3 ounces, not 2 to 3 ounces as in the Four Food Group Plan.
[b]Servings size is ¾ c.
[c]Whole-grain products only, not enriched.

Source: Designed to increase intakes of needed nutrients, especially iron, vitamin B_6, zinc, magnesium, and vitamin E, within about 2200 kcal/day, by J. C. King and coauthors, Evaluation and modification of the basic four food guide, *Journal of Nutrition Education* 10 (1978): 27–29.

Appendix D

Table of Infant Formula Composition

Table D–1 compares the nutrient composition of three milk-based infant formulas and three soy-based infant formulas. All infant formulas are designed to resemble breast milk and must meet an American Academy of Pediatrics standard for nutrient composition. Milk-based formulas are intended for full-term, healthy infants. Soy-based formulas are designed for infants with milk sensitivity or lactose intolerance. Special formulas are available for premature infants or infants with medical conditions requiring special nutrition treatment.

Table D–1 Comparison of Nutrients in Infant Formulas

Nutrient	Cow's Milk-Based Infant Formulas			Soy Protein Formulas		
	Enfamil[a]	Similac[b]	SMA[c]	Isomil[d]	Nursoy[e]	Prosobee[f]
Energy (kcal/100 ml)	68	68	68	68	68	68
Carbohydrate (g/100 ml)	6.9 (lactose)	7.2 (lactose)	7.2 (lactose)	6.8 (corn syrup solids, sucrose)	6.9 (sucrose)	6.8 (corn syrup solids)
Protein (g/100 ml)	1.5	1.5	1.5	1.8	2.1	2.0
Casein	40	82	40	—	—	—
Whey protein	60	18	60	—	—	—
Soy protein	—	—	—	100	100	100
Fat (g/100 ml)	3.8	3.6	3.6	3.7	3.6	3.6
Minerals (milligrams/liter)						
Calcium	460	510	420	710	600	630
Chloride	420	510	375	440	375	550
Iron	13	12	12	12	12	13
Phosphorus	320	390	280	510	420	500
Potassium	720	810	560	950	700	780
Sodium	180	220	150	320	200	290
Vitamins (per 100 ml)						
Vitamin A (IU)	200	250	200	250	200	200
Thiamin (μg)	50	65	67	40	67	50
Riboflavin (μg)	100	100	100	60	100	60
Niacin (mg)	0.8	0.7	0.5	0.9	0.5	0.8
Vitamin B_6 (μg)	40	40	42	40	42	40
Vitamin B_{12} (μg)	.15	.21	.13	.30	.20	.20
Folacin (μg)	10	10	5	10	5	10
Vitamin C (mg)	5.2	5.5	5.5	5.5	5.5	5.2
Vitamin D (IU)	40	40	40	40	40	40
Vitamin E (IU)	2.0	1.5	1.0	1.5	.95	2.0
Vitamin K (μg)	*	*	5.5	*	10	10
Pantothenic acid (mg)	.30	.30	.21	.50	.30	.30

* Not available
[a] Mead Johnson, *Pediatric Products Handbook* (Evansville, Ind.: Mead Johnson and Company, 1986), pp. 7–8.
[b] Ross Laboratories, *Milk-Based and Soy-Based Formulations* (Columbus, OH.: Ross Laboratories, 1979).
[c] Wyeth Laboratories, *Wyeth Hospital Infant Feeding System* (Philadelphia, PA.: Wyeth Laboratories, 1986), p. 20.
[d] Ross Laboratories, 1979.
[e] Wyeth Laboratories, 1986.
[f] Mead Johnson, 1986.

Appendix E

Vitamin/Mineral Supplements Compared

The following tables are useful for comparing the essential vitamin and mineral contents of prenatal, infant, and child supplements commonly available in the United States. Notice that a blank column has been provided for the addition of locally available products you may wish to compare with those shown here.*

Not all ingredients in vitamin/mineral preparations are of proven benefit. To facilitate meaningful comparison, the tables list only the nutrients known to be essential in human nutrition. Other nutrients and compounds found on the labels of these supplements are listed in the table notes.

When a supplement is needed that supplies certain nutrients, these tables will ease the task of selecting an appropriate one. Notice, for example, that the iron and calcium contents of the supplements listed here for children (Table E-2) vary considerably. Some contain no iron at all, while others provide more than 100 percent of a child's RDA. Many of the supplements contain no calcium either.

---

*These tables are reprinted with permission from L. K. DeBruyne and S. R. Rolfes, *Selection of Supplements,* a 1986 monograph in the *Nutrition Clinics* series available from Stickley Publishing Co., 210 Washington Sq., Philadelphia, PA 19106.

Table E–1   Supplements for Pregnant Women

Company	Bronson[a]	Lederle	Lederle	Lederle	Lederle
Product	Prenatal	Filibon F.A.	Filibon Forte	Filibon	Materna[b]
Vitamins					
Vitamin A (IU)	8000	8000	8000	5000	8000
Vitamin D (IU)	400	400	400	400	400
Vitamin E (IU)	50	30	45	30	30
Vitamin C (mg)	150	60	90	60	100
Thiamin (mg)	5	1.7	2	1.5	3
Riboflavin (mg)	5	2.0	2.5	1.7	3.4
Vitamin B_6 (mg)	15	4	3	2	10
Vitamin B_{12} (μg)	15	8	12	6	12
Niacin (mg)	30	20	30	20	20
Folacin (mg)	0.8	1	1	0.4	1
Minerals					
Calcium (mg)	250[ef]	250[e]	300[e]	125[e]	250[e]
Iron (mg)	60	45	45	18	60
Magnesium (mg)	75	100	100	100	25
Zinc (mg)	20[f]	0	0	0	25[h]
Copper (mg)	1[f]	0	0	0	2[h]
Iodine (μg)	150	150	200	150	150
Manganese (mg)	1	0	0	0	5

Cost per day*

*Divide the total retail price for the container by the number of doses per container. For example, XYZ Vitamins are sold in bottles of 100 tablets, and the recommended dose is 2 tablets per day; there are 50 doses in the bottle. At $5.00 per bottle, XYZ Vitamins cost $.10 per day.
[a]Bronson prenatals also contain 250 μg biotin and 20 mg pantothenic acid.
[b]Lederle Materna also contains 30 μg biotin, 10 mg pantothenic acid, 0.25 mg chromium, and 0.25 mg molybdenum.
[e]Carbonate salt.
[f]Sulfate salt.
[h]Oxide salt.

Table E–1 (continued)

Company	Mead-Johnson	Mead-Johnson	Mission	Mission	Mission	Mission
Product	*Natalins*	*Natalins Rx[c]*	*Prenatal[d]*	*Prenatal F.A.[d]*	*Prenatal H.P.[d]*	*Prenatal Rx[d]*
Vitamins						
Vitamin A (IU)	8000	8000	4000	4000	4000	8000
Vitamin D (IU)	400	400	400	400	400	400
Vitamin E (IU)	30	30	0	0	0	0
Vitamin C (mg)	90	90	100	100	100	240
Thiamin (mg)	1.7	2.6	5	5	5	4
Riboflavin (mg)	2	3	2	2	2	2
Vitamin B_6 (mg)	4	10	3	10	25	20
Vitamin B_{12} (μg)	8	8	2	2	2	8
Niacin (mg)	20	20	10	10	10	20
Folacin (mg)	0.8	1	0.4	0.8	0.8	1
Minerals						
Calcium (mg)	200[e]	200[e]	50[egi]	50[egi]	50[egi]	175[ej]
Iron (mg)	45	60	30	30	30	60
Magnesium (mg)	100	100	0	0	0	0
Zinc (mg)	0	15[h]	0	15[f]	0	15[f]
Copper (mg)	0	2[h]	0	0	0	2[h]
Iodine (μg)	150	150	0	0	0	300
Manganese (mg)	0	0	0	0	0	0

Cost per day*

[c]Mead-Johnson Natalins Rx also contains 50 μg biotin and 15 mg pantothenic acid.
[d]Mission prenatals (regular, F.A., and H.P.) also contain 1 mg pantothenic acid; Mission Prenatal Rx contains 10 mg pantothenic acid.
[e]Carbonate salt.
[f]Sulfate salt.
[g]Gluconate salt.
[h]Oxide salt.
[i]Lactate salt.
[j]Ascorbate salt.

Table E–1   (continued)

Company	Parke-Davis	Parke-Davis	Parke-Davis	Parke-Davis	Stuart	Stuart	Other
Product	Natabec F.A.	Natafort Filmseal	Natabec Kapseals	Natabec Rx	Prenatal	Stuartnatal	
Vitamins	Kapseals			Kapseals		1 + 1	
Vitamin A (IU)	4000	6000	4000	4000	4000	4000	
Vitamin D (IU)	400	400	400	400	400	400	
Vitamin E (IU)	0	30	0	0	12	12	
Vitamin C (mg)	50	120	50	50	100	120	
Thiamin (mg)	3	3	3	3	1.5	1.5	
Riboflavin (mg)	2	2	2	2	1.7	3	
Vitamin B_6 (mg)	3	15	3	3	2.6	10	
Vitamin B_{12} (μg)	5	6	5	5	4	12	
Niacin (mg)	10	20	10	10	18	20	
Folacin (mg)	0.1	1	0	1.0	0.8	1.0	
Minerals							
Calcium (mg)	600[e]	350[e]	600[e]	600[e]	200[f]	200[f]	
Iron (mg)	150	65	30	30	60	65	
Magnesium (mg)	0	100	0	0	0	0	
Zinc (mg)	0	25[h]	0	0	25[h]	25[h]	
Copper (mg)	0	0	0	0	0	2	
Iodine (μg)	0	150	0	0	0	0	
Manganese (mg)	0	0	0	0	0	0	

Cost per day*

[e]Carbonate salt.
[f]Sulfate salt.
[h]Oxide salt.

Source: Adapted from V. Newman, R. B. Lyon, and P. O. Anderson, Evaluation of prenatal vitamin-mineral supplements, *Clinical Pharmacy* 6 (1987): 770–777.

Table E–2   Supplements for Infants and Children

Company	Lederle[a]	Miles Laboratories	Mead-Johnson	Mead-Johnson	Radiance[b]	Chocks
Product	Centrum Jr.	Flinstones with Iron	Poly-Vi-Sol	Poly-Vi-Sol Iron and Zinc	Chewable for Children	Bugs Bunny plus Iron
Age of Intended Users	Children over 4	Children over 2	Infants	Children and Adults	Children 2 to 12	Children over 2
Recommended Daily Dose	1 Chewable	1 Chewable	1 ml Dropper	1 Chewable	1 Chewable	1 Chewable
Vitamins						
Vitamin A (IU)	5000	2500	1500	2500	4000	2500
Vitamin D (IU)	400	400	400	400	400	400
Vitamin E (IU)	15	15	5	15	3.4	15
Vitamin C (mg)	60	60	35	60	60	60
Thiamin (B_1) (mg)	1.5	1.05	0.5	1.05	2	1.05
Riboflavin (B_2) (mg)	1.7	1.2	0.6	1.2	2.4	1.2
Vitamin B_6 (mg)	2	1.05	0.4	1.05	2	1.05
Vitamin B_{12} (μg)	6	4.5	2	4.5	10	4.5
Niacin (mg)	20	13.5	8	13.5	10	13.5
Folacin (mg)	0.4	0.3	—	0.3	—	0.3
Minerals						
Calcium (mg)	—	—	—	—	19	—
Phosphorus (mg)	—	—	—	—	—	—
Iron (mg)	18	15	—	12	12	15
Potassium (mg)	1.6	—	—	—	4	—
Magnesium (mg)	25	—	—	—	22	—
Zinc (mg)	10	—	—	8	—	—
Copper (mg)	2	—	—	—	0.2	—
Iodine (μg)	—	—	—	—	—	—
Manganese (mg)	1	—	—	—	—	—
Cost per day*						

*Divide the total retail price for the container by the number of doses per container. For example, XYZ Vitamins are sold in bottles of 100 tablets, and the recommended dose is 2 tablets per day; there are 50 doses in the bottle. At $5.00 per bottle, XYZ Vitamins cost $.10 per day.
[a]Lederle chewables also contain 1.4 mg chlorine (recommended daily dose for children 2 to 4 is ½ tablet).
[b]Radiance chewables also contain 2 mg pantothenic acid, 10 mg biotin, 2 mg inositol, and 2 mg of a choline compound.

Table E–2   (continued)

	Neolife[c]	J. B. Williams[d]	Upjohn	Amway[e]	Shaklee[f]	Richardson Vicks[g]	Ross Labs	Miles Labs	Other
	Vita Squares	Popeye with Mins/ Iron	Unicap	Nutrilite	Vita–Lea Children	Life–Stage Children	Vi–Daylin with Iron	Flintstones Complete	
	Children over 2	Children	Children	Children	Children over 4	Children 4 to 12	Children under 4	Children over 4	
	3 Chewables	1 Chewable	1 Chewable	1 Chewable	2 Chewables	2 Chewables	1 Dropper	1 Chewable	
	3000	2500	5000	2500	2000	5000	1500	5000	
	400	400	400	400	400	400	400	400	
	9	15	15	10	10	30	5	30	
	60	60	60	40	60	60	35	60	
	1.5	1.05	1.5	0.7	1.1	1.5	0.5	1.5	
	1.5	1.2	1.7	0.8	1.2	1.7	0.6	1.7	
	1.2	1.05	2	0.7	1.5	2	0.4	2	
	3	4.5	6	3	3	6	1.5	6	
	10	13.5	20	9	14	20	8	20	
	0.2	0.3	0.4	0.2	0.3	0.4	—	0.4	
	—	—	—	—	130	—	—	100	
	—	—	—	—	100	—	—	100	
	3	15	—	5	10	9	10	18	
	—	—	—	—	—	—	—	—	
	—	40	—	—	60	—	—	20	
	—	12	—	—	1.5	—	—	15	
	0.002	1.5	—	—	0.2	—	—	—	
	75	105	—	—	15	—	—	150	
	1	—	—	—	—	—	—	2.5	

[c]Neolife chewables also contain 10 mg pantothenic acid, 0.075 mg inositol, 0.05 mg of a choline compound, 15 mg biotin, and 15 mg PABA.
[d]Williams chewables also contain 2.5 mg pantothenic acid and 37.5 mg biotin.
[e]Amway chewables also contain 5 mg pantothenic acid.
[f]Shaklee chewables also contain 4 mg pantothenic acid and 0.1 mg biotin.
[g]Richardson Vicks chewables also contain 10 mg pantothenic acid and 0.3 mg biotin.

Appendix F

Recommended Resources

Reliable nutrition information and support is not always easy to come by, especially if you do not know where to look. The agencies, groups, and organizations listed here can provide reliable information or offer support for those with problems related to specific topics.

General

To obtain a copy of the *Dietary Guidelines for Americans*, write to:

> Superintendent of Documents
> Government Printing Office
> Washington, DC 20402

To obtain a copy of *Exchange Lists for Meal Planning*, write to:

> The American Dietetic Association
> 430 North Michigan Avenue
> Chicago, IL 60611

The USDA's Food and Nutrition Service (FNS) administers the food stamp program; the national school lunch and school breakfast programs; the special supplemental food program for women, infants, and children (WIC); and the food distribution, child care food, summer food service, and special milk programs. Write to:

> FNS, USDA
> 500 12th Street SW
> Washington, DC 20250

The World Health Organization (WHO) is an independent agency of the United Nations concerned with the health of the world. The WHO and the Food and Agriculture Organization (FAO) of the United Nations have issued international dietary standards. The FAO has many publications about food safety and nutrition.

> World Health Organization
> 1211 Geneva 27
> Switzerland

Food and Agriculture Organization
North American Regional Office
1325 C Street SW
Washington, DC 20025

For information about Canada's food group system, write to:

The Canadian Dietetic Association
385 Yonge Street
Toronto, Ontario M4T 1Z5 Canada

Alcohol

The following organizations offer information, programs, and support for anyone concerned with alcoholism.

Alcoholics Anonymous World Services
P. O. Box 459
Grand Central Station
New York, NY 10017

Al-Anon Family Group Headquarters
P. O. Box 182 Madison Square Station
New York, NY 10010

National Council on Alcoholism
733 Third Avenue
New York, NY 10017

The National Clearinghouse for Alcohol Information maintains a state-by-state list of most private and public treatment facilities.

National Clearinghouse for Alcohol Information
Box 2345
Rockville, MD 20850

Anorexia Nervosa/Bulimia

The following organizations provide information and help people with anorexia nervosa or bulimia and their families to find qualified therapists and support groups:

American Anorexia/Bulimia Association, Inc.
133 Cedar Lane
Teaneck, NJ 07666

Anorexia Nervosa and Associated Disorders, Inc.
P. O. Box 7
Highland Park, IL 60035

Anorexia Nervosa and Related Eating Disorders, Inc.
P. O. Box 5102
Eugene, OR 97404

Bulimia/Anorexia Self-help
6125 Clayton Avenue Suite 215
St. Louis, MO 63139

National Anorexic Aid Society, Inc.
5796 Karl Road
Columbus, OH 43229

Breastfeeding

La Leche League was founded by a group of women who had successfully breastfed their infants and realized many mothers need someone to talk to about breastfeeding. There are more than 40,000 groups internationally.

La Leche League International, Inc.
9616 Minneapolis Avenue
Franklin Park, IL 60131

Bulimia (see Anorexia)

Children

The American Academy of Pediatrics establishes standards for infant formula composition and recommendations for feeding infants and children. Their address is:

The American Academy of Pediatrics
P. O. Box 1034
Evanston, IL

To find out how you can influence children's television, write to:

Action for Children's Television (ACT)
46 Austin Street
Newtonville, MA 02160

Children's Foundation
1420 New York Avenue, N. W. Suite 800
Washington, DC 20005

Dental

To obtain government publications on dental health, write to:

National Institute of Dental Health
9000 Rockville Pike
Building 31, Room 2C36
Bethesda, MD 20892

To obtain information from the dental professional organization, write to:

American Dental Association
211 East Chicago Avenue
Chicago, IL 60611

To find out how to initiate a fluoride tablet program in a school, write to:

National Caries Program
National Institute of Dental Research
Westwood Building, Room 549
5333 Westbard Avenue
Bethesda, MD 20205

Infant Formulas and Foods

Infant formula and food companies will provide nutrient composition information on all their products, as well as how-to information for feeding infants.

Gerber Products Company
445 State Street
Fremont, MI 49412

H. J. Heinz
Consumer Relations
P. O. Box 57
Pittsburgh, PA 15250

Mead-Johnson Nutritional Division
2404 Pennsylvania Avenue
Evansville, IN 47721

Ross Laboratories
Director of Professional Services
625 Cleveland Avenue
Columbus, OH 43216

Wyeth Laboratories
Philadelphia, PA 19101

Obesity

Overeaters Anonymous (OA) and Weight Watchers International offer nutritionally sound weight loss programs as well as information and support for anyone interested in losing weight and enhancing health.

Overeaters Anonymous (OA)
2190 190th Street
Torrence, CA 90504

Weight Watchers International
800 Community Drive
Manhasset, NY 11030

Pregnancy

The March of Dimes Birth Defects Foundation has offices in many cities around the country. Their goal is to fight birth defects through preventive care and education. They offer consumer and professional materials about the most common birth defects, as well as materials about prenatal care and breastfeeding. They also serve as a referral service for those needing prenatal care or genetic counseling.

March of Dimes Birth Defects Foundation (National Headquarters)
1275 Mamaroneck Avenue
White Plains, NY 10605

The Supplemental Food Program for Women, Infants, and Children (WIC), is a government program that provides nutritious supplemental foods and nutrition education to low-income pregnant and lactating women, and their infants and children. WIC is one of the most effective and successful government health and nutrition programs available. State and county health departments can provide information about the nearest WIC location. For more information write to:

FNS, USDA
500 12th Street SW
Washington, DC 20250

Prevention

The American Institute for Cancer Research publishes dietary guidelines for lowering cancer risk and is dedicated to funding research and education programs on the relationship of diet and cancer. For more information write to:

American Institute for Cancer Research
803 W. Broad Street
Falls Church, VA 22046

The American Heart Association publishes pamphlets and recipe booklets about controlling dietary fat and preventing heart disease. Their address is:

The American Heart Association
National Center
7320 Greenville Avenue
Dallas, TX 75231

Index

About the Authors

Linda Kelly DeBruyne, M.S., R.D., received her B.S. in 1980 and her M.S. in 1982 in Nutrition and Food Science from Florida State University. As a founding member of Nutrition and Health Associates, an information resource center in Tallahassee, she serves on the board of directors. She writes *Nutrition Clinics* for nutrition and health professionals on such topics as choosing vitamin supplements, nutrition and behavior, nutrition and fitness, and vegetarian diet planning. She has authored articles for the monthly newsletter, *Healthline* on such topics as fish oils and heart disease, and fasting. As a nutrition consultant for a group of Tallahassee pediatricians, she teaches infant nutrition classes to parents. She is currently writing *Life Cycle Nutrition: Conception through Life* and *The Health Triad: Stress Management, Diet and Fitness.*

Sharon Rady Rolfes, M.S., R.D., received her B.S. in Psychology and Criminology in 1974 and her M.S. in Nutrition and Food Science in 1982 at the Florida State University. She is a founding member of Nutrition and Health Associates and serves on the board of directors. Her publications include the second edition of *Understanding Normal and Clinical Nutrition and* and several *Nutrition Clinics* on topics such as cancer, heart disease, vegetarian diet planning, hypoglycemia, and dental health. As a contributing editor of the monthly newsletter, *Healthline,* she has written articles on bulimia, cancer, fish oils and heart disease, and fasting. She prepared the *Instructor's Manual* and *Student Study Guide* that accompany the textbooks *Understanding Nutrition, Nutrition Concepts and Controversies,* and *Understanding Normal and Clinical Nutrition.* Her current projects include the production of *Life Cycle Nutrition: Conception through Life* and the preparation of the fifth edition of *Understanding Nutrition.*

Eleanor Noss Whitney, Ph.D., R.D., the editor of this text, received her B.A. in biology from Radcliffe College in 1960 and her Ph.D. in biology with an emphasis on genetics from Washington University, St. Louis, in 1970. Formerly an associate professor at the Florida State University, she now devotes full time to research, writing, and consulting in nutrition and health. Her publications include articles in *Science,* the *Journal of Nutrition, Genetics,* and other journals, and the textbooks, *Understanding Nutrition, Nutrition: Concepts and Controversies, Life Choices: Health Concepts and Strategies,* and others. She is president of Nutrition and Health Associates.